Children with Hearing Loss
Developing Listening and Talking

Birth to Six

Second Edition

Elizabeth Cole, EdD
Carol Flexer, PhD

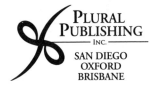

PLURAL
PUBLISHING
INC.
SAN DIEGO
OXFORD
BRISBANE

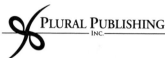

PLURAL PUBLISHING
INC.

5521 Ruffin Road
San Diego, CA 92123

e-mail: info@pluralpublishing.com
Web site: http://www.pluralpublishing.com

49 Bath Street
Abingdon, Oxfordshire OX14 1EA
United Kingdom

©

FSC

Mixed Sources
Product group from well-managed
forests and other controlled sources

Cert no. SW-COC-002283
www.fsc.org
© 1996 Forest Stewardship Council

Typeset in 11/13 Garamond by Flanagan's Publishing Services, Inc.
Printed in the United States of America by McNaughton & Gunn, Inc.

Library of Congress Cataloging-in-Publication Data

Cole, Elizabeth Bingham.
  Children with hearing loss : developing listening and talking, birth to six /
Elizabeth Cole and Carol Flexer. – 2nd ed.
    p. ; cm.
  Includes bibliographical references and index.
  ISBN-13: 978-1-59756-379-6 (alk. paper)
  ISBN-10: 1-59756-379-X (alk. paper)
  1. Hearing disorders in children. 2. Hearing disorders in infants. I. Flexer,
Carol Ann. II. Title.
  [DNLM: 1. Child. 2. Hearing Loss–therapy. 3. Hearing Aids. 4. Infant.
5. Language Disorders—rehabilitation. 6. Rehabilitation of Hearing Impaired.
7. Speech Disorders—rehabilitation. WV 271]
  RF291.5.C45C65 2011
  617.8'9–dc22
                                                    2010039054

Contents

Preface

Hearing loss is the most common birth defect. The National Institute on Deafness and Other Communication Disorders estimates that as many as 12,000 new babies with hearing loss are identified every year. In addition, estimates are that in the same year, another 4,000–6,000 infants and young children between birth and 3 years of age who passed the newborn screening test acquire late onset hearing loss. The total population of new babies and toddlers identified with hearing loss, therefore, is about 16,000–18,000 per year. Over the decades, numerous studies have demonstrated that when hearing loss of any degree is not adequately diagnosed and addressed, the hearing loss can adversely affect the speech, language, academic, emotional, and psychosocial development of young children.

There has been a veritable explosion of information and technology about testing for and managing hearing loss in infants and children. The vanguard of this explosion has been newborn hearing screening. As a result, in this day and age, we are dealing with a vastly different population of children with hearing loss, a population that never before in history have we had. With this new population, whose hearing loss is identified at birth, we can now prevent the developmental and communicative effects of hearing loss that were so common just a few years ago. With these babies and young children, we can now truly work from a developmental and preventative perspective rather than from a remedial, corrective one. What has happened in the field of hearing loss is revolutionary.

How do we understand and manage this new population of babies and their families? How do we revise our early intervention systems to respond to the desired outcomes of listening and talking that today's parents have a right to expect?

The second edition of *Developing Listening and Talking, Birth to Six* remains a dynamic compilation of crucially important information for the facilitation of auditorily based spoken language for infants and young children with hearing loss.

This text is intended for graduate level training programs for professionals who work with children who have hearing loss and their families (teachers, therapists, speech-language pathologists, and audiologists). In addition, the book will be of great interest to undergraduate speech-language-hearing programs, early childhood education and intervention programs, and parents of children who have hearing loss. Responding to the crucial need for a comprehensive text, this book provides a framework for the skills and knowledge necessary to help parents promote listening and spoken language development.

This second edition covers current and up-to-date information about hearing, listening, auditory technology, spoken language development, and intervention for young children with hearing loss whose parents have chosen to have them learn to listen and talk. Additions include updated information about hearing instruments and cochlear implants and about ways that professionals can support parents in promoting their children's language and listening development. The text also features a revised auditory development checklist.

A new appendix provides an important and useful tool for professionals who are interested in AG Bell Academy's Listening and Spoken Language Specialist Certification Program (LSLS)—LSLS Cert. AVT and LSLS Cert. AVEd. This appendix lists the competencies required for the LSLS, and references each chapter of the book with regard to those requirements.

This book is unique in its scholarly, yet thoroughly readable style. Numerous illustrations, charts, and graphs illuminate key ideas. The second edition should be the foundation of the personal and professional libraries of students, clinicians, and parents who are interested in listening and spoken language outcomes for children with hearing loss.

Accordingly, this text is divided into two sections. The first five chapters lay the foundation for listening and talking. They include neurological development and discussions of ear anatomy and physiology, pathologies that cause hearing loss, audiologic testing of infants and children, and the latest in amplification technologies. The second part of the book focuses on intervention; listening, talking, and communicating; through the utilization of a developmental and preventative model.

Acknowledgments

From both authors:
Thanks to the people at Plural Publishing for their help and guidance through the development process of this second edition.

Elizabeth Cole would like to express immense appreciation to Carol Flexer for enthusiastically embracing our collaboration on this second edition with such knowledge, savvy, and energy. Special thanks to Elaine Carroll, Ellen Gill, and Jacqueline St.Clair-Stokes for their ongoing inspiration, expertise, and wisdom, and to my wonderful Frank, Thea, and Ted for providing firsthand, endlessly rich, and ever-changing parent-child interactions to learn from.

Carol Flexer would like to express ongoing admiration, gratitude, and appreciation to Elizabeth Cole for her expertise, thoughtfulness, and professional aplomb. I am honored to share this second edition with her. A special acknowledgement needs to go to David Flexer and Hilary Krzywkowski Flexer for their diligent assistance with editing. And finally, I would like to deeply thank my dear husband, Pete, my amazing children Heather, Hillari, and David, and my 10 precious grandchildren for their consistent enthusiasm and love of life.

This second edition is dedicated to our children and grandchildren (present and future), and to all who access and develop a child's auditory neural centers for listening and talking.

1

Neurological Foundations of Listening and Talking

Key Points Presented in the Chapter

- Because they have had 20 weeks of auditory experience in utero, at birth, typical infants prefer their mother's speech and songs and stories heard before birth.
- We hear with the brain—the ears are just a way in. The problem with hearing loss is that it keeps sound from reaching the brain.
- In order for auditory pathways to mature, acoustic stimulation must occur early and often because full maturation of central auditory pathways is a precondition for the normal development of speech and language skills in children, whether or not they have a hearing loss.
- Neuroplasticity is greatest during the first 3½ years of life; the younger the infant, the greater the neuroplasticity.
- The highest auditory neural centers (called the secondary auditory association areas in the cortex) are not fully developed until a child is about 15 years of age. The less "intrinsic" redundancy, the more redundant the "extrinsic" signal must be.

- Skills mastered as close as possible to the time that a child is biologically intended to do so result in *developmental synchrony*.
- Hearing loss can be described as an *invisible acoustic filter* that distorts, smears, or eliminates incoming sounds, especially sounds from a distance—even a short distance.

Introduction

Everything that we thought we knew about deafness has changed in exciting and dramatic ways. Why? Newborn infant screening programs, new hearing aid and FM technologies, and cochlear implants have allowed access to critical auditory brain centers during times of maximum neuroplasticity. This early identification has enabled us to fit amplification technologies and cochlear implants on babies. We can now stimulate auditory brain centers that could not be accessed with previous, less effective generations of amplification technologies. Therefore, auditory language enrichment can be provided during critical periods of maximum brain neural plasticity—the first few years of life (Sharma, Dorman, & Spahr, 2002; Sharma et al., 2004; Sharma, Dorman, & Kral, 2005). Neuroplasticity refers to the brain's availability and malleability to grow, develop, and alter its structure as a function of external stimulation (Kilgard, Vasquez, Engineer, & Panda, 2007). As a result of neuroplasticity, today's babies and young children who are born deaf or hard of hearing have incredible possibilities for achieving higher levels of spoken language, reading skills, and academic competencies than were available to most children in previous generations (Nicholas & Geers, 2006; Yoshinaga-Itano, 2004). We are dealing with a new population of babies and children with hearing loss—a population that we have never experienced before.

There is substantial evidence that hearing is the most effective modality for the teaching of spoken language (speech), reading, and cognitive skills (Sloutsky & Napolitano, 2003; Tallal, 2004; 2005; Werker, 2006; Zupan & Sussman, 2009). Furthermore, with today's amplification technologies including cochlear implants and early identification and intervention, auditory brain access is available to babies with even the most profound deafness. This brain access allows us to utilize a developmental model of intervention that prevents the negative developmental outcomes so common a few years ago. The possibilities are startling (Haynes, Geers, Treiman, & Moog, 2009; Moog, 2002).

This chapter will begin at the beginning with a discussion of two lines of research that have direct relevance regarding the crucially important connection between listening abilities and speech and language development. Next, auditory neural development will be explored along with a discussion of neuroplasticity. A new context for describing deafness will be posited. An additional topic is the acoustic filter model of hearing loss. The chapter will conclude with the question to families that drives intervention.

Typical Infants: Listening and Language Development

Research on speech perception capabilities of typical neonates, using a non-nutritive sucking paradigm, confirms that infants acquire native languages by listening; they start life being prepared to speak (Werker, 2006; Winegert & Brant, 2005). At birth, infants prefer their mother's speech and they even prefer songs and stories heard *before* birth. How can this be? The fact is, infants are born with 20 weeks of listening experience because their cochleas are formed and functional by the 20th week of gestation (Gordon & Harrison, 2005). There is a great deal of sound available to the fetus in utero. That's why early identification and amplification and an enriched auditory-linguistic environment are essential. Newborns with hearing loss may have already missed 20 weeks of listening.

In the first 6 months of life, babies can discriminate many speech sounds, even those not heard in their home-spoken language(s). However, within a few months, the brain becomes a more efficient analyzer of speech. By the end of the first year, there is a functional reorganization of the brain to distinguish phonemes specific to language(s) heard daily. This neural reorganization improves and tunes the phonetic categories required for the infant's language and attenuates those phonemic distinctions not required for the infant's mother tongue (Vouloumanos & Werker, 2007; Werker, 2006).

Infants use their phonetic categories as the foundation for learning new words. Phonetic distinctions guide new word learning by 17 months of age. Thus, listening experience in infancy is critical for the development of both speech and language in young children, and a strong auditory language base is essential for reading (Sloutsky & Napolitano, 2003; Zupan & Sussman, 2009). Figure 1–1 displays this progression.

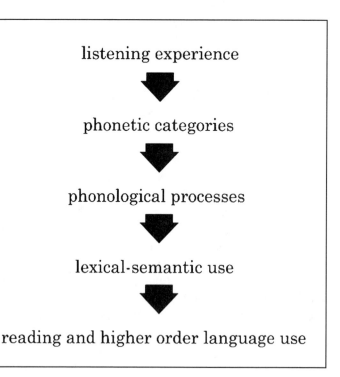

listening experience

phonetic categories

phonological processes

lexical-semantic use

reading and higher order language use

Figure 1–1. Listening experience in infancy is critical for adequate language development, and adequate language development is essential for reading.

Given that listening is the core event, how much listening experience is necessary for adequate language development? Hart and Risley (1999) explored this issue. They conducted an extensive, longitudinal study of person-spoken words heard by children ages birth to age 4 years. Electronic words (TV, books on tape, computer, etc) were not counted. Some of their results are as follows.

Average number of words per hour addressed to children by parents (Hart & Risley, 1999, p. 169):

- 2100 in a professional family
- 1200 in a working-class family
- 600 in a welfare family

Hart and Risley noted that, "The extra talk of parents in the professional families and that of the most talkative parents in the working-class families contained more of the varied vocabulary, complex ideas, subtle guidance, and positive feedback thought to be important to cognitive development" (Hart & Risley, 1999, p. 170).

They further explained that, "Parents who talked a lot about such things [ideas, feelings, or impressions] or only a little ended up with 3-year-olds who also talked a lot, or only a little" (Hart & Risley, 1999, p. xii).

Hart and Risley concluded that their data "show that the first 3 years of experience put in place a trajectory of vocabulary growth and the foundations of analytic and symbolic competencies that will make a lasting difference to how children perform in later years" (Hart & Risley, 1999, p. 193).

The bottom line is, all infants and children require a great deal of listening experience, about 20,000 hours in the first 5 years of life to create the neural infrastructure for literacy (Dehane, 2009). These data collected on typical infants and children have significant implications for children with hearing loss.

Human beings are organically designed to listen and talk if we do what it takes to access the brain with sound (through technology for children with hearing loss) and practice, practice, practice listening and reading.

Auditory Neural Development

The problem with hearing loss is that it keeps sound from reaching the brain (Figure 1-2).

The purpose of a cochlear implant (or a hearing aid) is to access, stimulate, and grow auditory neural connections throughout the brain as the foundation for spoken language, reading, and academics (Gordon, Papsin, & Harrison, 2004; Sharma & Nash, 2009). Due to the limited time period of optimal neural plasticity, age at implantation is critical—younger is better (Sharma et al., 2004; Sharma, Martin, Roland, Bauer, Sweeney, Gilley, et al., 2005; Sharma & Nash, 2009).

Studies in brain development show that sensory stimulation of the auditory centers of the brain is critically important and, indeed, influences the actual organization of auditory brain pathways (Berlin & Weyand, 2003; Boothroyd, 1997; Chermak, Bellis, & Musiek, 2007; Clinard & Tremblay, 2008). Furthermore, neural

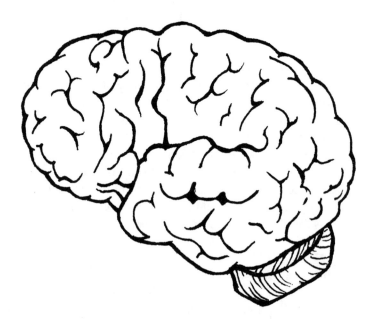

Figure 1-2. This is a picture of the "real ear." We hear with the brain—the ears are just a way in. Hearing loss is not about the ears; it's about the brain.

imaging has shown that the same brain area—the primary and secondary auditory areas—are most active when a child listens and when a child reads. That is, phonological or phonemic awareness, which is the explicit awareness of the speech *sound* structure of language units, forms the basis for the development of literacy skills (Pugh, 2005; Strickland & Shanahan, 2004; Tallal, 2004).

Clearly, anything we can do to access and "program" those critical and powerful auditory centers of the brain with acoustic detail will expand children's abilities to listen and learn spoken language. As Robbins, Koch, Osberger, Zimmerman-Philips, and Kishon-Rabin (2004) contend, early and ongoing auditory intervention is essential.

Important neural deficits have been identified in the higher auditory centers of the brain due to prolonged lack of auditory stimulation, and further, the auditory cortex is directly involved in speech perception and language processing in humans (Kretzmer, Meltzer, Haenggeli, & Ryugo 2004; Sharma & Nash, 2009; Shaywitz & Shaywitz, 2004). In order for auditory pathways to mature, acoustic stimulation must occur early and often because normal maturation of central auditory pathways is a precondition for the normal development of speech and language skills in children. Research also suggests that children receiving implants very early (in the first year of life) may benefit more from the relatively greater plasticity of the auditory pathways than will children who are implanted later within the developmentally sensitive period (Sharma, Dorman, & Kral, 2005). These results suggest that rapid changes in P1 latencies and changes in response morphology are not unique to electrical stimulation but rather reflect the response of a deprived sensory system to new stimulation. Gordon et al. (2003; 2004) concurred and reported that activity in the auditory pathways to the level of the midbrain can be provoked by stimulation from a cochlear implant (CI). The hypothesis that early implantation appears to be promoted by changes in central auditory pathways was supported by evidence provided by Gordon and colleagues.

Emerging data from the Colorado Project are showing that about 90% of children born with a profound hearing loss who obtain a CI before they are 18 months old attain intelligible speech. Further, if the cochlear implant is obtained between 2 and 4 years of age, about 80% of the children born with a profound hearing loss will attain intelligible speech (Yoshinaga-Itano, 1998; 2004; Yoshinaga-Itano, Sedey, Coulter, & Mehl, 1998). This outcome is based on having the CI mapped appropriately and worn consistently. Direct, repetitive auditory skills instruction as part of an effective family-based early intervention program also is critical. That is, the child must receive extra auditory exposure, stimulation, and practice (Nott, Cowan, Brown, & Wigglesworth, 2009). In con-

---

Acting in harmony with a structure can be illustrated by a child learning to pump on a swing. When they first begin to try to make the swing move without being pushed, children expend a great deal of energy but the swing moves only a little bit. Then something happens, and the child learns how to move in harmony with the swing. As a result of child and swing synchrony, a little bit of energy input by the child causes large movement by the swing (Figure 1–3). In an analogous fashion, a developmental model allows for synchrony of intervention and development, promoting large and rapid gains.

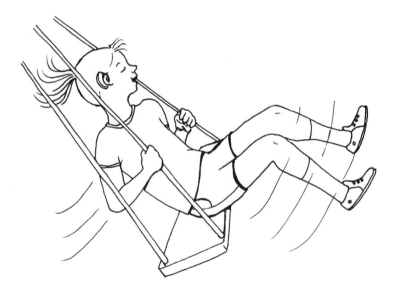

Figure 1–3. When the child learns how to act in harmony with the swing, a little bit of energy input leads to startling effects.

trast, only about 20% of children born with a profound hearing loss who wear hearing aids (and not a cochlear implant) attain intelligible speech.

Robbins et al. (2004) found that skills mastered as close as possible to the time that a child is biologically intended to do so result in *developmental synchrony*. As human beings, we are pre-programmed to develop specific skills during certain periods of development. If those skills can be triggered at the intended time, we will be operating under a developmental and not a remedial paradigm. That is, we will be working harmoniously within the design of the human structure. When we intervene later in a child's life, out of harmony with the typical developmental process, we are forced to work within a remedial model. A brain can only organize itself around the sensory stimulation that it receives. Remedial intervention means that we need to undo the neural organization that the brain has initially acquired and reorganize the brain around different stimuli. A remedial model takes longer and typically has reduced outcomes because the child is now neurologically and psychosocially out of synchrony with the typical developmental process. Think of how long it takes an adult to learn to ski. It's a very long and effortful time, compared with the amount of time that it takes a child to learn to zoom down the hill.

Mastery of any developmental skill depends on *cumulative practice;* each practice opportunity builds on the last one. Therefore, the more delayed the age of acquisition of a skill, the farther behind children are in the amount of cumulative practice they have had to perfect that skill. The same concept holds true for cumulative auditory practice. Delayed auditory development leads to delayed language skills which will necessitate using a remedial rather than a developmental paradigm.

No skill is acquired without practice. Children learn to walk by practicing walking. They learn to listen by practicing listening. They learn to talk by practicing talking. A great deal of practice is necessary for the acquisition of any skill. Learning following a developmental model allows for the necessary, substantial practice.

To summarize, neuroplasticity is greatest during the first 3½ years of life (Sharma & Nash, 2009). The younger the infant, the greater the neuroplasticity (Sharma et al., 2002, 2004; Sharma, Dorman, & Kral, 2005). Rapid infant brain growth requires prompt intervention, typically including amplification and a program to promote auditory skill development. In the absence of sound, the brain reorganizes itself to receive input from other senses, primarily vision; this process is called *cross-modal reorganization* and it reduces auditory neural capacity. Early amplification or implantation stimulates a brain that is in the initial process of organizing itself, and is therefore more receptive to auditory input, resulting in greater auditory capacity (Sharma & Nash, 2009). Furthermore, early implantation synchronizes activity in the cortical layers. Therefore, identification of newborn hearing loss should be considered a neurodevelopmental emergency! Please refer to Chapter 4 for more information about EHDI programs.

The popular book about change, Who Moved My Cheese? *by Spencer Johnson, M.D., is particularly meaningful in the world of hearing loss. Technology and early hearing detection and intervention (EHDI) programs have allowed outcomes of listening and talking only dreamed of a few years ago. It is important to realize that the new outcomes available today do not invalidate the decisions that we made for intervention in the past. We did what we did when that's what there was to be done. Because we now know more, we can offer better services. We do the best that we can in today's world. Tomorrow's world will bring new possibilities, and we need to "move with the cheese." Our job is to prepare today's babies to be the take-charge adults in the world of 2030, 2040, and 2050 . . . not in the world of 1970 or 1990 or even 2015. Because information and knowledge are the currencies of today's cultures, listening, speaking, reading, writing, and the use of electronic technologies must be made available to our babies and children to the fullest degree possible.*

New Context for the Word *Deaf*

Today, hearing aids and/or cochlear implants and FM and Blue-tooth technologies (wireless connectivity) can allow infants and children with even the most profound hearing loses/deafness access to the entire speech spectrum. Indeed, there is no degree of hearing loss that prohibits the brain's access to sound if cochlear implants are available. Degree of hearing loss as a limiting factor in auditory acuity is now an "old" acoustic conversation. That is, when one uses the word "deaf," the implication is that one has no access to sound, period. The word deaf in 1970 occurred in a very different context than the word deaf is used today. Today's child who is deaf without using technology may function as a child with a mild or moderate hearing loss when he or she is using hearing aids or cochlear implants—because the brain has been developed with meaningful sound. Therefore, the words used to express hearing loss convey different conditions as contexts change.

Hearing Versus Listening

There is a distinction between hearing and listening. Hearing is acoustic access to the brain; it includes improving the signal-to-noise ratio by managing the environment and utilizing hearing technology. Listening, on the other hand, is attending to acoustic events with intentionality.

> *Lack of high quality acoustic access to the brain is the biggest challenge worldwide. It is imperative to have very high expectations for today's technologies to make soft sounds available to the brain at a distance and in the presence of noise. Children must use technologies that enable them to overhear conversations and to benefit from incidental learning in order to maximize auditory exposure for social and cognitive development.*

Sequencing is important. *Hearing* must be made available before *listening* can be taught. That is, parents and interventionists can focus on developing the child's listening skills, strategies, and choices only after the audiologist channels acoustic events to the brain by fitting and programming technologies—not before.

A Model of Hearing Loss: The Invisible Acoustic Filter Effect

Hearing loss of any type or degree that occurs in infancy or childhood can interfere with the development of a child's spoken language, reading and writing skills, and academic performance (Davis, 1990; Ling, 2002). That is, hearing loss can be described as an *invisible acoustic filter* that distorts, smears, or eliminates incoming sounds, especially sounds from a distance—even a short distance. The negative effects of a hearing loss may be apparent, but the hearing loss itself is invisible and easily ignored or underestimated.

It is critical to note that as human beings we are neurologically "wired" to develop spoken language (speech) and reading skills through the central *auditory* system (Figure 1-4). Most people think that reading is a visual skill, but recent research on brain mapping shows that primary reading centers of the brain are located in the auditory cortex—in the auditory portions of the brain (Chermak et al., 2007; Pugh, 2006; Tallal, 2005). That is why many children who are born with hearing losses and who do not have brain access to auditory input when they are very young (through hearing aids or cochlear implants and auditory teaching) tend to have a great deal of difficulty reading even though their vision is fine (Robertson, 2009). Therefore, the earlier and more efficiently we can allow a child access to meaningful sound with subsequent direction of the child's attention to sound, the better opportunity that child will have to develop spoken language, literacy, and academic skills. With the technology and early auditory intervention available today, a child with a hearing loss *can* have the same opportunity as a typically hearing child to develop spoken language, reading, and academic skills.

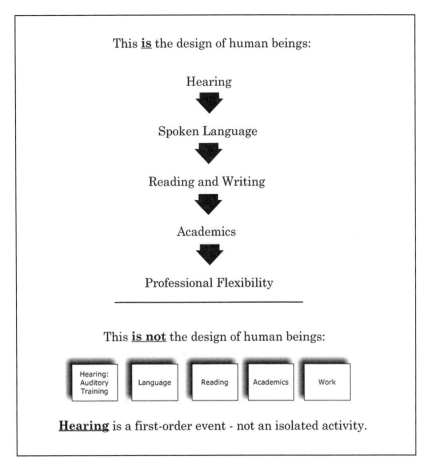

Figure 1–4. The design of human beings is such that hearing (auditory neural growth) is a first order event for the development of language, reading, and academic skills, not an isolated activity.

Summary: The Question That Drives Technological and Intervention Recommendations

The bottom-line question to ask families is: What is your vision for your child? Ninety-five percent of children with hearing loss are born into hearing and speaking families (Mitchell & Karchmer, 2004); they are interested in having their child talk. Once we know that listening and speaking are desired outcomes, the next conversation is centered around, what will it take?

To develop listening and talking, it takes (*Note:* see the second half of this book for detailed instruction in the development of listening and talking.):

- Early identification and intervention to take advantage of neuroplasticity and developmental synchrony.
- Vigilant, ongoing, and kind audiologic management.
- Immediate and consistent auditory brain access via technology—hearing aid loaner banks—to preserve and develop auditory neural capacity.
- Guidance from a professional who is highly qualified in the development of listening and speaking, through techniques of parent coaching.
- Following the professional's coaching with daily and ongoing formal and informal auditory, language, cognitive, and literacy enrichment.

What Will It Take?

Because early intervention is a family-focused strategy, it's necessary that families assist in formulating their role. A "what will it take" conversation with families is important to clarify the necessary steps to attaining the family's desired outcome of listening and talking. One strategy is to use the analogy of driving a car. What are the steps necessary to acquire the desired outcome of a driver's license? Well, to begin with, one needs to have access to a car. Then, a coach or driving instructor is sought. Most states then require up to 150 hours of supervised driving practice with a licensed, adult driver. Next is the necessity of passing a written exam and a vision exam, followed by a practical exam—the driving test. If all that is completed satisfactorily, one has a driver's license. If any requirement is deleted, the driver's license is not achieved no matter how badly one wants it or how sympathetic the excuses.

- Integration and use of auditory strategies into all-day, everyday interactions with the child to "grow the baby's brain." See Appendix 1 for a handout of How to Grow Your Baby's or Child's Brain.

2

The Auditory System

Key Points Presented in the Chapter

■ The subtle and often ambiguous functions of hearing can be divided into three levels: unconscious (primitive), signal warning, and spoken language.

■ The Ling 6-7 Sound Test allows parents, professionals, and teachers to know the child's distance hearing/"earshot" distance.

■ The human ear is an extremely sensitive and delicate yet amazing structure for sound and balance perception; therefore, it is important to note the significance of each function of the ear's many parts and the effects that environmental, physiological, and psychological factors have on the ability to hear and maintain equilibrium.

■ Sounds are received through the peripheral auditory system: the outer, middle, and inner ear.

■ Ossicles, the smallest bones in the body, are made up of the malleus, incus, and stapes, which are attached to two membranes: the tympanic membrane and the oval window.

■ The distinctions of the peripheral and central auditory systems include two general processes of hearing which are the transmission of sounds to the brain through the outer, middle, and inner ear; and learning the meaning of those sounds once they are transmitted to the brain. Therefore, auditory perception requires sensory evidence.

The Nature of Sound

In order to appreciate the impact of hearing loss and the benefits of hearing management strategies, it is useful to understand first the vital and often subtle role that sound plays in our physical and psychological lives. The functions of hearing can be divided, roughly, into three levels: unconscious (primitive), signal warning (environmental monitoring), and spoken language learning—communication (Northern & Downs, 2002).

Unconscious Function

The *unconscious level* distinguishes the most primitive function of hearing by carrying the auditory background and sounds that serve to identify a location. A hospital sounds different compared to a school, which sounds different from a department store. Typically, one does not notice these sounds; however, if a location does not produce the expected sound, one becomes uneasy. For example, entering an empty hospital or deserted school may evoke feelings of anxiety.

Also heard at the primitive level are one's own biological sounds such as breathing, swallowing, chewing, heartbeat, and pulse. All furnish proof that we are indeed alive and functioning. Some people

A new hearing aid, cochlear implant, or assistive listening device alters the wearer's auditory background because sounds not previously heard become amplified. A wearer's anxiety may reflect this change in auditory background, although he may be unable to understand why. Certainly, a baby or young child cannot explain that an altered auditory background may be a cause for resistance to amplification, which is expressed as an irritable disposition. Yet, as professionals, we should be mindful that there is an adjustment period to amplification as the wearer's brain reorganizes itself to the altered auditory background. One could also speculate about the effects of a hearing loss in constant fluctuation, like otitis media (ear infections), on a child's auditory background and subsequent emotional state.

who suddenly lose their hearing may experience acute psychosis due to feelings of disconnectedness from the environment, time, and their own bodies.

Signal Warning Function

The second level of hearing function, *signal warning*, is less subtle and pertains to monitoring the environment. Classified as distance senses, hearing and vision allow us to know what happens away from our bodies. However, we cannot always actually see events to know what occurs around us. A baby in bed at night can hear people talking, the television prattle, a computer's clatter, dogs barking, cars roaring, and so forth. Knowledge of what happens around us promotes feelings of security, whereas being uninformed about the environment may induce anxiety.

Unfortunately, persons with hearing loss of any degree, even while wearing suitable hearing aids, lack the ability to hear well over distances. Distance hearing becomes problematic because the speech signal loses both intensity and critical speech elements as the signal travels away from its sound source (Leavitt & Flexer, 1991). The greater the hearing loss, the greater the reduction in earshot or distance hearing (Ling, 2002). Said another way, the greater the hearing loss, the closer the listener must be to the talker for speech to be heard at levels loud enough and with sufficient redundancy to be understood.

A child with a hearing loss, whether mild or unilateral (hearing loss in only one ear), cannot casually hear what people are saying or the events that are occurring (Ling, 2002). Often, children with normal hearing seem to absorb passively information from the environment; they can learn from overhearing the speech of others. In contrast, children with hearing problems may seem distractible or oblivious to environmental events; they often experience a disconnection from the environment.

Because of the reduction in signal intensity and integrity with distance, children experiencing hearing problems have limitations in their access to auditory information in the environment. Therefore, these children may need to be taught directly the many skills that other children learn incidentally. Lack of access to social clues and the redundancy of spoken information that occurs in day-to-day transactions may also result from reduction of distance hearing.

> *Following is one example of how distance hearing and inci-*
> *dental learning impact day-to-day family life. A young child*
> *later discovered to have a moderate hearing loss would*
> *repeatedly take food from the kitchen without asking permis-*
> *sion, an activity that was viewed by the family as disruptive*
> *and rude. The family later recognized that while the child*
> *could observe his siblings taking food from the kitchen, because*
> *of his hearing loss, he could not overhear them first ask the*
> *parent's permission. The child's behavior improved dramat-*
> *ically once the family realized that the child needed to wear*
> *his hearing aids all of the time, not just at school. In addition,*
> *he required direct instruction of the family's social function,*
> *even though the other children learned social cues passively.*

Tangential information not directed to the child is important for learning. Listening in to others' conversations teaches children how to start a conversation, make a request, problem solve, negotiate, compromise, joke, tease, and use sarcasm.

Any degree of hearing loss presents a barrier to the casual acquisition of information from the environment.

Spoken Communication Function

Children learn to talk through listening (Werker, 2006). Therefore, spoken communication does not develop naturally or completely for infants and children who do not hear well, unless technology and specific auditory strategies are used to improve the quantity and quality of their auditory access.

Verbal language takes form after a great deal of hearing and active listening experience (Estabrooks, 2006; Hayes et al., 2009; Ling, 2002; Northern & Downs, 2002). Because the inner ear is fully developed by the 5th month of gestation, an infant with normal hearing potentially has 4 months of in utero auditory stimulation prior to birth (Simmons, 2003). At approximately 1 year of age, after 12 months (or maybe 16 months if we count before-birth listening) of meaningful and interactive listening, a normal hearing child begins to produce words. The point is that listening time cannot be skipped, and a child who misses months of brain access due

> *The brain benefits from practice listening to music as well as speech. Studies provide biological evidence that listening to music boosts the brain's ability to distinguish emotional aspects of speech by focusing on the paralinguistic (nonverbal) elements of speech (Sheridan & Cunningham, 2009).*

to hearing loss must make them up (Estabrooks, 2006). The brain requires extensive listening experience to properly organize itself around the speech signal.

Acoustics

In order to understand the causes of hearing loss it is first important to establish an appreciation of the human ear. Though this intricate and complex mechanism may not appear very impressive from the outside, the inner structures of the ear enable a person to access a 10,000-to-1 range of sensitivity from the softest sound that can barely be detected to one that is uncomfortably loud (Bess & Humes, 2003). The typical human ear has such amazing sensitivity that it can nearly detect random molecular movement.

When hearing sound, an individual interprets a pattern of vibrations initiated from a source in the environment. Vibrational energy produces the sound waves we can hear. Vibrations need two properties—mass and elasticity. Sound waves are very similar to ring patterns in water produced when a pebble is thrown into a pond, only with sound, the waves are formed by the vibration of air molecules. Much like the effect of water ripples, sound waves originate from a point where the sound is first generated and spread out in circles of waves.

The speed at which sound travels through the air is called velocity. Sound travels through the air as fast as 770 miles per hour at sea level, or 1,130 feet per second. Water waves travel much slower, only a few miles an hour.

Graphed as a circle on a flat plane plot, a *sine wave* is the simplest form of sound called simple harmonic motion; it is heard as a pure tone (Figure 2–1).

Our ability to hear sound is defined by the three characteristics of frequency, intensity, and duration. A hearing loss may affect one's ability to perceive one or all of these features.

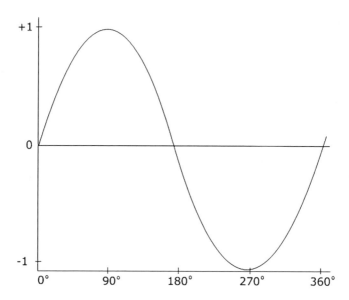

Figure 2–1. Graphed as a circle on a flat plane plot, a *sine wave* is the simplest form of sound.

The riddle, "If a tree fell in the forest and no one was around, would a sound still be made by the falling tree?" serves as a good example of whether one describes sound from a physical or psychological basis. The answer depends on one or the other. Existing independently of the observer are the physical parameters of intensity, frequency, and duration; these features can be measured by equipment. However, the psychological perceptions of loudness, pitch, and time require the presence of a person for interpretation.

The psychological attributes of sound are pitch and loudness. The physical parameter of frequency corresponds to the psychological attribute of pitch. The listener hears high-frequency sounds as high in pitch, whereas the perception of low-frequency sounds is that of a low pitch. The physical parameter of intensity is the psychological correlate of loudness. So, when a sound has more intensity the listener perceives it as louder.

The number of back-and-forth oscillations produced by a sound source in a given time period is called *frequency*. The terms *hertz*

(Hz) and *cycles per second* (cps) are measures of frequency. By counting the number of cycles per second of a sound wave, one can measure the frequency of sound. The distance between the top (crest) of one sound wave and the top of the next sound wave is one cycle. To have a frequency of 1000 Hz, a sound source would need to complete 1,000 back-and-forth cycles in one second. Low frequencies are characterized by fewer cycles per second, whereas many cycles per second indicate a higher frequency sound. In Figure 2–2 the frequency of the sound increases as the wavelengths become shorter and the number of cycles per second increases.

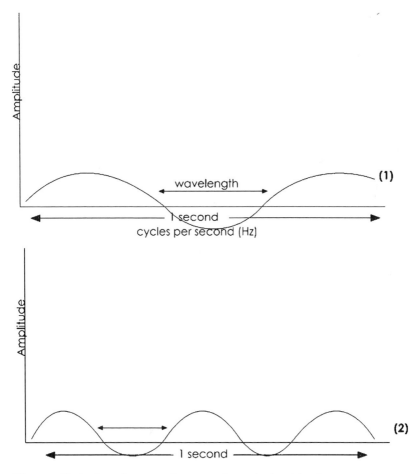

Figure 2–2. Low frequencies are characterized by fewer cycles per second, whereas many cycles per second indicate a higher frequency sound.

Although humans can hear frequencies ranging from 20 to 20000 Hz, frequencies between 250 and 8000 Hz are of particular importance for the perception of speech. Middle C on the piano corresponds to 250 Hz. Frequencies of 500 Hz and below are identified as low-pitched sounds and they have a bass quality. Relative to individual speech sounds (phonemes), those that are low-pitch carry melodies of speech, vowel sounds, and most environmental sounds (Ling, 2002). On the other hand, high-pitched sounds are 1500 Hz and above and they have a tenor quality. The high frequencies are important for understanding speech because they carry the energy that helps distinguish among the consonants. Put simplistically, the meaning of speech is carried by high frequencies whereas low frequencies carry the melody. The softest and loudest sounds in conversational speech are separated by approximately a 30 dB range. The *th* sound, as in *thin*, is the least intense speech sound. The most intense speech sound is /a/ as in *law*. Refer to Table 2–1 for a more detailed description of speech information carried by each relevant frequency.

A sound's intensity can be defined as pressure or power. Graphed as the amplitude of a sine wave caused by displacement of air molecules, intensity is measured in decibels (dB) and perceived as loudness (Figure 2–3). The degree of air particle displacement that occurs while a sound is made determines a sound's intensity. The abbreviation dB stands for decibel; the B is capitalized in honor of Alexander Graham Bell. The hearing level (HL), defined as 0 dB HL, is the softest sound a young adult with normal hearing can just barely detect. The loudness of a person whispering a few feet away is about 25 to 30 dB HL. Typical conversational speech in a quiet environment when the speaker is a few feet away is heard at 45 to 50 dB HL. City traffic is about 70 dB HL, a food blender is about 90 dB HL, an alarm clock is about 80 dB HL, a rock concert can be louder than 110 dB HL, a jet airport can produce sounds reaching an intensity as high as 120 dB HL, and a firecracker can produce a bang at approximately 140 dB HL (Berg, 1993).

Because the decibel has a logarithmic and not a linear scale, every dB counts a great deal. For example, if a sound increases or decreases 10 times in intensity, the change is only 10 dB. A 20-dB change means a sound is 10 × 10, or 100 times the intensity of the original sound. The average hearing loss caused from ear infections is about 20 dB—usually described as a slight or "minimal" hearing loss.

Table 2–1. Speech Information Carried by the Key Speech Frequencies of 250–4000 Hz (± one half octave)

250 Hz	500 Hz	1000 Hz	2000 Hz	4000 Hz
• First formant of vowels /u/ and /i/	• First formants of most vowels	• The important acoustic cues for manner of articulation	• The important acoustic cues for place of articulation	• The key frequency for /s/ and /z/ audibility that is critical for language learning:
• Fundamental frequency of females' and children's voices	• Harmonics of all voices (male, female, child)	• Second formants of back and central vowels	• The key frequency for speech intelligibility	– plurals – idioms
• Nasal murmur associated with the phonemes /m/, /n/, and /ng/	• Voicing cues	• Consonant-vowel and vowel-consonant transition information	• Second and third formant information for front vowels	– possessives – auxiliaries
• Prosody	• Nasality cues	• Some plosive bursts	• Consonant-vowel and vowel-consonant transition information	– third person singular verb forms
• Suprasegmental patterns (stress, rate, inflection, intonation)	• Suprasegmentals	• Voicing cues	• Acoustic information for the liquids /r/ and /l/	– questions
• Male voice harmonics	• Some plosive bursts associated with /b/ and /d/	• Suprasegmentals	• Plosive bursts	– copulas – past perfect
• Voicing cues		• Unstressed morphemes	• Affricate bursts	• Consonant quality
			• Fricative turbulence	

Source: Adapted from *Speech and the Hearing Impaired Child* (2nd ed.) by D. Ling, 2002, Washington, DC: Alexander Graham Bell Association of the Deaf and Hard of Hearing. Reprinted with permission.

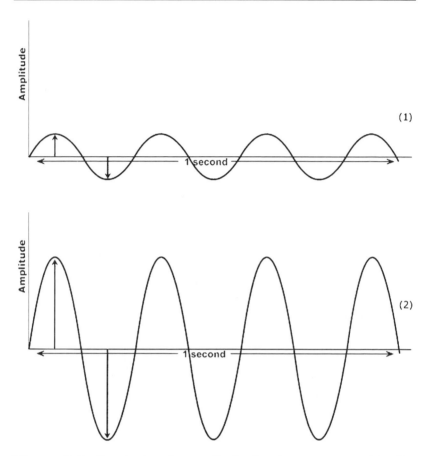

Figure 2–3. Graphed as the amplitude of a sine wave caused by displacement of air molecules, intensity is measured in decibels (dB) and perceived as loudness.

When understanding the dB scale as logarithmic, one recognizes that in reality, the child's "slight" hearing loss means that what is heard is approximately 100 times less intense when the fluid is present than can be heard when the fluid is cleared.

Most environmental sounds are complex in structure. Complex sounds are comprised of many frequencies with varying intensities occurring at the same time. Speech is one example of a complex sound. The spectrum of a speech wave specifies the frequencies, amplitudes, and phases of each of the waves' sinusoidal components.

In all learning domains—home, school, and community settings—there are a variety of sounds from many sources. Undesirable sounds typically are referred to as *noise*. Noise levels tend to be more intense in the low frequencies and less powerful at the high frequencies. The weaker consonant sounds (i.e., *th, s, sh, f, p*) are more affected by noise than are the louder vowel sounds. In noisy situations, the intelligibility of speech (the ability to hear word-sound distinctions clearly) is compromised even though the sounds might still be audible.

Audibility versus Intelligibility of Speech

There is a big difference between an *audible* signal and an *intelligible* signal. Speech is audible if the person is able simply to detect its presence. However, for speech to be intelligible the person must be able to discriminate the word-sound distinctions of individual phonemes or speech sounds. Consequently, speech might be very audible but not consistently intelligible to a child with even a minimal hearing loss, causing the child to hear, for example, words such as *walked, walking, walker,* and *walks,* all as "__ah."

Vowel sounds (such as *o, u, ee,* etc.) have strong low-frequency energy, about 250 to 500 Hz. They are the most powerful sounds in English. Vowels carry 90% of the energy of speech. On the other hand, consonant sounds (like *f* and *s*) are very weak high-frequency sounds, with energy focused at 2000 and 4000 Hz and above (see Table 2–1). Consonants carry only 10% of the energy of speech but 90% of the information needed to perceive the differences among the sounds. The octave band at 2000 Hz carries the greatest amount of speech information. For speech to be heard clearly, both vowels and consonants must be acoustically available. Persons with hearing losses typically have the most difficulty hearing the weak, unvoiced, high-frequency consonant sounds.

The Ling 6-7 Sound Test: Acoustic Basis and Description

The Ling sound test allows a quick and easy way to verify that a child detects the vowel and consonant sounds of spoken language

> *The Ling 6-7 Sound Test allows parents, professionals, and teachers to know the child's distance hearing or earshot. Knowing this information has vital instructional ramifications if one intends to use audition as a viable modality of reception. Sounds must first be detected before the brain can be stimulated. Frequent administration of this test can help parents, professionals, and teachers monitor for hearing aid malfunction and/or cochlear implant failure, changes in the child's hearing, or onset of middle ear conductive involvement that would be reflected by reduced earshot. Refer to Chapter 4 for a further discussion of distance hearing, and to Appendix 2 for specific Ling 6-7 Sound Test application and instructions.*

(Ling, 2002). The sounds used for this test were selected because they encompass the entire speech spectrum as noted below.

- ▪ /m/ corresponds to 250 Hz, plus and minus ½ octave.
- ▪ /u/ is like a narrowband of noise corresponding to 500 Hz on the audiogram, plus and minus ½ octave.
- ▪ /a/ corresponds to 1000 Hz, plus and minus ½ octave.
- ▪ /sh/ is a band of noise corresponding to 2000 Hz, plus and minus ½ octave.
- ▪ /s/ is a band of noise corresponding to 4000 Hz, plus and minus ½ octave.
- ▪ /i/ has a first formant (resonance of the vocal track) around 500 Hz, and a second formant around 2000 Hz; the second formant must be heard in order for the listener to be able to distinguish between front and back vowels.
- ▪ The silent interval is really a seventh "sound" that is necessary to track false positive responses.

Ear Mechanisms

At birth, the auditory system of a child with normal hearing is functioning and completely developed (Northern & Downs, 2002). Specifically, the middle ear structures are developed and functional by the 37th week of prenatal development. The inner ear mechanism is developed, adult size, and receiving sound by the 20th week of prenatal development. The external ear and auditory canal continue to grow as the child grows, up to the age of about 9 years (Simmons, 2003; Wright, 1997). Therefore, normal development of the auditory mechanism including neural enervation begins in the early weeks of embryological development. The ear develops from the same embryonic layer as the central nervous system (Gordon & Harrison, 2005).

The auditory system is an incredible structure. Figure 2–4 shows a cross section of the auditory system. The peripheral portion can

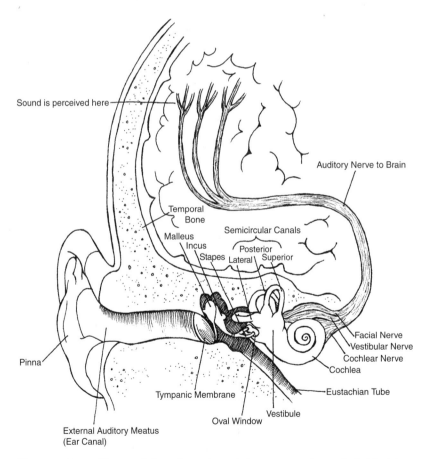

Figure 2–4. The peripheral portion of the ear can be subdivided into three general areas—the outer ear, the middle ear, and the inner ear; the central portion includes the brainstem and cortex.

be subdivided into three general areas: the outer ear, the middle ear, and the inner ear; the central portion includes the brainstem and cortex.

To understand how the auditory system breaks down resulting in hearing loss, it is first necessary to discuss how the ear is put together and how it normally functions.

Data Input Analogy

Together, the outer, middle, and inner ear are known as the *peripheral auditory system* and function to receive sounds. The brainstem and auditory cortex, called the *central auditory system*, take the sounds that are received through the peripheral system and code them for more complex, higher level auditory processes.

Therefore, two general processes of hearing exist: (a) transmission of sounds to the brain through the outer, middle, and inner ear; and (b) understanding the meaning of those sounds once they have been transmitted to the brain. Before understanding can take place, sounds must first be heard, similar to how computer data input precedes data manipulation. There can be no auditory perception without the sensory evidence of sound input (Berlin & Weyand, 2003; Boothroyd, 1997).

One way to illustrate the potentially negative effects of any type of a degree of hearing loss on a child's language and overall development and to further explain the peripheral-central distinction is to use a computer analogy. The primary concept is: *data input precedes data processing.*

An infant or toddler (or anyone) must have information/data in order to learn. A primary avenue for entering information into the brain is through the ears, via hearing. So, the ears can be thought of as analogous to a computer keyboard, and the brain could be compared to a computer "hard drive." As human beings we are neurologically wired to code and hence to develop spoken language and reading skills through the auditory centers of the brain, the hard drive (Pugh et al., 2006; Sharma et al., 2004). Therefore, auditory data input is critical, and it is worth our time and effort to make detailed auditory information available to a child with any degree of hearing loss. If data are entered inaccurately, incompletely, or inconsistently, analogous to using a malfunctioning computer keyboard or to having one's fingers on the wrong keys on a computer keyboard, the child's brain or hard drive will have incorrect or incomplete information to process. How can a child be expected to learn when the information that reaches his or her brain is deficient? The brain can organize itself only around the information that it receives.

Amplification technologies, such as hearing aids, personal FM systems, or sound-field systems, and biomedical devices such as cochlear implants can all be thought of as keyboards—as a means of entering acoustic information into the child's hard drive. So, technology is really a more efficient keyboard. Unfortunately, technology is not a perfect keyboard and it does not have a life of its own, any more than a car has a life of its own. Technology is only as effective as the use to which it is put, and only as efficient as the people who use it. Conversely, without the technology, without acoustic data input, auditory brain access is not possible for persons with hearing loss.

To continue the computer analogy, once the keyboard is repaired or the figurative "fingers" are placed on the correct keys of the keyboard—allowing data to be entered accurately, analogous to using amplification technology that enables a child to detect word-sound distinctions—what happens to all of the previously entered inaccurate and incomplete information? Is there a magic button that automatically converts inaccurate data to complete and correct information? Unfortunately, all of the corrected data need to be reentered. Thus, the longer a child's hearing problem remains unrecognized and unmanaged, the more destructive and far-reaching are the snowballing effects of hearing loss. *Early intervention is critical—the earlier the better!*

Hearing is only the first step in the intervention chain. Once hearing has been accessed as much as possible through appropriate amplification or biomedical technology, the child will have an opportunity to discriminate word-sound distinctions as a basis for learning language, which in turn provides the child with an opportunity to communicate and acquire knowledge of the world. All levels of the acoustic filter effect of hearing loss discussed previously need to be understood and managed. In other words, just medically managing/correcting a conductive hearing loss, or simply wearing hearing aids or a cochlear implant, does not ensure development of an effective language base.

The longer a child's peripheral auditory system remains unmanaged, the longer data entry to the central auditory system (the brain) will be incomplete and inaccurate, causing the snowballing effects of the acoustic filter to negatively impact the child's overall life development. Conversely, the more intelligible and complete the data entered are, the better opportunity the infant or toddler will have to learn language that serves as a foundation for later reading and academic skills. *It can't be said enough—the peripheral auditory system must be managed early to provide the best acoustic access to the central auditory network.*

The point is, from the inception of early intervention programming, comprehensive audiologic and hearing management is an absolutely necessary first step for a child of any age and with any type of hearing or listening difficulty to have an opportunity to learn.

Outer and Middle Ear

Except for the pinna portion of the outer ear, the structure of the human ear is located entirely inside the head and is well protected by the temporal bone which is the hardest bone in the body (Bess & Humes, 2003) (refer to Figure 2–4).

The conductive mechanism is comprised of the outer ear (pinna and ear canal) and the middle ear, which includes the eardrum and a tiny air-filled cavity containing the three smallest bones in the body—the malleus, incus, and stapes. The portion of each ear that is the most external and can be easily seen is a flap of skin and cartilage called the pinna. The pinnae are located on each side of the head, and they function to collect sound waves and focus them into the ear canal. In turn, the ear canal resonates critical high-frequency components of speech sounds. The resonant frequency of the typical ear canal is 2700 Hz; it is a crucial frequency for consonant intelligibility. Small hairs and ear wax within the ear canal function to protect the delicate tympanic membrane (eardrum) from debris. Located at the end of the inside portion of the ear canal (refer to Figure 2–4), the eardrum has a near-horizontal position within the ear canal at birth, making the eardrum difficult to view during infancy. The eardrum doesn't reach its more vertical position of 50–60 degrees from horizontal until the 3rd year of life (Wright, 1997). The eardrum marks the boundary between the outer and middle portions of the ear.

The middle ear is a very small cavity filled with air. Efficiently transmitting the airborne sound that hits the eardrum to the fluid-filled inner ear is the middle ear's primary function. Sound waves enter the ear canal and strike the eardrum causing it to vibrate. Next, vibrations travel from the middle to the inner ear through the three smallest bones in the body, known as the ossicles. The malleus, incus, and stapes are interconnected and attached to the tympanic membrane laterally, and oval window medially. The ossicular chain pumps this vibrational information to the oval window and then to the inner ear.

The eustachian tube passes air to the middle ear and runs from the back of the throat to the anterior (front) wall of the middle ear cavity. When the eustachian tube functions appropriately, the air that is used by the middle ear structures for metabolism is constantly replenished. If and when the eustachian tube does not open often enough to allow air into the middle ear, disease can develop from lack of sufficient oxygen. These diseases are discussed in the next chapter.

Inner Ear to the Brain

The organs of both hearing (cochlea) and balance and equilibrium (vestibular system—semicircular canals) are housed together deep within the temporal bone of the skull. Refer to Figure 2-4. It is not uncommon for an infant or toddler to evidence both a hearing and balance disorder, because the organs for vestibular and auditory detection are located together within the inner ear and have similar embryologic origins.

The sensorineural mechanism is comprised of the cochlea (sensory portion) and the eighth cranial nerve (neural portion). The highly specialized sense organ of the ear is called the organ of Corti, which acts as an acoustic intensity and frequency analyzer, all in the volume of a small grape.

The primary function of the inner ear structure is equilibrium as managed by the vestibular system. One can live without hearing, but actual survival is possible only if the organism can resist the pull of gravity.

The organ of Corti is contained within the cochlea, which is a small, snail-shell shaped, coiled tube that has approximately 2¾ turns and is about 3.5 cm long. The cochlea is a fluid-filled structure. Hair cells found in the organ of Corti contain stereocilia that project into a gelatinous structure that covers the specialized hair cells. The hair cells are the sensory receptors for sound. Vibrational movements generated from the middle ear ossicles instigate a wave complex in the cochlear fluids that displaces the inner ear fluid and hair cells. The hair cells function to transform the hydraulic movement of the inner ear fluids into electrical impulses. The electrical impulses generated from these hair cells stimulate nerve impulses in the auditory nerve. In turn, the auditory nerve transmits these neural impulses to the many auditory centers of the brainstem and brain.

The central nervous system is organized hierarchically. Neural structures become more complex as signals are transmitted from the brainstem to the cortex. Some scientists section the auditory cortex into primary and association areas. Others refer to the auditory cortex as those areas of the brain that are exceedingly receptive to various acoustic stimuli and have similar cell types (Musiek, 2009).

Sound enters the auditory neural system through approximately 16,000 hair cells in the cochlea; about 3,500 are the inner hair cells that are key for transmitting sound to the brain. From the hair cells, impulses are sent to the eighth cranial nerve that has both auditory and vestibular branches as it reaches the brainstem. There are approximately 25,000 afferent nerve fibers. Ultimately, auditory signals are processed by more than 200 million neurons in the brain.

This chapter has offered a brief overview of acoustics and the structure and function of the ear. The next chapter will discuss how these structures can break down.

3

Hearing and Hearing Loss in Infants and Children

Key Points Presented in the Chapter

- Hearing losses are classified as congenital or acquired depending on when they first occur in a child's life.
- Endogenous (genetic) or exogenous (environmental) factors may cause either congenital (early-onset) or acquired (later-onset) hearing losses.
- Genes may predispose a baby to develop a hearing loss when triggered by an environmental event; this is called a *multifactorial* situation.
- In addition to cause and time of onset, classification of hearing loss includes severity—from minimal to profound, depending on how much sound reception is blocked from reaching the brain.
- Every childhood hearing loss, no matter how slight, warrants auditory management.
- Today, the degree of hearing loss does not determine functional outcomes if we provide early use of technology and auditory habilitative services; there is no degree of hearing loss that precludes the primary use of audition if we do what it takes.

- Hearing losses also can be classified as conductive, sensori-neural, or mixed, depending on where they occur in the auditory system.
- Every hearing loss, whether or not it has a treatable medical cause, requires audiologic management to provide auditory access to the child's brain.
- Progressive sensorineural hearing losses may result from large vestibular aqueduct syndrome (LVAS), perilymphatic fistula (PLF), cytomegalovirus (CMV), meningitis, congenital syphilis, ototoxicity, endolymphatic hydrops, autoimmune disorders, delayed hereditary hearing losses, and unknown causes.
- Auditory neuropathy is a disorder of the auditory neural system, including the eighth cranial nerve (auditory nerve), in which cochlear amplification (outer hair cell function) is normal but conduction of sound to the brain is disordered.
- Among children with hearing difficulties, tinnitus affects as many as 24 to 29% to some degree.
- Studies show that at least 50% (and some say up to 90%) of children with sensorineural hearing loss also exhibit vestibu-lar/balance dysfunction.

Introduction

Infants and children require access to detailed sound for auditory learning. A primary problem with hearing loss is that it interferes with sound access to the brain, precluding or diluting auditory capabilities (Musiek, 2009). Neural development and organization of the auditory brain centers require sensory input and extensive auditory experience (Estabrooks, 2006; Kilgard et al., 2007; Sharma et al., 2004; Sharma, Dorman, & Kral, 2005).

Three general types of peripheral hearing loss interfere with acoustic access to the brain. Location of the damage in the auditory system, also called site of lesion, determines the classification of

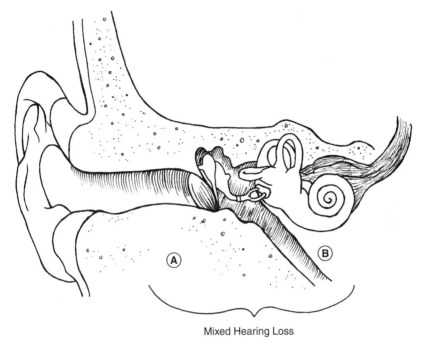

Mixed Hearing Loss

(A) Conductive Hearing Loss
(B) Sensorineural Hearing Loss

Figure 3–1. Location of the damage in the auditory system, also called site of lesion, determines the classification of hearing loss as conductive, sensorineural, or mixed.

hearing loss as conductive, sensorineural, or mixed (Bess & Humes, 2003; Northern & Downs, 2002) (Figure 3-1).

The purpose of this chapter is to provide an overview of the general classifications of hearing impairment, and then to detail some of the specific pathologies that can cause hearing loss.

Classifications

Degree (severity), timing of the onset, and overall cause comprise three general classification schemes for hearing loss.

Degree (Severity)—Minimal to Profound

An important classification of hearing loss is severity; how much sound reception is blocked from reaching the brain (Northern & Downs, 2002). Normal hearing sensitivity in children is 15 dB HL at all frequencies and in both ears with normal middle ear function. Anything less places the child at risk for spoken language learning problems and academic failure if we don't do what it takes to access and develop the auditory brain centers with enriched spoken language.

Please refer to Chapter 1 for a discussion of the distinctions between audiometric definitions of hearing loss and functional outcomes of hearing loss. Audiometric degree of hearing loss used to be a primary variable in functional outcomes—whether a child would likely be auditory or visual in orientation. Now, degree of hearing loss is not a variable if we do what it takes, technologically and habilitatively, to access and develop auditory brain centers. That is, a child with any degree of hearing loss, no matter how profound, can function like a child with a mild to moderate hearing loss who is well-managed if we access the brain with appropriate technology early on (hearing aids or cochlear implants) and provide enriched auditory language stimulation as discussed in the second part of this book.

Normal Hearing Sensitivity: 0 to +15 dB HL for Children

An adult with normal hearing sensitivity has a hearing threshold equal to or better than 25 dB HL. A child, in the unique situation of developing crucial word-sound distinctions of language, requires better hearing sensitivity. To receive the complete speech signal for even soft conversation, a child's hearing sensitivity must be 15 dB HL or better at all frequencies in both ears (Bess & Humes, 2003; Dobie & Berlin, 1979; Northern & Downs, 2002; Tharpe, 2006).

A baby or child may hear well in the perfect quiet of the audiologic test room or the quiet of a close, one-to-one conversation, but she will understand significantly less in the background noise of more public settings. Good hearing sensitivity does not always indicate effective auditory access in different auditory environments.

Minimal or Slight Hearing Loss: 15 to 25 dB HL for Children

A minimal, borderline, or slight hearing loss may cause difficulty for children in the following areas (Northern & Downs, 2002; Tharpe, 2006): distinguishing distant or soft speech (the child may miss at least 10% of classroom learning), responding appropriately to subtle conversational cues, keeping up to speed in rapid-paced interchanges, overhearing social exchanges, and detecting the subtle phonetic markers in grammar, such as those indicating plurality, possessives, or regular past tense.

The greater effort required for the child to hear may cause fatigue and create the appearance of immaturity (Anderson, 2004). Complete access to clear speech is essential, so a minimal hearing loss can have major negative consequences. Due to inadequate hearing screening environments and lack of information about the cornerstone role of hearing in the development of literacy and academics, many of these slight hearing losses fall under the radar.

Every childhood hearing loss, no matter how slight, warrants auditory management. A mild hearing loss (greater than 15 dB HL but less than 40 dB HL) or a unilateral hearing loss may not be problematic for a linguistically mature person who has sophisticated and disciplined attending skills; but even a "minimal" hearing impairment can seriously affect the overall development of an infant or child who is in the process of learning language and developing spoken communication skills as the basis for literacy and acquiring knowledge.

Unilateral Hearing Loss

A person with normal hearing in one ear and at least a mild permanent hearing loss in the other has a unilateral hearing loss. A unilateral hearing loss can cause significant trouble hearing, contrary to popular opinion. In fact, children with unilateral hearing losses are at 10 times greater risk for academic failure than are children with normal hearing in both ears (Bess, Dodd-Murphy, & Parker, 1998; Tharpe, 2006). Identifying speech in noise, localizing sound sources, and other important skills for classroom learning are difficult for the unilateral listener. A child with unilateral hearing loss has more difficulty discerning speech, even when directed into the good ear, than a child with two fully functional ears.

There are differences in behavior between children with normal hearing and children with unilateral hearing losses (Bess et al., 1998; English & Church, 1999; Tharpe, 2006). When compared to peers with normal hearing, children with unilateral hearing losses are described as more distractible, more frustrated, more dependent, less attentive, and appearing less confident in the classroom. Often, behavioral difficulties are more obvious than hearing difficulties in a child with unilateral hearing loss. The connection is rarely made between behavior and hearing because the child has one perfectly good ear and is thought to be able to hear when he or she wants to.

Due to newborn hearing screening programs, unilateral hearing losses are being identified in neonates for the first time, and professionals are wrestling with appropriate management strategies for this new population (Scholl, 2006). Below are some summary points (McKay, 2008).

Unilateral Hearing Loss in Infants—A Summary

- Definition of unilateral hearing loss in babies: good ear has pure tone average (PTA) of 15 dB HL or better; poor ear has PTA of 20 dB or worse or air conduction thresholds poorer than 25 dB HL at two frequencies above 2000 Hz.
- Newborn hearing screenings do not identify mild hearing losses—screenings usually are conducted at 35 dB.
- The biggest problems posed by unilateral hearing losses are difficulty localizing the sound source, poor understanding of speech in noise, and a reduction of distance hearing that interferes with incidental learning.
- There is not yet research to identify if hearing aid fitting before 12 months of age is better than waiting until that time, because it is possible to create a good signal-to-noise ratio (S/N ratio) by physical positioning of the baby close to the talker before 12 months of age.
- After 12 months of age, amplify a mild to moderately severe unilateral hearing loss having obtained the ear and frequency-specific air and bone thresholds that are required for accurate amplification. Use a hearing aid loaner bank initially to determine if a hearing aid is helpful before requiring parents to purchase a hearing aid.
- The goal of amplification for a unilateral hearing loss is to create more equal binaural hearing, with confidence in the results and evidence to justify the fitting.

- Extra and enriched auditory, language, and preliteracy stimulation must be provided to the infant from the beginning. Also, the parent ought to receive counseling about unilateral issues.
- Data show that the more severe the unilateral hearing loss, the greater the likelihood of academic failure if the child does not receive management.
- Right ear unilateral hearing losses seem to be more problematic than left ear losses.
- When retesting the hearing of the infant with unilateral hearing loss, test and monitor *both* ears often—unilateral hearing losses can progress to bilateral hearing losses.
- Possible causes of unilateral to bilateral hearing loss progression are: CMV, enlarged vestibular aqueduct, and genetics.
- See the Web site http://www.cdc.gov/ncbddd/ehdi for more information—this is the proceedings of a conference on mild and unilateral hearing loss.

Mild Hearing Loss: 25 to 40 dB HL

Depending on environmental noise level, distance from talker, and the configuration (pattern) of the hearing loss, a child who experiences a 30 dB hearing loss can miss 25 to 40% of the speech signal if she does not receive audiologic management (Killion & Mueller, 2010; Martin, 2008; Northern & Downs, 2002). The child likely also misses passive learning opportunities by being unable to overhear conversations.

A child with a 35 to 40 dB hearing loss without hearing technology can miss up to 50% of class discussions, especially with far-off or soft voices. Accusations of "daydreaming," "hearing when he or she wants to," or "not trying" may foster a negative self-image in a child (Estabrooks, 2006; Tharpe, 2006). The extra effort exerted to hear often leaves the child more fatigued or irritable than peers with normal hearing (Anderson, 2004).

Though this degree of hearing loss is labeled "mild," the repercussions are great in the life of the baby/child, especially the impact of not hearing clear speech. With a mild, unmanaged hearing loss, a child may be at least one grade level behind his or her peers (Northern & Downs, 2002; Tharpe, 2006). However, appropriate hearing aids/FM systems and auditory-based intervention can overcome the secondary negative effects of hearing loss.

Moderate Hearing Loss: 40 to 55 dB HL

If the content and vocabulary of the message are known, a child with a moderate, unmanaged hearing loss may understand face-to-face conversational speech from three to five feet away in a quiet room, causing the parent or teacher to vastly overestimate this child's auditory access. However, in typical classroom situations, with a 40 to 50 dB hearing loss, 50 to 75% of the speech may be missed, and with a 50 dB hearing loss, 80 to 100% might be missed (Killion & Mueller, 2010). The child often has impaired speech production, delayed or defective syntax, and limited vocabulary. Additional negative effects may include deficits in maturity, communication, and social interaction (Meyer, 2003). By fourth grade, children without appropriate early (and often continuing) intervention for their moderate hearing losses often fall at least two grade levels behind (Northern & Downs, 2002; Ross, Brackett, & Maxon, 1991). Therefore, it is critical to use appropriate hearing aids/FM systems and auditory-based intervention to overcome the secondary negative effects of hearing loss.

Moderately Severe Hearing Loss: 55 to 70 dB HL

One hundred percent of classroom content can be missed with an unamplified 55 dB hearing loss (Killion & Mueller, 2010), and spoken communication must be very close and loud to be minimally understood if amplification technologies are not worn. Without appropriate early and continual assistance, most children with this degree of hearing loss have significant difficulty in school and evidence delayed language, syntax, reduced speech intelligibility, and perhaps an atonal voice quality. Social interactions are, of course, likely difficult. Appropriate use of hearing aids/FM systems and in some cases cochlear implants along with auditory-based intervention can overcome the secondary negative effects of hearing loss.

Severe Hearing Loss: 70 to 90 dB HL

With appropriate amplification (hearing aids or, more likely, cochlear implants), a child with a severe hearing loss should be able to detect all speech sounds as well as environmental sounds, even though she cannot hear conversational speech at all without using technology (Ling, 2002). Spoken language will not develop well or at all without appropriate early use of technology (auditory brain access) followed by auditory language intervention. A child with appropriate auditory technology and auditory-based intervention can be functionally hard of hearing (see Chapter 1) and thus learn and live in a mainstreamed environment, perhaps with the assistance of some support services (Ling, 2002).

Profound Hearing Loss: 90 dB HL or Greater

A baby or child with a profound hearing loss cannot hear speech or environmental sounds without amplification. However, in this day and age, the degree of hearing loss does not determine functional outcomes when there is early use of technology and auditory habilitative services. Audiometric deafness does not preclude auditory brain access and auditory neural development when we use cochlear implants. That is, if the family has spoken language as a desired outcome for their baby who is born with profound deafness, that outcome is likely if we do what it takes, as detailed in this book.

Timing—Congenital or Acquired

The first occurrence of hearing loss in the child's life determines classification into congenital or acquired hearing loss. *Congenital hearing losses* typically occur before, at, or shortly after birth but prior to the learning of speech and language, usually before age 3 (Bess & Humes, 2003). In contrast, *acquired hearing losses* happen after speech and language develop. Because programming already took place in the auditory brain centers for language and spoken communication, the negative effects of an acquired hearing loss tend to be less severe.

The earlier the hearing impairment occurs, the more the hearing loss interferes with language, learning, and development of auditory brain function, unless the child receives effective intervention. Though an acquired hearing loss remains subject to the acoustic filter phenomenon discussed in Chapter 1, the consequences of an acquired hearing loss are not as pervasive if the child had already established a complex linguistic system and mature neural connections in the auditory cortex. Still, with a severe later-onset hearing loss the child's speech can degenerate if speech conservation therapy is not provided.

General Causes—Endogenous, Exogenous, or Multifactorial

Endogenous or exogenous factors may cause either congenital (early-onset) or acquired (later-onset) hearing losses.

Endogenous hearing losses have hereditary or genetic sources and different likelihoods of occurrence (Van Camp, 2006). In the case of a hearing loss being genetically dominant, even if one parent carries the gene, each child has a 50% chance of receiving the gene and the hearing loss. When the hearing loss is recessive, both parents must carry the gene and there is a 25% probability of each child receiving both genes and the resulting hearing loss. For an X-linked recessive hearing loss, each son has a 50% chance of inheriting the gene from his mother; the daughters will be unaffected. In a mitochondrial mutation, all children will receive the gene from the mother, but the father's sperm does not contribute mitochondria to the developing child (Rehm, Williamson, Kenna, Corey, & Korf, 2003).

In a multifactorial inheritance, the additive effects of several minor gene-pair abnormalities combine with nongenetic environmental factors or "triggers" (Rehm et al., 2003). When this happens, hearing loss may manifest in a child with a genetic predisposition for hearing impairment who experiences an environmental event such as a virus or lack of oxygen. Because of the complexity of genetic transmission, families requiring information about endogenous hearing losses should consult a genetic counselor. Of the 50% of congenital hearing losses that have no identifiable cause, it is speculated that 90% are of genetic origin (Northern & Downs, 2002; Van Camp, 2006).

There is increasing interest in a condition called *delayed hereditary sensorineural hearing loss*. Though the child has normal hearing at birth and passes a newborn hearing screening, a hearing loss develops in the first 12 months of life and may continue until about 6 years of age. The parents may experience their baby responding to their voice and saying some words, only to have the child later stop hearing and talking altogether. Even if the hearing loss ultimately progresses to profound in degree, because of the early listening experience, the child typically responds well to auditory-based intervention because the brain was initially organized around auditory input. Delayed hereditary sensorineural hearing loss may affect more than one child per family, though the genetic transmission seems to be recessive in nature (Pappas, 1998; Van Camp, 2006).

In contrast, when external events cause hearing loss the classification is exogenous. Because exogenous hearing loss comes from environmental events, such as lack of oxygen, bacterial or viral infection (such as meningitis, measles, chickenpox, influenza, encephalitis, mumps), noise exposure, head injury, and medications that damage the inner ear, this kind of hearing loss is not transmitted from parents to offspring.

Genetics, Syndromes, and Dysplasias

Connexin 26

In the past few years, many genes have been identified as causing hearing loss. The most common one is connexin 26. Mutations in the connexin 26 gene, on chromosome 13, are believed to be responsible for up to half of recessive nonsyndromic hearing losses. Connexin 26 is a protein that is a critical part of the potassium exchange that occurs in the organ of Corti (inner ear). Hearing loss is caused when a connexin 26 protein cannot be produced during embryological development.

Connexin 26 hearing loss is most often seen in a baby or child with a mild, moderate, severe, or profound congenital hearing loss without any other medical problems and with no identified cause for the hearing loss; more than 50% will experience some hearing loss progression, usually gradually but sometimes precipitously (Kenna et al., 2010). Because the hearing loss is recessive (both parents must carry the gene), no other family member may have a hearing loss. Certain connexin 26 mutations are more common in specific populations such as Caucasians and Ashkenazi Jewish populations (Rehm et al., 2003).

Genetic testing has been successful in identifying connexin 26 as the cause of a baby's hearing loss. Genetic testing is the process of comparing the sequence of a child's gene with that of the regularly occurring gene sequence; the comparison might detect mutations that could make the gene stop functioning. The test is performed by taking a blood sample. Note that genetic testing can be performed only if the gene that is altered is known. There are many forms of hearing loss where the responsible gene remains unknown.

The value of genetic testing is that knowing the cause of a baby's hearing loss can lead to better treatment and management decisions. For example, children with profound hearing losses caused by connexin 26 tend to do very well with cochlear implants because the underlying auditory neural tissue is intact.

Syndromes

A set of symptoms that together characterize a disease or disorder comprise a *syndrome*. *Phenotype* is the word used to identify the outward, physical manifestation of the organism—anything that is part of the observable structure, function, or behavior of a person (Van Camp, 2006). On the other hand, *genotype* is the internally coded, inheritable information found in almost all cells that store the blueprint for building and maintaining a living organism. All syndromes can be described in terms of their phenotype (how they look) and genotype (how they are coded inside cells).

An associated hearing loss accompanies over 200 syndromes; many of them are rare or affecting only single families. For a detailed listing and discussion of syndromes that often include hearing loss, please refer to Northern and Downs (2002), Rehm and Madore (2008), and Shprintzen (2001), and to numerous Web sites, including: National Institutes of Health, Medline Plus, Harvard Medical School Center for Hereditary Deafness, and Boystown National Hospital in Omaha.

A single structural abnormality raises the probability of additional abnormalities. Therefore, the presence of any structural abnormality in a child warrants investigation of the child's hearing. Conversely, a child diagnosed with a hearing loss should be monitored for additional abnormalities (Schein & Miller, 2010). In about 30% of babies with hearing loss, the hearing loss is part of a syndrome; the baby has other problems. Pigmentation abnormalities, such as a white forelock or eyes of different colors, for example, often accompany sensorineural hearing losses (Waardenburg syndrome). Middle ear malformation caused by skeletal abnormalities can cause a congenital, conductive hearing loss. Sensorineural hearing loss may accompany significant visual deficits.

> *In one family, the grandmother had a unilateral, profound hearing loss and no other anomalies. The father had a white forelock and one blue eye and one brown eye, but normal hearing. The baby had a bilateral, profound sensorineural hearing loss and no other stigmata. Their phenotypes differed, but genetic testing revealed that all had variable expressions of Waardenburg syndrome.*

The most common disorders that coincide with hearing loss include asthma, vision disturbance, neuropsychiatric problems, arthritis, heart trouble, mental retardation, cerebral palsy, and cleft palate (Raphael, 2006). Often the number and severity of symptoms vary from person to person and from family member to family member; this is called *variable expression.*

Below are four of the most common dominantly transmitted syndromes; only one parent has to carry the gene for the traits to be expressed, often in a variable fashion (Van Camp, 2006).

- *Alport's syndrome.* Hearing and vision problems are associated with this renal (kidney) disorder. Females tend to be less severely affected than males, and the accompanying sensorineural hearing loss is usually bilateral, high frequency, ranges from mild to severe, and appears in 40 to 60% of the cases. The hearing loss usually begins in adolescence and is progressive.
- *Crouzon's syndrome.* Primary diagnostic features include an abnormally shaped head characterized by a central prominence in the frontal region and a nose resembling a beak. The premature closing of the cranial sutures causes the abnormal shape of the skull. Pinna may be low-set, and in a third of the cases structural abnormalities occur in the middle ear, causing conductive hearing impairment.
- *Treacher Collins syndrome.* Prominent diagnostic features include facial bone abnormalities like deformed pinna, receding chin, depressed cheek bones, and large fishlike mouth with dental abnormalities. Atresia (absence or closure) of the ear canal, malformation of the middle ear ossicles, and cleft palate commonly appear. The manifestation of these

features in persons with Treacher Collins syndrome varies in severity and appearance. A sensorineural component may be present, but the hearing loss is primarily conductive.

■ *Waardenburg syndrome.* Primary diagnostic characteristics include a white forelock, lateral displacement of medial canthi, prominence of the root of the nose, and occasionally cleft palate. Fifty percent of the children have congenital sensorineural hearing impairment ranging from mild to profound, and the hearing loss may be unilateral, bilateral, and/or progressive.

Below are three of the most common recessively transmitted syndromes; both parents need to carry the gene for the traits to be expressed in offspring:

■ *Jervell and Lange-Nielsen syndrome.* Also known as Long Q-T syndrome (LQTS), this cardiovascular disorder correlates with severe to profound, symmetrical, congenital hearing loss. The child may experience fainting attacks or seizures in which no blood leaves the heart. The health of the child appears normal except for two abnormalities in electrocardiogram readings. Thinking it to be a seizure disorder, LQTS often gets treated improperly. Death can result without treatment. Therefore, an electrocardiogram is an important test to perform for a child with profound, congenital sensorineural hearing loss who experiences any fainting spells or seizures. Cardiac events may be precipitated by exercise or emotion, and vestibular dysfunction often is a part of this syndrome (Siem et al., 2008).

■ *Pendred's syndrome.* This endocrine-metabolic disorder includes goiter (an enlarged thyroid gland). Moderate to profound hearing loss usually appears in the first 2 years of life. Large vestibular aqueduct often is part of this syndrome.

■ *Usher syndrome.* This major syndrome involves both hearing and vision disorders. Vision deteriorates beginning in the early teens or twenties, narrowing the visual field until blindness occurs. This sensorineural hearing loss varies in age of onset, severity, and speed of progression. It is bilateral and moderate to severe in degree. There are three clinical types of Usher syndrome: Type I, Type II, and Type III distinguished primarily by severity of hearing loss, presence or absence of vestibular function, and time of onset of vision loss (Wallber, 2009).

Another syndrome that refers to children with a specific set of birth defects is CHARGE syndrome. Babies with CHARGE syndrome are often born with life-threatening birth defects, including complex heart defects and breathing problems. They usually spend many months in the hospital and undergo many surgeries and other treatments. The name originally came from the first letter of some of the most common features seen in these children, although a gene has since been identified:

- <u>C</u> = coloboma of the eye
- <u>H</u> = heart defects
- <u>A</u> = atresia of the choanae, passages that go from the back of the nose to the throat
- <u>R</u> = retardation of growth and development
- <u>G</u> = genital and urinary abnormalities
- <u>E</u> = ear abnormalities and/or hearing loss

The diagnosis of CHARGE is based on finding several of these and possibly other features in a child. The diagnosis should be made by a medical geneticist who has ruled out other disorders that may have similar phenotypes.

Inner Ear Dysplasias

Malformations or incomplete development of the inner ear/cochlea is called a dysplasia. The inner ear has many anatomic abnormalities that are associated with hearing loss. The three most common include (Stach & Ramachandran, 2008):

- *Scheibe.* Scheibe is incomplete development, malformation, or degeneration of the membranous cochlea, and is the most common dysplasia. A CT scan will not identify this dysplasia since the osseous cochlea is normal.
- *Mondini.* A child with Mondini dysplasia has incomplete development or malformation of the inner ear, including the osseous cochlea, and has increased susceptibility to a

perilymphatic fistula (PLF), large vestibular aqueduct (LVAS), and endolymphatic hydrops (Holden & Linthicum, 2005). The hearing loss may be fluctuating or progressive, and the malformed cochlea may cause some difficulty inserting a cochlear implant. A CT scan can identify this dysplasia.

■ *Michel's aplasia.* Michel's is actually an aplasia which means an absence of an organ or tissue. This relatively rare aplasia is the total absence of differentiated inner ear structures, leaving absolutely no residual hearing. Michel's also may be described as a common cavity inner ear deformity. A CT scan can identify Michel's aplasia.

Medical Aspects of Hearing Loss

Conductive Pathologies and Hearing Loss

The outer and/or middle ear is the location of damage (also called site of lesion) that causes conductive hearing loss. The conductive mechanism transmits sound to the inner ear and thus does not contain irreplaceable nerve endings, enabling this part of the auditory structure to respond to treatment by medical or surgical interventions.

Both medical and educational issues and treatments need to be considered for a baby/child with a conductive hearing loss; one treatment does not substitute for the other. The pathology that causes the hearing loss may affect the child's general health, and medical treatment often restores the hearing that is caused by disease in the outer and/or middle ear. Any potential impact on language acquisition and educational performance is also crucial to address when treating conductive hearing loss. That is, physicians are trained to deal with medical and surgical management of disease, and audiologists are skilled to deal with diagnosis and treatment of the resultant hearing loss. Both professionals must be involved in managing conductive hearing losses.

The most common conductive hearing losses in infants and toddlers are: otitis media (middle ear infection), collapsed ear canals, abnormalities of the middle ear ossicles, atresia, stenosis, cerumen impaction, otitis externa, perforated tympanic membrane, objects in the ear canal, cholesteatoma, and mastoiditis.

Baby Alice was identified at birth with a moderate, bilateral sensorineural hearing loss. Subsequently, she was fitted with hearing aids that allowed detailed access to her brain of the complete speech spectrum. At 6 months of age, she began experiencing upper respiratory infections followed by ongoing bouts of otitis media. The added conductive hearing loss caused by otitis media caused her hearing to intermittently progress from a moderate sensorineural hearing loss to a severe mixed hearing loss. The initial fit of her hearing aids was no longer adequate to provide acoustic access to her brain; the aids needed to be readjusted (made stronger) if her early intervention program was to be effective. At the very least, her hearing aids must have an external volume control to allow more or less gain (amplification) depending on the status of her middle ears. In addition, more aggressive medical management was needed.

Otitis Media (Commonly Called Middle Ear Infection)

For children, ear infections are the most common cause of conductive hearing loss and hearing problems. Otitis media needs to be considered from two perspectives. The first is when otitis media occurs in the absence of other disabling conditions. The second is when otitis media is added to a preexisting sensorineural hearing loss, adding to the degree of hearing loss and the difficulty of appropriately managing the hearing loss. For children with coexisting sensorineural hearing losses, therefore, more aggressive medical management for ear disease is warranted to preclude adding to the child's hearing problem and perhaps sabotaging intervention.

Otitis media is an inflammation of the middle ear. Otitis media with effusion (OME) is an inflammation of the middle ear that includes fluid in the normally air-filled middle ear space (Northern & Downs, 2002; Stach & Ramachandran, 2008). Although this fluid can occur with or without the presence of an active infection, it can almost always cause hearing maladies. Acute otitis media (AOM) indicates a middle ear infection of recent onset, characterized by symptoms and signs of infection which include fever, pain, and irritability that can last as long as 2 to 3 weeks. Subacute otitis media indicates a chronic ear infection that fails to clear and can last anywhere from 3 weeks to 3 months, usually with effusion (fluid). Chronic otitis media indicates otitis media of more than 3 months' duration with or without perforation of the tympanic membrane (hole in the eardrum) and drainage.

Approximately one half of the episodes of OME are classified as "silent" and are undetected by parents because the child often does not appear to be sick. Noninfectious fluid, one cause for hearing difficulty, gathers in the middle ear. Therefore, when a baby visits the pediatrician for a general check-up, it is a shock to find that OME is discovered nearly 50% of the time (Northern & Downs, 2002). These unrecognizable bouts of OME often indicate that parents are not necessarily accurate reporters of a child's history of a dysfunctional middle ear.

Unfortunately, if the first bout of OME occurs in a baby, the likelihood of recurrent and severe episodes increases (Cook & Walsh, 2005), because the disease process of OME alters the structure of the middle ear lining. Recovery occurs more slowly with younger age and each additional ear infection.

Ear Infections: Causes and Effects

Malfunctioning eustachian tubes are the cause of OME—viral upper respiratory infections are the typical precursors of that malfunction. After the onset of a cold or other upper respiratory infection, the usual pattern is for an ear infection to occur a few days later because the eustachian tube's function becomes obstructed by infectious mucus. The prevalence of OME increases during the winter months (Kouwen & DeJonckere, 2007).

Comprised of cartilage and muscle along with a flutter valve opening, the eustachian tube is a tiny structure (1 cm long) that connects the back of the throat to the middle ear. The three main functions of the eustachian tube are: equalizing air pressure differences between the middle ear and the environment, protection of the delicate middle ear from nose and throat secretions, and draining normal secretions from the middle ear cavity into the throat (Stach, 1998). The most important function is pressure regulation. When the eustachian tube fails, normal atmospheric pressure cannot be maintained within the middle ear, resulting in negative pressure that can often lead to fluid buildup from the near vacuum "sucking" fluid out of the mucous lining of the middle ear cavity. Fluid can exist "silently," resulting in decreased hearing, or it can also contain infection from bacteria and/or viruses.

To reiterate, conductive hearing loss will typically accompany an ear infection. It is possible for hearing loss to occur even when fluid is not present but negative pressure occurs. On average, hearing loss is 25 dB, but it can increase up to 50 dB (Northern & Downs, 2002). Hearing loss may be more severe at some frequencies than others. Fluid and/or negative pressure in the middle ear, coupled with coexisting hearing loss, may persist from 2 weeks to 3 months following a single bout of OME (Waseem & Aslam, 2006). If and when a child is otitis-prone (has recurring ear infections), the child may experience the effects of constant middle ear fluid. Therefore, some children with OME may suffer temporary, fluctuating hearing impairment, whereas others will endure long-term hearing losses (Stach & Ramachandran, 2008).

High Incidence Populations

The peak prevalence of otitis media is between 6 and 18 months of age, and there is a second, lower peak between 4 and 5 years of age corresponding to entering school. One in four children with learning disabilities, twice the number as in the non–learning-disabled population, has recurrent OME. The following conditions and situations predispose a baby or child to otitis media (Waseem & Aslam, 2006):

- Congenital abnormalities such as cleft palate (*even after repair*), congenital cytomegalovirus (CMV), perinatally acquired HIV infection, and other immune deficiencies.
- Down syndrome and other genetic factors.
- Specific infections, especially those of the upper respiratory tract—incompletely treated sinusitis and purulent conjunctivitis. Both bacteria and viruses are seemingly involved.
- Environmental factors: attendance at day care centers and exposure to passive smoking.
- Allergies are a factor in 30 to 40% of recurring OME cases.
- Immune deficiency that does not permit the body to fight the resultant bacterial or viral infection.
- Children in neonatal intensive care units (NICUs) as infants have an incidence of around 80%.

Even temporary hearing loss during the first year of life may have associated attention and language learning problems (Northern & Downs, 2002). According to Nozza (2006), children who experience OME during their first year may experience difficulty learning to discern individual phonemes because the presence of even a slight hearing loss necessitates a more favorable speech-to-noise ratio than exists in typical communication environments.

Medical Diagnosis and Treatment of OME

The use of pneumatic otoscopy, an otoscope with a bulb and tube attached that blows small puffs of air through the ear canal to cause eardrums to move, is the most reliable method to diagnose ear infections (Waseem & Aslam, 2006). The mobility of the eardrum and its color and shape are keys to accurate medical diagnosis. The eardrum will not move well with the middle ear filled with fluid. Compared to adult eardrums, those of infants are more horizontal and thus more difficult to see (Wright, 1997).

Behavioral symptoms and other case history information also aid in diagnosis (Northern & Downs, 2002). Irritability (the most common symptom), listlessness, and distractibility are some general symptoms as well as pulling the ears, head banging, and rolling the head from side to side.

The most common bacterial pathogen in AOM is *Streptococcus pneumoniae,* followed by nontypeable *Haemophilus influenzae* and *Moraxella catarrhalis.* These three organisms are responsible for more than 95% of all OME cases with a bacterial etiology.

The recommended medical treatment for OME is no treatment—watchful waiting to avoid antibiotic resistance because in otherwise healthy children, OME will resolve itself (Finkelstein, Stille, Rifas-Shiman, & Goldmann, 2005). If a decision is made to treat with an antibacterial agent, amoxicillin is prescribed for most children. When amoxicillin is used, the dose should be 80 to 90 mg/kg/d. Studies of other adjunctive therapy for AOM and OME have shown that decongestants and antihistamines provide no obvious benefits.

The surgical intervention, called tympanostomy, entails making an incision through the eardrum, suctioning the fluid out of the middle ear, then inserting tympanostomy tubes (also called ventilation tubes or PE tubes) through the tympanic membrane (Oomen et al., 2005). These tubes provide air to the middle ear space by functioning as a substitute for the malfunctioning eustachian tubes. The procedure is regarded as very safe, takes about 10 minutes, and requires a general anesthetic. The possibility of scarring exists with repeated tube insertions. The tubes require careful management to prevent infection, and one should keep the ear canal clean and dry. After 6 to 18 months, the tympanostomy tubes usually fall out naturally. If infections continue, the tubes may need replacement.

Following are indications for tympanostomy tube insertion in children (Waseem & Aslam, 2006):

■ Chronic OME: Tube insertion is recommended in children when OME is unresponsive to a trial of antibiotic therapy and has persisted for at least 3 months when bilateral, or at least 6 months when unilateral.

■ Recurrent AOM: Tube insertion is recommended in children with recurrent acute otitis media, especially when antibiotics fail. A minimum frequency of AOM of three or more episodes during the previous 6 months, or four or more episodes (one of which is recent) during the previous year, indicates tube insertion.

■ Recurrent OME: Tube insertion is recommended in children with recurrent OME in which the duration of each episode does not meet criteria for chronic disease; however, the cumulative duration is considered excessive, for example, 6 of the previous 12 months.

■ Eustachian tube dysfunction: Tube insertion is recommended in children with eustachian tube dysfunction even in the absence of middle ear fluid when the child has persistent or recurrent signs, and symptoms are not relieved by medical treatment. Signs and symptoms include hearing loss (usually fluctuating), dizziness or balance problems, tinnitus, autophony, and severe retraction pocket in the tympanic membrane.

In recent years, there has been research into vaccinations for children with OME. The Red Book Report (2006) of the Committee on Infectious Diseases states the following about immunization of children with severe or recurrent otitis media: "Pneumococcal polysaccharide vaccines that are not conjugated to carrier proteins have not decreased the incidence of AOM in children of any age; therefore, PPV23 is not recommended for prevention of AOM. For children younger than 2 years of age, PCV7 provides a modest decrease in AOM and recurrent AOM (as defined by 3 or more episodes in 6 months, 4 or more episodes in 1 year, or in placement of tympanostomy tubes)" (p. 535).

Visit the following Web sites for additional and updated medical information about OME: KidsHealth, NIDCD, eMedicine, the American Academy of Pediatrics, and MedlinePlus.

Audiologic Diagnosis and Treatment of Otitis Media

Pediatric audiologic evaluation has three main goals: (a) to evaluate hearing sensitivity, (b) to evaluate auditory behaviors (Does the child's response to sound correspond to her particular developmental age?), and (c) to make sure that necessary treatment is provided to allow sound to reach the child's brain.

Since the prerogative to diagnose middle ear disease is medical and not audiologic, the audiologic diagnosis of hearing loss caused by otitis media does not differ from the diagnosis of hearing loss from any other pathology. The audiologist deals with audiologic treatment of the hearing loss, not medical treatment of the ear disease. The audiologist does, however, make sure that appropriate medical referrals are made and that medical management is received.

Though the outcomes of continuing, persistent, and current hearing losses are more definite, the negative repercussions of early and fluctuating hearing loss stem from many factors. Some factors are: irregular medical management, low socioeconomic level, large family size, multiple languages spoken to the child, general malaise caused by diseases, effectiveness of the child's cognitive style, and reduced parental linguistic interaction due to nonresponsiveness of the child (Northern & Downs, 2002). Accurate prediction of how devastating a fluctuating hearing loss will be on the child's later verbal and academic performance becomes difficult because of these factors. Golz et al. (2005) found that children with recurrent AOM during the critical early years are at greater risk for delayed reading than aged-matched peers with no history of middle ear problems. Therefore, rather than wait to see whether difficulties develop and then attempt to remediate, it seems prudent to always initiate early intervention for any hearing loss in order to prevent later speech, language, literacy, and academic deficits.

Following are some additional causes of conductive hearing losses in infants and children (Stach & Ramachandran, 2008).

Kouwen and DeJonckere (2007) found that the probability of children having OME is reduced by 40% if they chew gum daily or several times a week. It appears that chewing and swallowing activities activate jaw movements, increase salivary flow, and increase the chance of the eustachian tube opening to allow ventilation of the middle ear space.

Collapsed Ear Canals

If external earphones are used during hearing tests, the pressure caused by their placement can close or collapse the ear canal if the infant's or child's ear canal is very soft and small. An erroneous conductive hearing loss results from a collapsed ear canal. Therefore, insert earphones are recommended for all audiologic testing of infants and children (see Figure 4–3 in Chapter 4).

Ossicular Abnormalities

Ossicular abnormalities mean that the tiny middle ear bones did not develop appropriately embryologically. The resultant conductive hearing loss is usually treated very successfully with hearing aids rather than with surgery. The nature of conductive hearing loss is that the sound needs only to be made louder without having to deal with the distortion caused by a sensorineural hearing loss.

Atresia and Microtia

Atresia is a type of birth defect that causes a complete closure of the ear canal. Obviously, sound cannot travel through an absent or blocked ear canal. Atresia is often accompanied by microtia—an abnormally small external ear/pinna. Through CT scans, Mayer, Brueckmann, Sigert, Witt, and Weerda (1997) identified a variety of external, middle, and, less frequently, inner ear changes in connection with microtia.

Because cases of atresia feature an unknown position of the facial nerve, fear of facial paralysis typically precludes surgical opening of the ear canal until the child becomes an adult and an informed decision of risk can be made. Bone conduction amplification, including the bone anchored hearing aid (Baha), is typically used. Chapter 5 will discuss amplification possibilities.

Stenotic Ear Canal

The stenotic ear canal is abnormally small and narrow. Hearing loss can result from small amounts of cerumen or earwax plugging the small canal, acting like an earplug. Comfortable fitting of earmolds for hearing aids and physical examination of the eardrum are very difficult. This seemingly minor problem can thus become a source of constant discomfort for the child and a cause of fluctuating or even continual hearing loss.

Cerumen, or Earwax, Impaction

Earwax is a normal secretion of the body that functions to protect and cleanse the delicate ear canal (Oliveira et al., 2006). Its color and consistency may vary and look like blood clots, black tar, yellow crayon, white rocks, or amber liquid. The appearance may be dark due to the oxidation that comes with age, or gold if the cerumen is relatively new.

Normally, the cells lining the ear canal move the earwax down the ear canal to the opening in the pinna where it dries and flakes away. Using Q-tips and other foreign objects to remove wax is potentially dangerous because the objects interfere with the ear canal's natural cleansing process by forcing wax back into the ear canal.

Wax production varies from person to person, and a large producer may make enough to block the ear canal. This wax needs to be removed, often by a physician, although the audiology scope of practice does include routine cerumen removal. Genetic makeup, emotional states, and medications can influence the amount of secretion due to cerumen glands' similarity to sweat glands.

High frequency hearing loss may result from a partial cerumen impaction, where the mass of the earwax narrows the ear canal diameter, but does not totally block the opening. Complete cerumen impaction or blockage may result in a 30 to 50 dB HL hearing loss across all frequencies (Northern & Downs, 2002). Approximately 10% of children and about 30% of persons with developmental disabilities have cerumen problems that cause hearing loss until the cerumen is removed. Impacted cerumen may also result in tinnitus (ringing in the ears), dizziness, itching, earache, otitis externa (infection in the ear canal), cardiac depression, and chronic cough.

Hearing aids can interfere with the natural cleansing process of the ear canal, and may even push the wax back into the ear.

> *Because the pinna and ear canal have very thin skin with little subcutaneous tissue, skin lesions can be quite painful; most are easily treated by a physician (Garvey, Garvey, & Hendi, 2008).*

Because the excess cerumen can block the ear canal or the earmold, infants and toddlers who wear hearing aids should be monitored carefully for excess cerumen.

Otitis Externa

An infection of the ear canal is called otitis externa; one example is swimmer's ear. Bacterial or fungal infections many prosper due to collected moisture in the ear canal, and result in pain, swelling, and drainage. Excessive moisture is a problem because it removes cerumen and increases the pH of the ear canal, providing a good setting for bacterial growth. The infection requires medical treatment, typically with topical medication applied directly to the ear canal.

Earmolds cause discomfort and impede healing of otitis externa, making the infection a big problem for wearers of hearing aids. The child loses valuable educational time when amplification is discontinued to allow air into the ear canal until the infection is cleared. Prevention is the key. Keep the ear canals clean and dry and wash the earmolds regularly in mild soapy detergent.

Perforated Tympanic Membrane

A hole in the eardrum, often caused by ear infection or trauma, is called a tympanic perforation. The eardrum may rupture from a sharp blow to the ear, and the ossicles behind it may receive damage, also. Natural healing may occur or surgical repair may be necessary. The perforation causes varying degrees of hearing loss depending on its size and location (Stach & Ramachandran, 2008).

Object in the Ear Canal

Small children have been known to push objects into their ear canals, such as hairpins, cereal, marbles, rocks, earrings, small hearing aid batteries, bugs, beads, and other food and toys. The objects can cause discomfort, infection, and/or hearing loss. Usually, a physician removes them.

Cholesteatoma

A nonmalignant tumor that grows from a perforated eardrum is called a cholesteatoma. The tumor usually results from chronic ear infections, though a child may also be born with it. Cholesteatomas often take the form of a cyst or pouch that sheds layers of old skin that builds up inside the ear. Over time, it can increase in size and destroy the tiny ossicles of the middle ear. A cholesteatoma poses a threat to health and can cause hearing loss, dizziness, and facial muscle paralysis; it must be surgically removed. Desire to prevent such a tumor should strengthen diligent medical management of ear infections. Children with cholesteatomas typically require temporary amplification while they undergo a series of middle ear surgeries.

Mastoiditis

An infection of the mastoid process, the bony projection behind the pinna, is called mastoiditis. Ear infection spreading from the middle ear space to the mastoid was common before the discovery of antibiotics. Mastoidectomy, a surgery that literally cleared out the entire middle ear space and caused significant hearing loss, was often a necessary treatment. In this day and age, mastoiditis is easily avoided with good medical management of otitis media.

Sensorineural Pathologies and Hearing Loss

The inner ear/cochlea is that part of the ear that houses thousands of tiny sensory receptors called hair cells that currently cannot be repaired once they are damaged or destroyed. Thus, injury or pathology in this area causes a sensorineural hearing loss that is permanent. To mitigate the effects of sensorineural hearing loss, hearing aids, cochlear implants, or assistive listening devises are employed. Amplification does not correct damage to the inner ear; rather, sound is amplified and shaped to make sounds audible to an ear that could not otherwise detect them.

The following are common causes of sensorineural hearing losses in children: noise, viral and bacterial infections such as cytomegalovirus and meningitis, anoxia, ototoxicity, large vestibular aqueduct, perilymphatic fistula, and Rh incompatibility (Raphael, 2006). Genetic/endogenous/syndromic hearing losses were discussed earlier in this chapter.

All children with sensorineural hearing loss should be screened for vestibular dysfunction because many experience undiagnosed problems. Unlike adults, vestibular dysfunction does not show as dizziness or vertigo in children—it manifests itself as balance problems. If a child has no vestibular function in either ear, intervention needs to focus on compensatory strategies such as physical therapy to strengthen core muscles and lower extremities (for balance), occupational therapy to enhance eye coordination, and, above all, safety issues because a child without vestibular function cannot function in the dark.

Tinnitus

Tinnitus, often associated with sensorineural hearing loss, involves hearing ringing, buzzing, roaring, or chirping sounds, and can occur in children. The sounds range from being hardly perceptible to very distracting, and from being infrequent to constant. The onset of tinnitus or the increase in severity of tinnitus has been associated with progressive hearing loss. In addition, tinnitus may co-occur with hyperacusis, a condition characterized by an abnormally strong reaction or reduced tolerance to typical environmental sounds (Sun, 2009). Baguley and McFerran (2002) have summarized the following points about childhood tinnitus:

- Between 6 and 13% of children with normal hearing experience tinnitus from time to time.
- Tinnitus may be caused by ear infections, noise exposure, and head injuries in children, just like in adults.
- Among children with hearing difficulties, tinnitus affects as many as 24 to 29% to some degree.
- There appears to be greater prevalence and severity of tinnitus in children with moderate to severe sensorineural hearing losses than in children with profound sensorineural hearing losses.
- An acquired (later onset) sensorineural hearing loss is more likely to be associated with tinnitus than a congenital hearing loss.
- A child with sensorineural hearing loss rarely complains of tinnitus if not asked about it.

> *Noise exposure at young ages can negatively affect the auditory cortex. Moreover, diet, stress, and genetics all influence the child's susceptibility to drug- or noise-induced hearing loss (Campbell, 2009).*

Noise-Induced Hearing Losses

Permanent inner ear damage caused by prolonged exposure to loud noises constitutes noise-induced hearing loss, and it can occur in infants and children. In addition to loud music, parents need to be aware that many toys are louder than a chainsaw when held close to a baby's ear, and can potentially cause or worsen hearing loss (Sylvester, 2006). Parents should listen to the toy before they buy it, or put masking or packing tape over the speaker of the toy to reduce its volume.

Some studies have found that antioxidants have been effective in reducing hearing loss caused by noise, but other studies have found no benefit (Kramer et al., 2006). More research exploring antioxidant use in different noise conditions needs to be conducted.

For more information about noise induced hearing loss in children and school hearing conservation programs, refer to the "Wise Ears!" Web site of the National Institute on Deafness and Other Communication Disorders.

Viral and Bacterial Infections

Some infections are transferred through the placenta to the fetus from the mother. Whether or not the mother feels ill herself, the effects of the infection on the fetus vary. Infections may cause mild to profound hearing losses and minimal to serious additional abnormalities. Blood tests can usually identify exposure to infections such as cytomegalovirus, rubella, herpes, toxoplasmosis, and syphilis. Infections that occur in the child after birth also might cause hearing loss, with bacterial meningitis being the worst.

Refer to the Centers for Disease Control and Prevention (CDC) Web site for more information about bacterial and viral infections.

Meningitis

Meningitis is primarily a disease of the central nervous system, causing inflammation of the coverings (meninges) of the brain and its fluids. Historically, meningitis has been the most common cause of hearing loss in infants and children (Stach & Ramachandran, 2008). Symptoms include high fever, headache, and stiff neck in anyone over the age of 2 years. These symptoms can develop over several hours, or they may take 1 to 2 days. Other symptoms may include nausea, vomiting, discomfort looking into bright lights, confusion, and sleepiness. In newborns and small infants, the classic symptoms of fever, headache, and neck stiffness may be absent or difficult to detect (Raphael, 2006). The infant may only appear slow or inactive or be irritable, have vomiting, or be feeding poorly. As the disease progresses, patients of any age may have seizures.

Making a definite diagnosis should occur quickly and requires a lumbar puncture (spinal tap). The hearing loss that results from meningitis is caused by inflammation of the membranous structures of the cochlea from the spreading of the infection from the meninges (Stach & Ramachandran, 2008). Complete hearing loss may occur if the cochlea ossifies over time, as revealed by a CT scan. Therefore, if listening and talking are desired outcomes for the baby or child, a cochlear implant must be inserted quickly before cochlear ossification occurs. Chapter 5 discusses cochlear implants.

Postmeningitic children have varying amounts, symmetries, and configurations of hearing loss. Commonly, patients possess fluctuating but progressive hearing loss (Northern & Downs, 2002). All children who experience bacterial meningitis, especially *H. influenzae*, require careful and ongoing audiologic monitoring and management.

There are several vaccines against meningitis that are safe and highly effective. They are recommended for all children, and especially for children who are going to receive a cochlear implant (Cohen, Roland, & Marrinan, 2004). Postimplant meningitis has been found to be related to patient, surgical, and (implant) device factors, but by adhering to sound surgical principles, vaccinating patients and eliminating potentially traumatic electrode arrays, the incidence of meningitis has been significantly diminished in this population (Cohen et al., 2004).

Cytomegalovirus (CMV)

Congenital CMV is the primary cause of viral-type sensorineural hearing losses in the United States (Wills & Goodrich, 2006). Hearing losses range from stable to fluctuating and progressive and bilateral to unilateral, and vary in severity from mild to profound (Fowler, 2008). Consistent audiologic evaluations and flexible amplification fittings are a must for a child suspected of having CMV. When severe to profound hearing loss exists, cochlear implants can provide useful auditory input even though the child with CMV may have additional medical and cognitive deficits (Ramirez & Nikolopoulos, 2004).

Along with herpes simplex virus (cold sores), varicella-zoster virus (chickenpox and shingles), and Epstein-Barr virus (mononucleosis), CMV is a member of the herpes family and thus can cause latent infections by persisting in the body indefinitely (Wills & Goodrich, 2006). CMV infects almost everybody at some point without negative consequences. However, 1 in 10 cases of acute CMV during pregnancy are estimated to result in congenital CMV disease.

Only 10% of infants with CMV show symptoms at birth, such as central nervous system disabilities, hearing loss, visual disorders, developmental delay, psychomotor retardation, enlarged liver and spleen, decreased platelet count in the blood, inflammation of the retina, cerebral palsy, and language or learning disorders. CMV appears in the saliva, urine, blood, tears, stool, cervical secretions, and semen of an infected person for many months or years with or without obvious symptoms. Though an infant appears healthy, she can still secrete CMV. When working in clinical/educational settings, infection control procedures, like regular handwashing, are very important.

Anoxia

Lack of oxygen before, during, or shortly after birth, causes anoxia. Respiratory problems are often associated with low birth weight (less than 1,500 grams). Anoxia has a unique audiometric configuration, with essentially normal low frequency hearing, but more severe hearing loss in the high frequencies. The infant or toddler can thus hear sounds (mostly vowels), but individual speech sounds

> *Any child with a history of anoxia, prematurity, or low birth weight needs repeated hearing tests focusing on high frequency hearing. Be sure to start testing and conditioning in the low frequencies where hearing is likely to be better.*

like consonants remain difficult or impossible to distinguish. Because the child responds to low frequency sounds, hearing loss may be overlooked. This severe to profound high frequency sensorineural hearing loss may be difficult to fit with hearing aids. That is, if the high frequency hearing loss is beyond the reach of conventional amplification, cochlear implantation ought to be considered to allow the baby/child access to the critical consonant sounds.

Ototoxicity

High doses of certain drugs can cause ototoxicity, a poisoning of the delicate inner ear. These drugs can also cause vestibulotoxicity, poisoning of the vestibular/balance system with symptoms of imbalance, unsteadiness, and severe fatigue. Problem drugs include mycin drugs (kanamycin, gentamicin, tobramycin, amikacin, and neomycin), some diuretics, quinine, cisplatin (a chemotherapeutic agent effective in the treatment of cancer), and aspirin. Mycin drugs in conjunction with loop diuretics appear especially problematic. The term *high dose* is relative; a normal dose for a 130-pound woman is very high for a 1-pound fetus. A baby or child can receive ototoxic drugs directly (usually as a life-saving measure), or the fetus can receive them in utero through medications that the mother takes. Interestingly, mutations in a mitochondrial gene can cause hearing loss that begins after antibiotic therapy in an infant (Campbell, 2009; Rehm et al., 2003).

Ototoxic hearing losses are usually high frequency and permanent, but some fluctuate, such as those caused by aspirin. Most important, delayed onset hearing loss frequently occurs with ototoxicity, so even after discontinuing medications, monitoring hearing sensitivity must continue. Specifically, children treated for malignancies with cisplatin require long-term surveillance to avoid missing hearing deficits (Bertolini et al., 2004).

Large Vestibular Aqueduct Syndrome (LVAS)

A vestibular aqueduct diameter larger the 1.5 mm to 2.0 mm (identified in CT scan) usually constitutes this congenital malformation of the temporal bone, predisposing the affected person to early onset, high frequency, fluctuating, or progressive sensorineural hearing loss as well as vestibular dysfunction (Wu, Chen, Chen, & Hsu, 2005). Arjmand and Webber (2004) found that almost 50% of the children that they studied who had unilateral LVAS had bilateral, asymmetrical sensorineural hearing loss. LVAS also is called "enlarged vestibular aqueduct" (EVA) syndrome (Dabrowski, Myers, & Danilova, 2009).

Clark and Roeser (2005) noticed that a conductive component may co-occur in some people, perhaps due to decreased mobility of the stapes or incomplete bone formation around the inner ear. Note that a medical misdiagnosis of otitis media with effusion can easily delay the eventual finding of LVAS.

There are several different theories proposed to explain the progressive hearing loss associated with LVAS; most are related to the architectural changes in the cochlea (Clark & Roeser, 2005). Reportedly, events like minor head trauma can trigger decreases in hearing. Positive medical diagnosis requires a CT scan, and because CT scans are not routine, LVAS may be more common than initially expected.

Audiologists should be aware that children or adolescents who have a sensorineural hearing loss of unknown cause, with or without accompanying dizziness, may have LVAS, especially if their hearing loss is progressive. A decrease in sensitivity at 500 Hz is a prognostic factor for progression of the hearing loss (Lai & Shiao, 2004). Hearing loss requires close monitoring. If hearing loss progresses to the severe to profound range, a cochlear implant should be considered sooner rather than later in order to advance listening, talking, and literacy skills (Clark & Roeser, 2005).

Perilymphatic Fistula (PLF)

A perilymphatic fistula is an abnormal communication between the fluid-filled perilymphatic space of the inner ear and the air-filled middle ear cavity, usually through the round or oval windows, resulting in sensorineural hearing loss and/or vestibular symptoms.

The existence of PLF was proposed more than a century ago, yet it remains a topic of controversy, especially regarding the existence of "spontaneous" etiologies. The diagnosis is made by clinical history and otoneurological tests with a definitive diagnosis being made at surgery, although the use of surgical findings as a criterion standard for PLF has been questioned.

In the absence of prior surgery or definite traumatic event, it may be difficult to distinguish a perilymphatic fistula from Ménière's disease. Fitzgerald (2001) wrote that the issue is not whether the patient has PLF or Ménière's disease, but whether the Ménière's disease is primary, or the PLF is primary with a secondary Ménière's disease. Both conditions have various presenting symptoms of fluctuating hearing loss, often spinning vertigo, feelings of fullness, and tinnitus.

PLF can have many causes, such as a congenital weakness or defect in the bony partition between the perilymphatic compartment of the inner ear and the middle ear, or a traumatic event like a head injury or sudden barometric change. Sudden and dramatic hearing loss or increase in severity of an existing hearing loss can result from a fistula (Alexiades & Hoffman, 2008).

To preserve hearing, diagnosis and surgical repair of a PLF must be virtually immediate. Weber, Bluestone, and Perez (2003) found that surgical repair, including packing the oval and round windows even if a leak is not visualized, may prevent further deterioration of hearing loss, may alleviate symptoms, and does not result in significant risk for postoperative hearing loss or additional complaints of vertigo.

Acoustic Neuroma

When the main nerve trunk that carries auditory sensations from the inner ear to the brain grows a nonmalignant tumor, it is called acoustic neuroma, or eighth nerve tumor. If not diagnosed and surgically removed, a neuroma can grow into a brainstem tumor that causes hearing loss and ultimately could be fatal. The hearing loss is usually unilateral, high frequency, progressive, and may have accompanying facial nerve involvement and dizziness. The tumor is usually slow-growing, diagnosed best with an MRI, and surgically removed if it becomes large. Sometimes, surgery is not recommended for a small, slow growing tumor. Monitoring is done using periodic MRIs.

Rh Incompatibility

Rh incompatibility occurs when maternal antibodies from her Rh negative blood destroy the Rh positive blood cells of the fetus. Hearing loss, jaundice, and possible brain damage can result. Thanks to medical advances, Rh incompatibility, like rubella, is no longer a primary cause of sensorineural hearing loss in children.

Mixed, Progressive, Functional, and Central Hearing Losses

Mixed Hearing Loss

Two or more ear pathologies occurring at the same time can cause both conductive and sensorineural hearing losses; it is identified as a *mixed hearing loss*. For example, a child with a congenital, genetic sensorineural hearing loss could also have ear infections. Another child might have stenotic ear canals blocked by wax, a cholesteatoma (tumor in the middle ear), and a sensorineural hearing loss from anoxia (lack of oxygen at birth). The hearing loss becomes the sum of each individual component, and all pathologies and sites of lesion need to be identified and managed.

Unfortunately, conductive hearing losses often obscure coexisting sensorineural losses (Clark & Roeser, 2005). For example, once otitis media is diagnosed, the ear infection is often considered the cause of the child's entire hearing problem. A careful audiologic assessment should identify all locations in the auditory system where pathologies occur, and appropriate medical (for the conductive component) and audiologic management (for the hearing loss) must occur (Northern & Downs, 2002).

Progressive Hearing Losses

A hearing loss that gets worse over time is said to be *progressive*. The way to identify if a hearing loss is stable or progressive is to compare all previous audiograms (graphs of hearing sensitivity), not just the most recent two audiograms.

Progressive sensorineural hearing losses may result from large vestibular aqueduct, perilymphatic fistula, cytomegalovirus, meningitis, congenital syphilis, ototoxicity, endolymphatic hydrops, autoimmune disorders, delayed hereditary hearing losses, and unknown causes (Northern & Downs, 2002; Stach & Ramachandran, 2008). The child needs an immediate medical referral to an otologist whenever the hearing loss appears to be progressive. A CT scan often aids medical diagnosis. In some cases, medical treatment may halt or slow progressive hearing losses if the cause is identified. Children with progressive hearing losses may be candidates for cochlear implants sooner rather than later; each case needs to be individually evaluated (Sweetow, Rosbie, Philliposian, & Miller, 2005).

Functional Hearing Loss

If a child claims to have a nonexistent hearing loss or exaggerates an existing one, the child is said to be experiencing a *functional auditory disorder.* The child may be using the fabricated hearing loss as a call for help, a bid for attention, or an excuse for poor performance at home or at school. The true extent of the hearing problem needs to be carefully identified and managed by an audiologist along with an appropriate supportive team of professionals and family members.

(Central) Auditory Processing Disorder (C)APD

Central auditory processing disorder impairs the understanding of meaning for incoming sounds, as opposed to a peripheral hearing loss of auditory sensation. As early as 1954, Myklebust identified a child experiencing a central auditory problem as one who could "hear," but lacked the ability to structure the auditory world and select immediately relevant sounds. Some causes are congenital brain damage, head trauma, and stroke, which often show as problems understanding speech.

When a child fails to respond to sounds, an audiologist must determine whether the cause is (a) a function of not detecting the sound (peripheral hearing loss), (b) not being able to interpret the meaning of the sound that is "heard" (central auditory processing problem), or (c) a combination of these problems.

Please refer to Chermak and Musiek (2007a, 2007b) for detailed information about (central) auditory processing disorder.

What Are the Behaviors of Children with (C)APD?

Children who have auditory processing disorders may behave as if they have a hearing loss. Following are some examples of behaviors displayed by children with (C)APD. Note that not all children present with the same behaviors.

- Normal audiogram but difficulty on tests of speech perception
- Frequent requests for repetition
- Parent, clinician, or teacher reporting that the child does not seem to hear consistently
- Making mistakes in sound vocalization

- Appearing to become confused when several people are talking or in the presence of noise
- Appearing to have more problems understanding speech directed to one ear than the other
- Weak short-term auditory memory
- Difficulty localizing the sound source
- Poor expressive and receptive language abilities
- Poor reading, writing, and spelling skills
- Poor phonics and speech sound discrimination
- Difficulty taking notes
- Difficulty learning foreign languages

Note that all of these behaviors and characteristics can also be displayed by a child with a peripheral hearing loss, especially if that child had not had early and effective amplification and auditory intervention to strengthen and program the auditory neural centers. A child who does not receive clear and complete sounds will certainly have limited information to process—muddled information into the brain, muddled information out (Doidge, 2007). Therefore, it is extremely difficult to separate peripheral hearing loss from a (central/neurological) auditory processing disorder.

Synergistic and Multifactorial Effects

Two or more conditions occurring together may increase or magnify the effect of each condition. For example, a low-birth-weight baby with some difficulty breathing may be placed in an incubator with safe noise levels, but with some noise and impulse sounds. The baby also may receive medication, like a mycin drug for possible infection, but in small, safe doses not associated with ototoxicity. Though each condition by itself has minimal to no risk for hearing loss, together they can work *synergistically* to cause hearing impairment. Added to the previous scenario is the current knowledge that genes may predispose a baby to develop a hearing loss when triggered by an environmental event; this is called a *multifactorial* situation (Rehm et al., 2003; Rehm & Madore, 2008).

Predicting or proving synergistic effects is difficult. It is important to recognize when taking a case history that risk factors can act together and cause a result that seems unlikely when each factor is considered individually.

Auditory Neuropathy/Dyssynchrony (AN/AD)

A neuropathy is a disease of the nervous system, so auditory neuropathy is a disease or disorder of the auditory neural system, including the eighth cranial nerve (auditory nerve), in which cochlear amplification (outer hair cell) function is normal but afferent neural conduction in the auditory pathway is disordered (Rance, McKay, & Grayden, 2004). Berlin et al. (2005) state that the condition is better named *auditory dyssynchrony* because it is a disorder of the timing of the auditory nerve. More recently, the term auditory neuropathy spectrum disorder (ANSD) has been proposed due to the broad and variable nature of presenting symptoms; however, most professionals continue to use the shorter, simpler term of auditory neuropathy (Hood, 2009). There are many possible causes but in newborns the most common is a mild hyperbilirubinemia (12–16 cc/dl). AN/AD is indicated when the auditory brainstem response (ABR) looks absent or abnormal but the otoacoustic emissions (sounds that come from the ear) are normal if not robust.

Auditory neuropathy was first identified in the 1980s when advanced testing procedures became available to measure the action of the cells in the cochlea. Some auditory neuropathies are caused by a genetic disorder, but many are idiopathic (of unknown cause); usually they are not tumors. Most children's hearing loss appears on the audiogram, and the audiometric configuration could be flat or rising with absent acoustic reflexes. The hearing loss may progress, improve, or fluctuate. Based on the child's pure-tone thresholds, the ability to recognize words generally is poorer than expected. The child typically has normal otoacoustic emissions (OAEs), but auditory brainstem responses (ABRs) and acoustic reflexes are elevated or absent (Berlin et al., 2005).

Defining, describing, and managing auditory neuropathies is controversial (Price, Hitchcock, Breneman, Peterson, & Shallop, 2005). To protect hair cells in the cochlea, some professionals recommend that patients not be amplified, whereas others suggest FM systems or compression hearing aids. Sometimes cochlear implants are recommended to restore synchrony in the auditory system. One should expend every effort to provide input to the critical auditory brain centers.

Summary of Auditory Neuropathy

The following are the facts as we know them so far; information is changing with ongoing research (Berlin et al., 2009). Possible mechanisms that produce AN/AD are:

- Inner hair cell loss
- Pre- or postsynapse disorder
- Auditory nerve disorder
- Myelin or axonal disorder

Characteristics of AN/AD are variable across patients and over time:

- Characterized by absence or gross abnormality of short-latency evoked potentials (CAP and ABR)
- Elevation or absence of acoustic reflexes
- Presence of otoacoustic emissions (OAEs)—showing normal outer hair cell function
- Poor speech discrimination, inconsistent with degree of hearing loss
- Difficulty understanding speech in noise
- Moderate or greater pure-tone hearing loss
- Hearing loss may appear to fluctuate from day to day or from hour to hour
- Additional peripheral neuropathies (in some children) that may affect coordination for activities like walking, talking, and writing
- Incidence: about 11% of children with moderate or greater hearing losses also have AN/AD; 50% of children with AN have at least a moderate hearing loss
- Screening with OAEs alone will miss AN/AD; ABR is needed
- Recommend to screen NICU babies with ABR since they are at greater risk for AN/AD due to higher incidence of (mild) hyperbilirubinemia (12–16 cc/dl); OAEs will not identify potential AN/AD

As many as 50% of infants with AN/AD may experience improvement in their hearing thresholds over time (12–18 months), especially if their AN is associated with hyperbilirubinemia/jaundice.

What can be done about AN/AD?

- Early identification
- Family-focused intervention
- Watchful waiting
- Provision of hearing aids or cochlear implants—50 to 60% have improved speech perception abilities with hearing aids, so try hearing aids first. Base the gain (amplification) of the hearing aid on the behavioral audiogram, as opposed to fitting only a mild gain hearing aid, as was the trial amplification recommended in the past for children with AN/AD. A trial with hearing aids is recommended prior to determining if a cochlear implant would be appropriate.
- Careful monitoring of functional hearing and emerging language and speech perception abilities
- Treatment is controversial regarding communication mode and cochlear implantation—evaluate the child's progress over time and be flexible!
- Cochlear implantation (CI) of children with AN/AD has resulted in synchronous neural firing and similar benefits as those received by age-matched children with sensorineural hearing loss who have received a CI.
- Be sure to evaluate the needs of child and family before treatment is determined; treatment and technological recommendations may change over time.

Please refer to the Web site of the National Institute on Deafness and Other Communication Disorders (NIDCD) for further, up-to-date information.

Summary

The purpose of this chapter has been to describe and discuss the types and degrees of hearing loss along with various auditory pathologies. If listening is to be a vital part of intervention, we need to first understand and manage all hearing problems that prevent full acoustic access to the brain.

Hearing loss happens for a reason; there is disease or damage somewhere in the auditory pathway that causes the problem. All aspects of the hearing loss need to be diagnosed and understood before effective treatments can be initiated.

4

Diagnosing Hearing Loss

Key Points Presented in the Chapter

- Infants of any age can have their hearing screened, assessed, and managed.
- Newborn hearing screening has changed everything that we used to know and believe to be true about hearing loss.
- EHDI programs have made possible new paradigms in service delivery and expectations.
- Today, degree of hearing loss is no longer a factor in determining the functional outcome for infants and children who are young enough to have brain neural plasticity; these children's auditory brain centers can be accessed, stimulated, and developed through the early use of amplification or cochlear implant technologies.
- The primary job of a pediatric audiologist is to diagnose a baby's or child's peripheral hearing loss and to evaluate the maturity of his auditory behaviors; these tasks typically require several test sessions.
- Making a differential diagnosis, which is the separation of hearing loss from other problems that display symptoms similar to hearing loss, requires collaboration between the audiologist and other professionals such as physicians and psychologists.

- An accurate audiologic diagnosis requires a test battery approach (using several tests) that consists of both behavioral and objective (also called electrophysiologic) tests appropriately selected on the basis of a child's developmental age.
- Parents should be included in all hearing test sessions (especially behavioral tests) and participate in the diagnosis. Inclusion promotes parents' acceptance of hearing loss and helps make them partners in intervention procedures from the very beginning.
- Even though objective tests such at OAEs, ABR, and immittance provide important data about physiological function, these tests do not provide information about how the child will actually process speech; behavioral speech perception tests are necessary for this information.

Introduction

A hearing loss must be identified before intervention can take place. Hearing screening programs indicate that a hearing loss likely is present, and an audiologic diagnostic assessment specifies the nature, type, and degree of the hearing loss. The purpose of this chapter is to discuss issues and procedures for audiologic screening and diagnosis.

Newborn Hearing Screening and EHDI Programs

Universal newborn hearing screening has reinforced everything that we used to know about and believe to be true about hearing loss. We believed that the earlier we diagnosed hearing loss the better, and we believed that early intervention was important, but we had no real data to substantiate those assumptions. Now we do, as detailed in Chapter 1 of this book (Halpin, Smith, Widen, & Chertoff, 2010; Nicholas & Geers, 2006; Robbins et al., 2004; Sharma et al., 2004; Sharma, Dorman, & Kral, 2005; Sininger et al., 2009; Yoshinaga-Itano, 2004). The key issue concerns neuroplasticity. The earlier the brain is stimulated with sound, the more complete will be the auditory brain development.

The National Institute on Deafness and Other Communication Disorders estimates that as many as 12,000 new babies with hearing loss are identified every year. In addition, estimates are that in the same length of time, another 4,000 to 6,000 infants and young children between birth and 3 years of age who passed the newborn screening test acquired late onset hearing loss. The total population of new babies and toddlers identified each year with hearing loss, therefore, is about 16,000 to 18,000.

Statewide programs to screen every newborn were prompted by the research of Marion Downs in the 1960s (Northern & Downs, 2002). Finally, in March of 1993, the NIH Consensus Development Conference recommended that all babies be screened for hearing loss before being discharged from the hospital. More recently, the Joint Committee on Infant Hearing's Year 2007 position statement continued to emphasize that all infants should be screened for hearing loss prior to leaving the hospital. Further, the degree, type, and configuration of the hearing loss should be identified by 3 months of age, and intervention begun by 6 months of age.

All states require establishment of state-based systems, with various levels of funding, for early identification of newborns with hearing loss. We are now screening between 90 and 98% of all infants. Unfortunately, even though states are becoming more efficient with their screening paradigms, follow-up diagnostic evaluations and early intervention services lag far behind in many locations (Krishnan, 2009; Tharpe, 2009; Windmill & Windmill, 2006).

An effective and complete *Early Hearing Detection and Intervention* (EHDI) program should have three basic components: newborn hearing screening, audiologic diagnosis, and early intervention. These three components also should contain within each item culturally competent family support, a medical home, data management, legislative mandates, and program evaluation tools. See Web sites for the Centers for Disease Control and Prevention (CDC) and http://www.infanthearing.org for more and updated information about EHDI programs.

Current hearing screening tools include otoacoustic emissions and auditory brainstem response testing (Figure 4–1). Both assessment tools are objective, safe, and noninvasive and have a relatively high degree of accuracy. A description of these tests is provided later in this chapter.

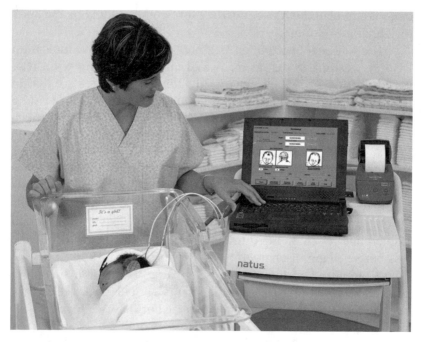

Figure 4–1. A neonate is being screened using automated ABR equipment as part of an EHDI program. (The ALGO3i Newborn Hearing Screener; image is courtesy of Natus Medical Incorporated.)

Below are some facts about infant hearing:

- Hearing loss is the highest incidence birth defect/difference.
- The incidence is 1–3/1,000 births; each well baby has a 1 in 600 chance of having a hearing loss.
- There is a 1 in 20 chance of having a hearing loss if a baby fails even one newborn hearing screening test.
- Ninety-five percent of babies with hearing loss are born to hearing and speaking families.
- ABR (auditory brainstem response, testing is used for NICU (neonatal intensive care nursery) screening to identify auditory neuropathy.
- OAEs (otoacoustic emissions testing can be used for well babies who have a much lower risk of auditory neuropathy.
- Refer an infant for diagnostic evaluation after failing two screenings; do not keep rescreening. Multiple rescreening sessions increase the possibility of false negative results

(identifying hearing as normal when there really is a hearing loss present).

■ Only 10% of babies with hearing loss have profound hearing losses, and only 10% of these babies are born to parents who are profoundly deaf.

Following are some interesting discoveries about infant hearing:

■ Unilateral hearing loss isn't benign; a unilateral hearing loss can cause later language, learning, psychosocial, and attention problems. See Chapter 3 for more information about unilateral hearing losses.
■ A mild hearing loss is not mild relative to impact. See Chapter 3 for a discussion of the potential implications of an untreated mild hearing loss in infants and children.
■ Screening at 35 dB misses a 30 dB hearing loss; normal hearing for children is 15 dB HL but we do not screen infant hearing at this level. Consequently, mild hearing losses are not identified at birth.
■ All babies, at-risk or not at-risk, can have later onset hearing losses.
■ Early rescreening is better than later rescreening; it is easier to screen a younger baby/child. So, don't wait to confirm a possible hearing loss.

Key risk factors for later onset hearing loss include: a family history of childhood hearing loss, CMV (cytomegalovirus) infection, unilateral hearing loss, and ECMO—extracorporeal membrane oxygenation. Extracorporeal life support (ECLS) is used when a baby or child has a condition that prevents the lungs from working properly, that is, transferring oxygen into the blood and removing carbon dioxide. Many illnesses may result in lung failure.

EHDI programs have made possible the following new paradigms in service delivery and expectations (Fitzpatrick et al., 2008; Sininger et al., 2009):

■ We can now implement a developmental rather than a remedial model of intervention.
■ As a result of newborn hearing screening and early intervention, 90% of children with hearing loss should be going into general education rather than into special education classrooms by kindergarten.

■ The emphasis is family-child with interventionist as coach, rather than a teacher-child dyad; early intervention focuses on adult education.

■ Degree of hearing loss is no longer a factor in outcome; there is *no* degree of hearing loss that precludes auditory access because we are not limited to acoustic input if cochlear implants are used.

■ The audiologist is a key player—the professional who makes auditory brain access possible.

■ An accessible auditory world (rather than a visual world) is now possible for children with all degrees of hearing loss— if we do what it takes.

To conclude, current research confirms several facts for families who desire a spoken language outcome for their infant or toddler who experiences profound deafness. Families need to know that very early use of hearing aids or insertion of a cochlear implant for severe to profound degrees of hearing loss (to access, stimulate, and grow auditory centers of the brain during times of critical neuroplasticity), followed by thoughtful, intense, and ongoing auditory skill development activities (to take advantage of developmental synchrony and cumulative practice), offers a high probability of reaching their desired outcome. Thanks to EHDI programs, we live in a time of exciting new possibilities for infants and children with hearing loss.

Test Equipment and Test Environment

To ensure accurate results, hearing testing must be performed in a sound-isolated booth. Therefore, an audiologic assessment cannot be conducted in a classroom, therapy room, or physician's office, unless a sound-isolated booth is used because any noise can interfere with a child's ability to detect very soft sounds.

A specialized piece of test equipment known as an audiometer is used to present controlled and calibrated sound stimuli to the child (Figure 4–2). If the child will tolerate them, earphones also are used to test each ear separately. Although supra-aural earphones that fit over the ear were used in the past, ear-insert earphones are the standard today (Figure 4–3). Insert earphones are desirable

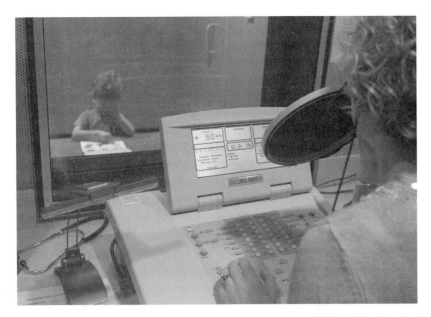

Figure 4–2. An audiometer is used to present controlled and calibrated sound stimuli to the child.

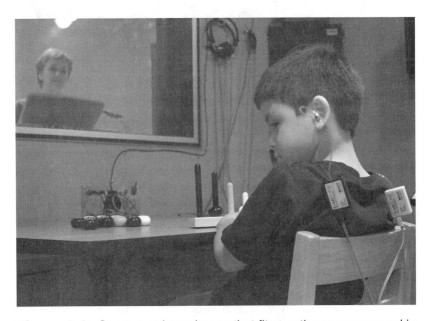

Figure 4–3. Supra-aural earphones that fit over the ear were used in the past; however, ear-insert earphones are the standard today even when obtaining ear-specific responses from babies.

because they have eliminated the possibility of collapsed ear canals caused by the weight and placement of supra-aural earphones. Additionally, insert earphones are more comfortable; they have reduced the need for masking and have improved the stability of sound relayed to the ear. Conditions preventing the use of insert earphones include atresia (absent or closed ear canal), stenosis (an abnormally small ear canal), and discharge from the ear canal as a result of an infected outer or middle ear.

Sound field results are obtained when earphones are not or cannot be used due to the young age of the child or the child's resistance to having something in the ears. Test stimuli are presented through the loudspeakers located in the sound room (Figure 4–4). Testing in a sound field can measure only the response of the better ear; a difference in sensitivity between the ears cannot be identified unless earphones are used.

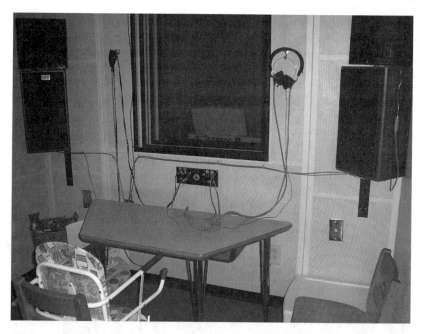

Figure 4–4. Sound field testing is performed when test stimuli are presented through the loudspeakers located in the sound room; earphones are not used.

Audiologic Diagnostic Assessment of Infants and Children

The American Speech-Language-Hearing Association has developed *Guidelines for the Audiologic Assessment of Children from Birth to 5 Years of Age* (ASHA, 2004a). ASHA has also identified the roles, knowledge, and skills that pediatric audiologists need to have (ASHA, 2006). Refer to the ASHA Web site and to the American Academy of Audiology Web site for continued updating of pediatric assessment issues and guidelines.

The ASHA guidelines (2004a) discuss the personnel, facilities, and equipment necessary for effectively evaluating infants and children. The document also includes issues such as universal precautions to prevent injury and transmission of infectious disease, the moderate sedation necessary to test some infants or children, equipment calibration, evidence-based practice, cultural competence, family-centered service provision, documentation, informed consent, terminology, and audiologic assessment procedures. A thorough assessment of infants and young children likely will require multiple test sessions in order to obtain ear-specific results with frequency-specific stimuli.

All infants who have failed a newborn hearing screening should be seen for a complete audiologic diagnostic evaluation before they are 3 months of age. It is recommended that audiologic assessments of infants and young children include a thorough case history, otoscopy, and both behavioral and physiologic measures. A description of specific pediatric behavioral and electrophysiologic tests will be presented in a following section.

The recommended test protocol will vary according to the chronological and developmental age of the child.

Test Protocols

There are four main purposes for a pediatric audiologic assessment: (a) to obtain a measure of peripheral hearing sensitivity that rules out or confirms hearing loss as a cause of the baby or child's problem; (b) to confirm the status of the baby's middle ear, on the day of test; (c) to obtain frequency-specific information through testing the pure tones that comprise speech sounds; and (d) to observe and interpret the baby's auditory behaviors.

To this end, the use of a test battery approach is standard. Several appropriate behavioral and electrophysiologic tests are utilized to determine the extent of a child's auditory function (Baldwin, Gajewski, & Widen, 2010). A test battery approach furnishes detailed information, avoids drawing conclusions from a single test, allows for the identification of multiple pathologies, and provides a comprehensive foundation for observing a child's auditory behaviors. Refer to Tables 4–1, 4–2, and 4–3 at the end of this chapter for a summary of audiologic diagnostic information and pediatric audiology test procedures.

ASHA (2004a) recommends the following test protocols according to the chronological/developmental age of the child:

1. *Birth through 4 Months of Age* (age is adjusted for prematurity). When very young or when experiencing severe developmental disabilities, the testing of infants or children should rely primarily on physiologic measures of auditory function, such as ABR using frequency-specific stimuli to estimate the audiogram. In addition, OAEs and acoustic immittance measures should be used to supplement ABR results. Case history, parent/caregiver report, behavioral observation of the infant's responses to a variety of sounds, developmental screening, and functional auditory assessments (see Chapter 5) should also be performed. Refer to Madell and Flexer (2008) for detailed information about how to behaviorally assess an infant using a sucking paradigm.

> *Observe and ask parents and teachers how the child responds to sounds outside of the audiologic test suite. Our audiological results need to be reconciled with the baby's real-world behaviors. For example, if the child is audiometrically hard of hearing, some unamplified behaviors to sound ought to have been observed at home. Conversely, if the child is audiometrically deaf, there would be no access to unamplified sound. The baby's behaviors should reflect that fact.*

2. *Five through 24 Months of Age.* At these ages, behavioral assessments should be performed first, with VRA (visual reinforcement audiometry) being the behavioral test of choice. OAEs and ABRs should be assessed only when behavioral audiometric tests are unreliable, ear-specific thresholds cannot be obtained, behavioral results are inconclusive, or auditory neuropathy is suspected. Developmental screening and functional auditory assessments also should be performed (see Chapter 5).

3. *25 to 60 Months of Age.* Behavioral tests (VRA or conditioned play audiometry [CPA]) and acoustic immittance tests are usually sufficient. Speech perception tests also should be performed in combination with developmental screening and functional auditory assessments.

The expected outcomes of audiologic protocols include: identification of hearing loss, auditory neuropathy, or a potential central auditory processing/language disorder; quantification of hearing

---

Begin the audiological diagnostic assessment by using appropriate speech material rather than pure tones. If the child stops responding to stimuli during the test session, return to a stimulus type and intensity where you are certain that the child responded. (a) If the child responds again, we can draw the inference that his or her later lack of response occurred because the stimuli were not heard. (b) However, if the child does not respond to a stimulus that he or she previously gave a response to, we can infer that the child may have habituated (become bored with the procedure).

Use warble tones instead of pure tones to obtain frequency-specific data because they are easier to hear and more interesting to babies and children. Narrowband noise, the Ling 6-7 Sound Test, or both can be used to obtain some frequency specificity if the child does not respond well to warble tones. Begin testing at 250 Hz (low frequencies) rather than at 1000 Hz when testing with warble tones or narrowband noise, especially if the child has a history of anoxia.

status based on electrophysiologic tests; development of a comprehensive report of history, physical and audiologic findings, and recommendations for treatment/management; implementation of a plan for monitoring, surveillance, and habilitation of the hearing loss; and provision of family-centered counseling and education.

The next section contains a brief summary of pediatric test procedures, both behavioral and objective. For detailed discussions of administration, methodology, and interpretation of pediatric assessments, refer to Baldwin, Gajewski, and Widen (2010), Madell and Flexer (2008), Northern and Downs (2002), and Roeser and Downs (2004).

Pediatric Behavioral Tests: BOA, VRA, CPA, Speech Perception Testing

Test procedures in which a response to sound is elicited and measured, and the function of the auditory system is subsequently inferred, are known as behavioral audiometric tests. The auditory system is not measured directly. For example, a child's localization behavior to a sound source might be observed with the subsequent inference that the child "heard" the sound. The actual function of the organ of Corti was not measured.

The ability of an infant or toddler to perform the tasks required determines the behavioral tests that are selected. Pediatric behavioral tests include, in the order of task complexity from the least to the most complicated: Behavioral Observation Audiometry (BOA), Visual Reinforcement Audiometry (VRA), and Conditioned Play Audiometry (CPA). Other behavioral tests such as Tangible Reinforcement Operant Conditioning Audiometry (TROCA) and Puppet in Window Illuminating (PIWI) are not commonly used (Madell & Flexer, 2008; Northern & Downs, 2002).

It is advisable to use the highest developmental pediatric test that a child is capable of performing, due to the potential for obtaining more precise results through strong stimulus-response conditioning bonds. Additionally, the tester must be mindful of appropriate positioning of the baby or child during the test session to allow the child to display a variety of response behaviors. Appropriate positioning is especially important for a child who experiences motoric disabilities. Parents should be included in all test sessions.

> *Before entering the sound room, begin the test session with noisemakers or the Ling 6-7 Sound Test. Observe the infant or child's auditory behaviors, first unaided, and then with hearing aids. The baby's or child's responses will give an indication of the level of behavioral test to be used (i.e., can the child localize a sound?) and the loudness level of where to begin testing (does the child respond to softer noisemakers, or must the noisemakers be very loud and very close to the child?).*

Pediatric behavioral tests also require the help of a *test assistant*. The test assistant is a trained observer who is in the test room with the baby or child and the parent. The test assistant's job is to observe and interpret auditory behaviors; to keep the baby or young child quiet, alert, and focused; and to reinforce responses when appropriate (Madell & Flexer, 2008).

Behavioral Observation Audiometry (BOA)

The simplest procedure in terms of the child's task requirements is BOA, where a selected test stimulus is presented through loudspeakers in a sound-isolated room and a baby's unconditioned response behaviors are observed. BOA is used from birth until a child can be conditioned to a lighted toy reinforcer (VRA) at about 5 months of age.

A baby's responses to BOA are not obtained at threshold—the point where the individual can just barely hear a sound 50% of the time—but rather at what is called *Minimum Response Level* (MRL). MRL is the minimal or softest level where a baby displays identifiable behavioral changes to sound. In general, these behavioral changes are observed at levels considerably louder than the baby's actual threshold.

There are several concerns, as discussed below, in interpreting BOA results. These include the infant's state, methodology of stimulus presentation, stimulus parameters, specific responses displayed by the baby, and control of observer bias. When BOA is used as the test procedure, each of these areas should be addressed in an audiometric report. Refer to Madell and Flexer (2008) for information about the use of a sucking paradigm to obtain BOA results.

An infant or toddler's behavioral state is a key variable that influences the responses they will make to sound (Bench, Hoffman, & Wilson, 1974; Northern & Downs, 2002). Behavioral state is the physical level of awareness of the child. Examples of these varying states include deeply sleeping, light sleeping, quiet awake, active awake, fussy, crying, and so forth. If a baby is deeply asleep, he or she can respond only to very loud sounds followed by reflexive behaviors such as startle or limb movement. This of course does not mean that he or she cannot respond to softer signals. If a baby is quietly awake and alert, then there exists the likelihood of obtaining meaningful, attentive-type behavioral responses to softer sounds. The belief that neonates are reflexive responders maintains popularity. However, if one reads carefully, reports typically note that very intense stimuli were used while the infant was fast asleep. If the same neonate had been awake and alert and had essentially normal hearing, it is likely that one would notice some attentive type behaviors to softer sounds. Thus, BOA responses become a function of an infant or child's state, which should be described in the audiologic report.

The Law of Initial Value (LIV) can provide valuable clues for the interpretation of an infant's behavioral changes to sound (Bench et al., 1974). LIV means that the auditory behaviors displayed in response to a sound are in the opposite direction of the infant's pre-stimulus behavior. For example, if the baby was active before the presentation of the stimulus, his or her post-stimulus behavior would be in the opposite direction—the baby would quiet if the sound was heard. If the baby did in fact hear the sound and was very quiet before its presentation, then afterwards, his activity would increase.

Attentive and Reflexive Auditory Behaviors

Provided below is a listing of behaviors that an infant or child could exhibit in response to speech and/or environmental sounds. Take note of the specific speech and environmental sounds that appear to elicit responses. Additionally, observe the sounds that the child can detect without amplification, compared to sounds that are detected only when the child wears amplification or a cochlear implant.

Consider the influence that background noise, distance from the source, competing sensory stimuli, ability to move, behavioral state, and attention all can have on a child's auditory behaviors.

Because distance, environment, and infant positioning are controlled during audiologic tests, the audiologist may elicit behaviors that are not apparent to parents or teachers in other learning situations.

The following attentive-type behaviors often suggest learning:

- When sleeping, the child awakens to sudden noises.
- Mother's voice soothes the child (quieting).
- The child's eyes widen, expressing a "What is it?" type of response.
- The infant's or child's eyes are observed to search for the sound but the head is held still.
- The eyes appear to localize directly to the sound.
- The child exhibits head searching, sometimes a rudimentary head turn towards the sound.
- The child localizes directly when sound is presented to the side, below, and/or above.
- The infant or child responds to the sound by smiling.

The following *reflexive behaviors*, typically elicited at the level of the lower brainstem, do not imply learning: the infant or child startles when sound is presented in a quiet room; the child's arms or legs move when sound is presented; the eyes blink when sound is presented in a quiet environment; the baby starts or stops sucking when sound is presented; the child's breathing rate changes when sound is presented; facial twitches, frowns, or grimaces are noted when sound is presented; or the child starts or stops crying to loud sounds.

Notice that arousal and quieting behaviors may be interpreted as either reflexive or attentive behaviors.

Although an infant or child initially may respond to sound with reflexive behaviors, he deserves an opportunity to learn to respond more meaningfully. Current auditory function does not always predict future auditory potential.

Even though conditioned audiometric procedures are preferred, conditioning is not always a possibility. BOA can provide a wide range of information about a baby's auditory ability, information that can be used in planning effective habilitative strategies. MRLs can be obtained to different types of stimuli, including the Ling 6-7 Sound Test and narrowband signals, to provide some frequency-specific information. Behavioral responses, therefore, can serve as a gauge for estimating auditory function.

Visual Reinforcement Audiometry (VRA)

VRA (Liden & Kankkunen, 1969) and Conditioned Orientation Reflex Audiometry (COR) (Suzuki & Ogiba, 1961) are the two visual reinforcement tasks most commonly used. A child's head turning response is rewarded with a visual display, usually a lighted, moving mechanical toy like a dancing bear or a running dog. The more complex the reinforcer, the more appealing it likely will be for the child. Typically, a baby is conditioned to *localize* to a toy every time a sound is presented (Figure 4-5). Because the baby is now older in addition to being awake and alert, auditory responses are elicited to softer sounds than those obtainable with BOA—usually within standard limits for babies with normal hearing. VRA procedures are used until about 2½ to 3½ years of age when play audiometry can

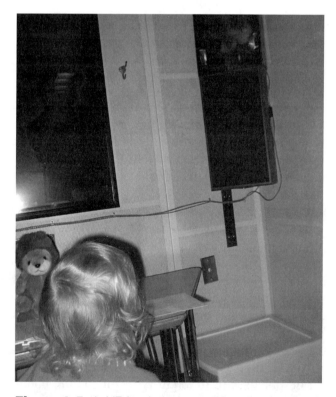

Figure 4–5. In VRA, a baby is conditioned to *localize* to a toy every time a sound is presented in the sound room.

> *There are substantial issues with state and insurance reimbursement for most audiologic tests. For example, the average Medicaid reimbursement for VRA, a task that takes about $50,000 worth of equipment, a highly trained pediatric audiologist, and a test assistant, and 1 to 2 hours test time per session, is only $14.20.*

be introduced. A test assistant is essential for the effective implementation of VRA.

Conditioned Play Audiometry

Conditioned play audiometry, also known as the "listen and drop" task (Lowell, Rushford, Hoversten, & Stoner, 1956), is described as the most sophisticated pediatric task. CPA demands the active cooperation of the child in dropping a block in a bucket or putting a ring on a peg (Figure 4-6). Have a variety of fun and interesting toys available (Scholl, 2007). Little boys might enjoy dropping plastic spiders, and little girls like to arrange "fairy wings." Most children are near 2 or 2½ years of age before they are able to participate in play audiometry, consistently. Conditioning may not be possible for some children with disabilities until an even older age. Threshold information can be obtained when the child is mature enough to employ active listening strategies and to maintain attention to task.

The hand raising or button pushing response used by older children and adults is a more abstract task. Some 3-year-olds and almost every child 5 years and older can raise his or her hand. However, in a relatively long test session where each ear is tested twice (by air and bone conduction), operant and social reinforcement can help maintain the child's attention throughout the procedure. A test assistant is also extremely helpful in varying operant reinforcers, and in keeping the child conditioned and focused.

Speech Perception Testing

The goal of audiologic practice is to assist infants and children in hearing typical and soft conversational speech in both quiet and

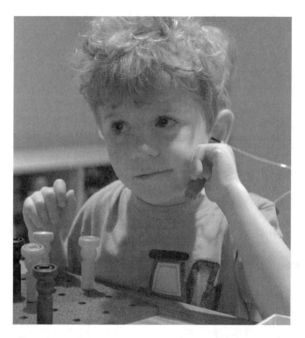

Figure 4–6. CPA, the "listen and drop task," demands the active cooperation of the child in dropping a block in a bucket or putting a ring on a peg. This toddler is wearing ear-insert earphones for testing in a pediatric sound suite.

noisy situations. Speech perception measures must be obtained regularly to: demonstrate hearing aid and cochlear implant benefit; demonstrate improvement and progress over time; identify equipment and child development problems; identify the child's speech perception errors; and assist in selecting the most appropriate educational environment (Madell & Flexer, 2008).

Speech perception testing should be performed when hearing loss is first identified, at reevaluations, and when selecting or altering technology. Test materials should be linguistically appropriate and should be presented at levels that can assess daily functioning. Functional presentation levels include the average level for conversational speech (50 dB HL) and also soft conversational levels (35 dB HL), in quiet and in noise (+5 S/N).

Following are some factors that can affect a child's speech perception capabilities:

Children speak what they hear, and how they hear. Therefore, while performing speech perception tests, one also should listen carefully to the child's speech or prespeech utterances. Based on how the child sounds, an audiologist ought to be able to plot the child's audiogram.

- Degree of hearing loss
- Length of time that the child has had the hearing loss
- Cause of the hearing loss
- The child's language level
- The child's experience with his technology including length of use
- The appropriateness of technology fit and settings
- Experience of the audiology or implant team
- The nature and quality of the intervention and education that the child has been receiving

There are many closed and open set speech perception tests that can be used. For very young children, informal speech perception measures can be obtained by using body parts, familiar toys or objects, and Mr. Potato Head. For detailed information about speech perception tests, please see Estabrooks (2006), Madell (2008), Northern and Downs (2002), and Roeser and Downs (2004).

An additional reason for audiologists to perform speech tests is to document acoustic accessibility issues in order to assist the child in qualifying for services under the new regulations for Part B of IDEA. That is, if we perform early intervention correctly, the child may not enter school with deficits that can be quantified using existing measures. Keep in mind that the special education system operates using a failure model (Ackerhalt & Wright, 2003). The child must demonstrate deficits in order to qualify for services. If we can't qualify the child for services under Part B due to academic deficits, then we need to show eligibility under Section 504 of the Rehabilitation Act by focusing on acoustic accessibility (Rehabilitation Act, 1973; Rehabilitation Act Amendment, 1992). Unfortunately, 504 may be a poor substitute for obtaining services because it is not funded by state educational agencies; local districts must assume the cost.

Electrophysiologic Tests: OAE, ABR/ASSR, and Immittance

Outer hair cell function, neural responses in the lower brainstem, and eardrum and middle ear mobility are examined through objective/electrophysiologic tests that provide some direct measurement of the auditory system. It is important to note that objective tests do not evaluate hearing, cognitive function, or the central processing of sound. Therefore, even though they provide important data about physiological function, these tests do not provide information about how the child will actually process speech; behavioral speech perception tests are necessary for this information.

Three main objective/electrophysiologic tests used with infants and young children are Otoacoustic Emissions (OAE), Auditory Brainstem Response (ABR) and Auditory Steady State Response (ASSR), and immittance—middle ear assessment. Please see Hall and Swanepoel (2010) and Madell and Flexer (2008) for more information about objective assessments.

Otoacoustic Emissions

OAEs evaluate outer hair cell integrity. The cochlea (inner ear) actively produces energy during the hearing process (Lonsbury-Martin, & Feeney, 2009). These emissions are a normal byproduct of micro-mechanical actions of the cochlear amplifier that is thought to be located in the outer hair cells. OAEs, therefore, assist in the differentiation between sensory and neural components of a sensorineural hearing loss. Because they are noninvasive, easy to set up, and can be obtained quickly, OAEs have been used extensively in screening for the very beginning stages of hearing loss, especially in newborns and in other difficult-to-test patients (Prieve, Hancur-Bucci, & Preston, 2009).

Otoacoustic emissions are separated into two general categories: spontaneous and evoked. Spontaneous emissions are detected in approximately half of the persons with normal hearing sensitivity and they occur in the absence of deliberate acoustic stimulation of the ear. Conversely, evoked otoacoustic emissions necessitate acoustic stimulation of the ear. If a child has normal OAEs but lacks ABRs, auditory neuropathy may exist (Berlin et al., 2005; Hood, 2009).

A small probe is inserted in the ear canal, sounds are presented, and response tracings are recorded in order to measure

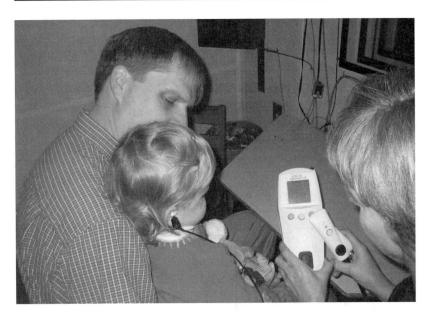

Figure 4–7. A small probe is inserted in the ear canal, sounds are presented, and response tracings are recorded in order to measure evoked otoacoustic emissions.

evoked otoacoustic emissions (Figure 4–7). The child feels no discomfort and is not required to cooperate beyond holding still. Evoked emissions are present in the ears of persons possessing normal hearing sensitivity and are systematically reduced or absent in the ears of persons who have a sensorineural hearing loss (Bess & Humes, 2003).

The procedure also has limitations. For example, the middle ear must be essentially normal for otoacoustic emissions to be measured.

Auditory Brainstem Response and Auditory Steady State Response

Proven a safe, noninvasive test, ABR does not require a child's voluntary cooperation. Several electrodes, attached to the top of the head as well as on or near each ear, measure the very tiny electrical signal caused by the nerves' respondent firing to click sound stimuli presented through earphones or a bone oscillator (refer back to Figure 4-1). Although not a hearing test per se, an ABR's tracing represents the synchronous discharge of first- through sixth-order neurons in the eighth cranial nerve (auditory nerve) and brainstem. If appropriately performed, the procedure provides some information about the auditory sensitivity of each ear that can be inferred from the resultant tracing.

Patients undergoing ABR must be very still because the slightest movement can invalidate the test. Therefore, in the case of young children, a mild sedation can be administered by a physician just before the test.

Determining ABR thresholds requires skill on the part of the observer because responses are small and are embedded in a background of ongoing brain activity and muscle activity (Gorga et al., 2004). In addition, middle ear pathology complicates results and damage to the brainstem can affect or obscure ABR responses. If a child has normal bilateral ABR tracings, one can be confident that the child has normal peripheral hearing. However, if the ABR responses are abnormal, the interpretation of hearing loss remains more ambiguous.

Because of these problems with ABR, an alternative, more robust technique often is used for predicting behavioral hearing thresholds—the auditory steady-state response (ASSR) (Cone & Garinis, 2009). The ASSR response is elicited by a modulated pure tone and it does not rely so much on the experience and expertise of the observer. Even though ASSR can better differentiate between severe and profound hearing losses than can ABR, Gorga et al. (2004) caution that reliable ASSR measurements cannot be made for stimulus levels at and above 100 dB HL.

Immittance (Impedance) Testing

Immittance, also called aural immittance measures, consists of an estimation of external ear canal volume, documentation of the integrity of the eardrum, and a description of mechanical properties of a normal or abnormal middle ear. Aural immittance testing also typically includes acoustic reflex testing. It is important to recognize that immittance *is not* a test of hearing. A child can have normal immittance results and still have a significant sensorineural hearing loss.

Immittance measures are predicated on the principle that when acoustic energy (sound) is presented to the ear, a certain quantity of the sound energy is reflected back from the eardrum. The amount of energy that is reflected is based on the stiffness or flaccidity of the middle ear system.

To take immittance measures, a small rubber plug is inserted in the child's ear canal (Figure 4–8). Small air pressure changes that cause the eardrum to move accompany the continuous tone relayed to the ear. Patterns of eardrum movement as well as protective muscle reflexes in the ear are measured. If the child remains still so that test results are not compromised, immittance measures may take only 1 to 2 minutes to obtain.

Because it often provides primary evidence of middle ear pathology (mostly fluid or ear infection), immittance audiometry functions as an important part of the audiologic test battery (Hall & Swanepoel, 2010). Tympanometry shows the eardrum's range of mobility from normal, to abnormally stiff, to abnormally compliant. In regards to otitis media, middle ear function may not always be stable. A child may experience negative pressure in the middle ear one day and fluid the next. Therefore, interpretation of immittance results only applies to the "day of test."

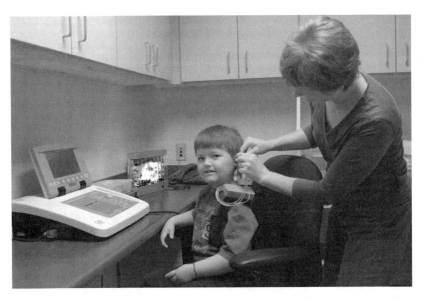

Figure 4–8. To take aural immittance measures, a small rubber plug is inserted in the baby's or child's ear canal to evaluate middle ear function; fluid in the middle ear is the most common reason for abnormal immittance results.

> *Because some babies and young children resist having the probe inserted in their ear canal, conduct immittance testing as the last procedure in the test session—unless the child is older or you know that the child will not be frightened or annoyed by the procedure.*

Interpretation of immittance results from babies under approximately 7 months of age can be difficult unless multifrequency tympanometry is employed. Specifically, a probe-tone frequency of 1000 Hz is recommended for tympanometry in neonates and young infants, and ear canal volume measurements should be conducted with a low-frequency probe tone—226 Hz (Joint Committee on Infant Hearing, 2007). Especially for the otitis-prone child, immittance is most meaningful when multiple measures are performed over time, providing a long-range picture of the child's middle ear function (Mazlan, Kei, & Hickson, 2009).

The Audiogram

An audiogram is a simple graph that charts the softest sounds that a person is actually able to hear. The audiogram is obtained by testing a person in a sound-isolated booth using pure tones that are presented to each ear through earphones.

The audiogram shows the type of hearing loss, whether it is conductive, sensorineural, or mixed; the degree of hearing loss, whether it ranges from minimal to profound; and the pattern of the hearing loss, how much hearing loss exists at different frequencies.

Frequencies (pitches) from 250 Hz through 8000 Hz are shown along the horizontal dimension. Displayed along the vertical dimension is intensity (loudness) in dB HL, showing the amount of the hearing loss (Figure 4–9). The higher the number of decibels, the louder is the sound and the greater the hearing loss.

Threshold is defined as the softest sound that a person can just barely hear. All sounds greater than threshold are audible and located towards the bottom of the graph. Sounds softer than threshold are inaudible and are found toward the top of the audiogram.

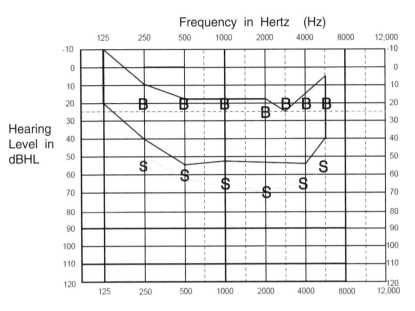

B = binaural aided thresholds
S = binaural unaided sound field thresholds

LEGEND

MODALITY	EAR		
	LEFT	UNSPECIFIED	RIGHT
AIR CONDUCTION EARPHONES UNMASKED MASKED	x □		○ △
BONE CONDUCTION MASTOID UNMASKED MASKED	>]	∧	< [
SOUNDFIELD THRESHOLDS		S	
BINAURAL AIDED THRESHOLDS		B	
COCHLEAR IMPLANT THRESHOLDS		C	

Figure 4–9. This audiogram (graph of a person's hearing sensitivity) shows binaural aided thresholds (B), which are the softest tones that the child can hear while wearing both of her hearing aids, compared to unaided sound field thresholds (S), which show the softest sounds that the child can hear with both ears when not wearing hearing aids.

Measuring a child's response to an array of distinct frequencies allows us to study the relationship between speech sounds and test frequencies. The typical tones presented in hearing tests are spaced in octave intervals from 250 Hz, which is about middle C on the piano, through 8000 Hz. These particular frequencies are used because together they comprise speech sounds much like individual threads weave a cloth (Ling, 2002). One is not consciously aware of the individual pure tones contained in someone's speech, any more than one is aware of each individual thread contained in a dress. However, each individual tone makes a precise and important contribution to speech detection and understanding, as discussed in Chapter 2 of this book.

The threshold of sensitivity for each ear is displayed on an audiogram using the following symbols:

1. O = the softest sound a person can hear with his or her right ear under headphones.
2. X = the softest sound a person can hear with his or her left ear under headphones.
3. ^ = the softest sound a person can hear while being tested by bone conduction; the test ear is not specified. Figure 4-10 shows a photograph of a bone conduction transducer.

All the above audiometric symbols specify that the non-test ear was not masked or removed from the test situation by having a static noise "keep it busy." Different symbols designate when masking has been used. For example, a triangle is used when testing the right ear by air conduction while masking the left ear. When the left ear is being tested by air conduction and the right ear is masked, an open box is used. A left bracket ([ ) means the right ear was tested by bone conduction while the left ear is masked. And a right bracket ( ]) means the left ear was tested by bone conduction while the right ear was masked. Masking is used when there is a possibility that the ear not being tested responds instead of the test ear, thereby contaminating the test results. Masking is then used to ensure that the ear being tested is indeed the ear responding to the test signal.

A legend that defines all symbols used should be included on the audiogram. Additional audiometric symbols include *S* which represents sound field thresholds—the tones are presented through loudspeakers directly into the sound room. Sound field thresholds are often obtained when a baby or young child will not wear earphones or when a comparison is needed between hearing aided and unaided stimuli. *A* or *B* (binaural hearing aids) represents

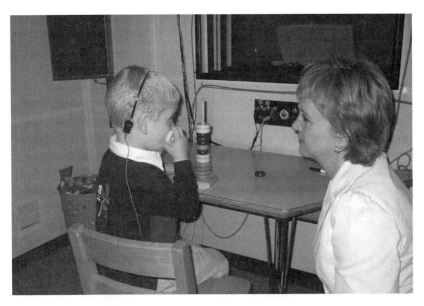

Figure 4–10. A bone oscillator is a piece of audiometric equipment that looks like a small black box attached to a headband, as seen on this child. It is used to measure bone conduction thresholds.

hearing aid sound field thresholds, which are the softest sounds that a person can hear while wearing their hearing aids. *C* represents cochlear implant sound field thresholds, which are the softest sounds that a person can hear while wearing a cochlear implant. Whenever a child wears hearing aids or a cochlear implant, aided or cochlear implant measurements must be made to determine how the child functions with amplification. A child's ability to detect soft tones while wearing technology cannot be determined without obtaining data. Therefore, it is important to include aided or implant as well as unaided sound-field thresholds on a child's audiogram in order to compare, according to acoustic phonetics, speech sounds that are audible with and without amplification.

Note the example in Figure 4-9 and the relationship shown between thresholds obtained with and without the hearing aid. The young child depicted on the audiogram has a moderately severe to severe hearing loss as measured in sound field. Average conversational speech would not be audible to this child, though some environmental sounds could be heard without amplification. When wearing her hearing aids, all of conversational speech and all speech

> *Plot all unaided, aided, FM, and cochlear implant thresholds on a Familiar Sounds audiogram to assist in parent and teacher counseling.*

sounds would be acoustically available if the talker is close to the child, the environment is relatively quiet, the child is attending, and many meaningful listening opportunities are presented.

The child's amplification (see Figure 4-9) provides a wonderful "keyboard" through which data can be entered into her brain. What if this child was brought to your early intervention program without wearing her hearing aids? What if the battery died during therapy? What if the parents put the hearing aids on her for only a few hours each day? This child possesses a great deal of very usable residual hearing; however, it is of no significant value unless and until it can be accessed via appropriate amplification that maximizes the brain's opportunity to receive speech.

Configuration (Pattern) of Thresholds on the Audiogram

The pattern formed when pure-tone thresholds are plotted and connected on an audiogram can give an indication of the etiology/cause of the hearing loss. The shape formed by the pattern is called the configuration or profile of the hearing loss (Baldwin, Gajewski, & Widen, 2010; Bess & Humes, 2003). Configurations can be described as follows:

- Bilateral—hearing loss is present in both ears.
- Unilateral—one ear has normal hearing and the other ear has at least a mild hearing loss.
- Symmetrical—the degree (severity) and configuration of the hearing loss are about the same for both ears.
- Asymmetrical—the degree and/or the configuration is different for each ear.
- Notched—there is a specific frequency or frequencies on the audiogram where hearing loss exists; all other frequencies show better hearing.

■ Stable—hearing loss is about the same over time; it does not seem to be getting worse.

■ Progressive—hearing loss becomes worse over time.

■ Fluctuating—hearing loss varies over time.

■ Sloping hearing loss—hearing loss is worse in the high frequencies; low frequencies show better hearing sensitivity.

■ Falling—hearing loss is substantially worse in the high frequencies.

■ Rising—hearing loss is worse in the low frequencies, becoming better as the frequencies get higher.

■ Cookie-bite (also called saucer-shaped)—hearing sensitivity is poorest in the mid-frequencies, with better hearing in the low and high frequency region.

Some configurations or audiometric profiles of hearing loss are suggestive of particular etiologies. Said another way, some patterns are rarely associated with certain etiologies. For example, large vestibular aqueduct syndrome—LVAS (see Chapter 3), almost always presents as an asymmetrical, fluctuating, and progressive sensorineural hearing loss. It rarely, if ever, presents as a symmetrical, stable hearing loss. A cookie-bite configuration is usually symmetrical, often progressive, and suggestive of a recessive genetic etiology. A bilateral, symmetrical, rising, sensorineural hearing loss typically is genetic and may be progressive. A hearing loss caused by anoxia typically shows as symmetrical, sharply falling (with relatively good low frequency hearing), and stable. A hearing loss caused by noise exposure often presents with a "noise notch" at 4000 Hz. That is, the worst hearing is shown at 4000 Hz with all other frequencies having better hearing sensitivity. The conductive hearing loss caused by otitis media (ear infections) may by asymmetrical, and most often presents with a rising pattern. Please see Madell and Flexer (in press) *Pediatric Audiology: Cases in Childhood Hearing Loss* for detailed information about pediatric audiometric profiles.

The audiogram depicted in Figure 4–9 presents as a moderately severe to severe cookie-bite-shaped hearing loss, suggestive of a genetic etiology. Past audiograms need to be evaluated carefully for evidence of progressive hearing loss, and future monitoring of the hearing loss must be responsibly maintained because this configuration usually is not associated with a stable hearing loss.

An example of configuration interpretation occurred in the following scenario. A young mother brought her 22-month-old to the clinic for hearing aids after the toddler had been diagnosed with a hearing loss. The mother sobbed that the hearing loss was her fault because the baby had fallen out of his high chair while the mother was talking on the phone with her back to the child. The child had suffered a bump to the head and a slight concussion. The mother stated that she had been told by the physician that the hearing loss was probably caused by the fall because it was identified after the fall, and the baby had passed his newborn hearing screening. Following testing using a combination of Visual Reinforcement Audiometry and Conditioned Play Audiometry with insert earphones, a bilateral, symmetrical, mild hearing loss in the low frequencies, sloping to moderate hearing loss in the mid-frequencies, and rising again to a mild hearing loss in the highest frequencies was noted. Tympanometry revealed normal middle ear function on the day of test, ruling out a conductive component to the hearing loss. This symmetrical, cookie-shaped, bilateral hearing loss had a very low chance of being caused by a fall. If the hearing loss was caused by a concussion, it likely would not be symmetrical and saucer shaped. It is far more likely that the hearing loss was progressive and genetic; it probably was not present at birth. The fall did not cause the hearing loss. Rather, the fall caused the physician and family to test the child to make sure that he was okay. When the hearing loss was revealed, a cause-effect relationship was inferred, when really the relationship likely was coincidental.

Formulating a Differential Diagnosis

The separation of a hearing loss from other problems that have effects similar to those of hearing loss is known as a *differential diagnosis*. Certainly, a *peripheral hearing loss* should always be ruled out first as a primary or contributing cause of a child's lack of or inconsistent auditory responses and/or difficulty developing spoken communication skills. Conditions such as general developmental delay, autism, childhood psychosis, and central auditory processing problems may resemble hearing loss by showing a similar lack of response to sound and/or lack of speech and language development.

A central auditory processing problem may be present when sounds get into the auditory system, but the brain is unable to interpret efficiently, or at all, the meaning of the sounds due to some degree of brain damage. In an extreme case, meaningful sounds cannot be differentiated from nonmeaningful sounds. See Chapter 3 for more information about auditory processing issues, including how these issues relate to peripheral hearing loss. With *general developmental delay*, a child experiences delay or retardation in many developmental areas including auditory behaviors. A child with autistic spectrum disorder (ASD) may appear unresponsive to most sensory stimuli. *Childhood psychosis* may elicit reactions in the child that did not appear to be present at birth, such as deviant responses to sounds.

All of these conditions can occur separately or in combination. Therefore, it is not always easy to identify a hearing loss; careful case histories, observations, and multiple hearing tests often are required. Making a differential diagnosis requires collaboration between the audiologist and other professionals such as teachers, speech-language pathologists, early interventionists, physicians, and psychologists.

Sensory Deprivation

The phenomenon of sensory deprivation is another factor that may complicate the diagnosis of hearing loss in children. Sensory deprivation is characterized by a lack of sensory stimulation to the brain as a result of a hearing loss that can cause delayed and/or deviant behaviors. As mentioned in Chapter 2, hearing functions on three levels: the unconscious, signal warning, and spoken language levels. A peripheral hearing loss can eliminate the environmental auditory background and deny a child access to his own biological sounds. The resultant delayed and/or atypical behaviors displayed by the child may resemble other developmental problems due to this lack of sensory input to the auditory centers of the brain.

> *Due to sensory deprivation, an infant's or young child's development can look very limited at the first visit to an audiologist, but that same child could end up functioning at a much higher level than we would initially predict. Therefore, beware of allowing our initial impression of the child to limit our prognosis and expectations.*

An example of sensory deprivation was seen in a 16-month-old girl who was referred for a hearing test. She did not yet walk or make any speech sounds, would not make eye contact, and wanted only to nurse and rub her mother's clothing. Completely unresponsive to sound, the baby also had a family history of childhood hearing loss. Through multiple behavioral and electrophysiologic tests, a severe to profound sensorineural hearing loss was revealed. Following the fitting of her hearing aids and meaningful auditory stimulation, the child's unusual behaviors declined. Professionals initially were uncertain as to the co-occurrence of other developmental problems. Two months after powerful hearing aids and auditory enhancement had alleviated the child's sensory deprivation, the auditory centers of her brain were stimulated and she was walking, listening, interacting, and finally beginning to vocalize. Subsequently, she received a cochlear implant at 24 months of age with excellent results. This particular case serves as one example of how hearing loss does not necessarily manifest itself in a straightforward manner.

Ambiguity of Hearing Loss

The very ambiguity of hearing loss poses yet another factor that complicates a differential diagnosis. The notion of "all or none" cannot be applied to hearing loss because a child might hear some sounds but not others. The audibility and intelligibility of speech for a child with a hearing loss are influenced by many factors such as the distance from a talker, background noise, room reverberation, and attention.

One uninformed therapist, upon removing a toddler's hearing aids, found this ambiguous nature of hearing loss to be confusing.

The therapist stated that for a period when the hearing aids were removed, the child still turned his head when his name was called. From this observation the therapist believed that if the toddler could hear his name, he must be able to hear everything, so the hearing aids were probably a mistake. From there, the conclusion was drawn that the toddler's speech and language delay must be linked to causes other than hearing loss. Although this particular child might have multiple difficulties, his moderate degree of hearing loss allowed audibility, even without amplification, but not intelligibility of consonant sounds. Without hearing aids the child certainly was not "deaf." However, he could not hear well enough to identify the word-sound distinctions necessary for the establishment of competent spoken communication. He could not hear details.

Therefore, making an accurate differential diagnosis of hearing loss in children is not a simple matter. Other problems can arise with symptoms that are similar to hearing loss, or that can coexist with the hearing loss. In addition, sensory deprivation can cause the hearing loss to appear to be more than a simple lack of response to sound. Finally, the ambiguity of hearing loss relative to type and degree, stability, noise, and distance can cause one to misinterpret a child's auditory responsiveness.

Measuring Distance Hearing

Subjective measures of distance hearing, using the Ling 6-7 Sound Test, are a vital part of audiologic assessments and validation of technology function.

Children with hearing losses, even minimal ones, cannot receive intelligible speech well over distances. This reduction in "earshot" has tremendous negative consequences for life and classroom performance because distance hearing is linked to passive/casual/incidental listening and learning (Ling, 2002). Research in the field of developmental psychology tells us that about 90% of what very young children know about spoken language and the world they learn incidentally. That is, young children learn a great deal of information unintentionally because they have access to overhearing conversations that occur at distances (Akhtar, Jipson, & Callanan, 2001). Thus, any type and degree of hearing loss can present a

> *Because of reduced bandwidth of acoustic stimuli caused by hearing loss, children with hearing loss need about three times the exposure to new words and concepts in order to learn them (Pittman, 2008). Extension of acoustic bandwidth and distance hearing therefore is critical for maximizing the child's exposure to linguistic and social information in the home, playground, and classroom.*

significant barrier to an infant's or child's ability to receive information from the environment.

Because of the reduction in acoustic signal intensity and integrity with distance, a child with a hearing problem has a limited range of distance hearing; that child may need to be taught directly many skills that other children learn incidentally. Refer to Chapter 2 for a discussion of the acoustic basis of Ling 6-7 Sound Test, and to Appendix 2 for instructions for the administration and application of the test.

Summary

The purpose of this chapter has been to discuss issues, descriptions, and procedures involved in the audiologic assessment of infants and young children with hearing loss. Test protocols were presented, and behavioral and objective tests were described. The next chapter will discuss the technological management of identified hearing loss.

Refer to Table 4-1 for a summary of audiologic tests included in a basic audiologic test battery.

Refer to Table 4-2 for a summary of specific pediatric audiology test procedures.

Refer to Table 4-3 for a listing of common abbreviations used by audiologists on reports.

Table 4–1. Summary of Audiologic Tests in a Basic Test Battery

Test	Measurement	Purpose
Pure-Tone Thresholds on an Audiogram	Hearing sensitivity; symbols are plotted in dB HL from 250 Hz through 8000 HZ on the audiogram	• Degree of hearing loss • Type of loss: conductive, sensorineural, or mixed • Shape of loss; i.e., falling, rising, saucer-shaped • Ear symmetry
Aided or CI Thresholds Ling 6-7 Sound Test	Access to sound while wearing hearing aids or CI; obtained in the sound field; recorded as dB HL on the audiogram	• Access to speech sounds when amplified • Access to environmental sounds when amplified • Benefit of technology
Speech Awareness Threshold; also known as Speech Detection Threshold (SAT or SDT)	Hearing sensitivity for speech; noted in dB HL	• The softest level that speech can be detected—not necessarily understood • Provides mostly low frequency cues
Speech Reception Threshold (SRT)	Hearing sensitivity for speech recognition using spondee words such as baseball, hotdog; noted in dB HL	• The softest level that speech can just barely be recognized; focuses on vowels; closed-set task • SRT should agree with low and mid-frequency pure-tone thresholds
Word Discrimination Score	Identification of speech by distinguishing single-syllable words; recorded as percent correct as a function of presentation level	• Tests the child's ability to identify both vowels and consonants of test words; open-set task • Identifies differences in word recognition ability between ears • Words are presented at an average conversational level (50 dB HL) and again at a level loud enough to overcome the hearing loss
Immittance Testing	Objective measure of middle ear function	• Identifies a need for medical intervention • Abnormal immittance could explain a temporary shift in hearing sensitivity • Abnormal results could signify that the hearing aid volume setting should be increased

Table 4–2. Pediatric Audiology: Test Procedures

Test	Expected Infant/Child Response	Cognitive Age Range Necessary for the Child to Engage in the Test	Benefits of the Test	Challenges to Performing the Test
Behavioral Observation Audiometry (BOA)	Change in sucking in response to auditory stimulus; other behavioral changes are not accepted for the test procedure, because they usually indicate supra-threshold responses. Refer to Madell and Flexer (in press) for details about BOA testing. Reflexive and attentive responses also can be noted as indicators of the infant's state and auditory development.	Birth–6 months	Enables audiologists to obtain valuable behavioral responses in infants; part of a complete diagnostic assessment. Testing can be conducted in sound field, with earphones, bone oscillator, hearing aids, or cochlear implants. Can reinforce accurate fitting of technology because minimal response levels (MRL) can be obtained.	Requires careful observation of infant sucking on the part of the audiologist, as well as noting other auditory developmental behaviors. BOA testing can be performed only when the infant is in a calm awake, or light sleep state. BOA has not been generally accepted in the audiology community as a reliable way to obtain MRLs because audiologists typically have not been trained to use a sucking response paradigm.

Test	Expected Infant/Child Response	Cognitive Age Range Necessary for the Child to Engage in the Test	Benefits of the Test	Challenges to Performing the Test
Visual Reinforcement Audiometry (VRA)	Conditioned head turn to a visual reinforcer, usually a lighted, animated toy.	5–36 months	Enables the audiologist to obtain valuable behavioral responses in infants and young children. Because responses are conditioned, more responses can be obtained during one test session. Testing can be conducted in sound field, with earphones, bone oscillator, hearing aids, or cochlear implants. Enables accurate fitting of technology because minimal response levels (MRL) can be obtained. The state of the infant or child is less problematic because the child can be more easily engaged.	Some children will not accept earphones, so obtaining individual ear information can be challenging.

continues

Table 4–2. *continued*

Test	Expected Infant/Child Response	Cognitive Age Range Necessary for the Child to Engage in the Test	Benefits of the Test	Challenges to Performing the Test
Conditioned Play Audiometry (CPA)	Child performs a motor act in response to hearing a sound (e.g., listen and drop task).	30 months to 5 years	Accurate responses can be obtained at threshold levels. Testing can be conducted in sound field, with earphones, bone oscillator, hearing aids, or cochlear implants.	Keeping the child entertained and involved long enough to obtain all the necessary information can be challenging. Multiple reinforcers, computer programs, etc., are often needed.
Immittance	None	All	Provides information about middle ear functioning and about the intactness of the auditory system (acoustic reflex arc).	The child must sit still and not speak during the test battery.

Test	Expected Infant/Child Response	Cognitive Age Range Necessary for the Child to Engage in the Test	Benefits of the Test	Challenges to Performing the Test
Otoacoustic emissions (OAE)	None	All	Measures cochlear outer hair cell function. If OAEs are present, they suggest no greater than a mild to moderate hearing loss. Contributes to the evaluation of the overall function of the auditory system.	The infant or child must sit still, not speaking during testing. Cannot rule out a mild-moderate hearing loss.
Auditory Brainstem Response Testing (ABR)	None	All	Tonal ABR provides frequency-specific threshold information. Click ABR provides information about the intactness of the auditory pathways, including measures contributing to the diagnosis of auditory neuropathy.	The infant or child must be asleep, sedated, or very still for the duration of testing. ABR testing is not a direct measure of hearing and is not a substitute for behavioral audiological testing.

Note: Adapted from *Pediatric Audiology: Diagnosis, Technology and Management,* by J. R. Madell and C. Flexer, 2008, New York, NY: Thieme.

Table 4–3. Common Abbreviations Used by Audiologists on Reports

BOA: Behavioral Observation Audiometry; method of assessment used with babies where a sound is presented and the baby's unconditioned behavioral responses are observed

CNT: Could not test (tried, but the audiologist could not obtain information; child was unable or unwilling to perform the task)

CPA: Conditioned Play Audiometry; method of assessment used with children with cognitive ages of 2–5 years where a sound is presented and child is taught to perform some play activity each time he or she hears the sound; also called the *listen and drop game*

DNT: Did not test—did not even attempt a test or a specific procedure

MCL: Most comfortable loudness level

MRL: Minimal response level—the softest level that a baby responded to the test signal; usually louder than actual threshold

NBN: Narrowband noise; noise bands centered at frequencies of 250–8000 Hz used in masking and in obtaining some frequency specificity for unaided and aided sound field testing

NR: No response; no measurable hearing when the test signal was presented at the loudest limits of the audiometer

PTA: Pure-tone average; average of the pure-tone thresholds at 500, 1000, and 2000 Hz in each ear; these are viewed as the key speech frequencies that give an indication of hearing sensitivity in the mid range; a high frequency hearing loss is not identified by the PTA:

PTA = −10 to 15 dB:	Normal PTA for children
PTA = 15 to 25 dB:	Minimal hearing loss
PTA = 26 to 40 dB:	Mild hearing loss
PTA = 41 to 55 dB:	Moderate hearing loss
PTA = 56 to 70 dB:	Moderately severe hearing loss
PTA = 71 to 90 dB:	Severe hearing loss
PTA ≥ 91 dB:	Profound hearing loss
PTA ≥ 15 dB in one ear:	Unilateral hearing loss

SAT: Speech Awareness Threshold, sometimes called *Speech Detection Threshold*; the faintest level where the child can just detect the presence of speech 50% of the time but did not indicate that the speech was understood

S: Sound field testing; refers to the way sound is presented to the child (e.g., through loudspeakers rather than earphones in a sound treated suite) in unaided and aided and cochlear implant testing; results always reflect hearing in the better ear

Table 4–3. *continued*

SRT: Speech Recognition Threshold; the faintest level where the child can repeat familiar two-syllable words, like baseball, cowboy, etc. (or point to pictures of them), 50% of the time

VRA: Visual Reinforcement Audiometry; method of assessment where the child is conditioned to localize to a toy each time she hears the sound; used with children with cognitive ages of 5–8 months to 3 years

WDS: Word Discrimination Score; the percentage score obtained by repeating open-set, one-syllable words (or pointing to pictures of them) in a 25- or 50-item list; interpretations of the scores vary; e.g:

90–100%:	Excellent word discrimination ability
75–89%:	Slight difficulty
60–74%:	Moderate difficulty
50–60%:	Poor word discrimination ability

5

Hearing Aids, Cochlear Implants, and FM Systems

Key Points Presented in the Chapter

- The purpose of all environmental and technological management strategies is to enhance the reception of clear and intact acoustic signals in order to access, develop, and organize the auditory centers of the brain.
- Speech intelligibility is based on the science of signal-to-noise ratio (S/N ratio)—the relationship of the desired signal to all background/competing noise; children need the desired signal to be 10 times, or approximately 15 to 20 dB, louder than background noise in order to clearly discriminate words.
- One strategy for improving the S/N ratio is to move closer to the infant's or child's ear so that the talker's voice will take precedence over all background sounds.
- Hearing aids (also called hearing instruments) are typically the initial technology used to access sound for a baby or child who experiences a hearing loss, and the hearing aid fit needs to be evaluated functionally (speech perception) as well as electroacoustically (real-ear measurements).
- The bone anchored hearing aid (Baha), an alternative to a traditional bone conduction hearing aid, is suitable for

children with a conductive or mixed hearing loss or single-sided deafness.

■ Traditionally, personal-worn FM systems coupled to hearing aids have been used for school-aged children in school settings, but growing evidence suggests that infants and toddlers also can benefit from personal FM systems used at home to increase auditory exposure to direct and overheard conversations.

■ Sound field amplification technology is an effective educational tool that allows control of the acoustic environment in a classroom, thereby facilitating acoustic accessibility of teacher instruction for all children in the room.

■ The cochlear implant is very different from a hearing aid; hearing aids amplify sound, but cochlear implants compensate for damaged or nonworking parts of the inner ear.

■ Efficacy of technology use may be measured through educational performance, behavioral speech perception tests, direct measures of changes in brain development, or functional assessments.

■ If the infant/child is not performing or progressing as expected, suspect equipment problems first.

Introduction

Sound has to reach the brain before learning can occur. All hearing losses in infants and children involve developmental and educational issues requiring auditory intervention. Some hearing problems also involve medical issues. Medical treatment, including medications and surgeries, was discussed in Chapter 3. Note that some children require both medical and audiologic/educational management, and one form of intervention cannot substitute for the other.

The components of technological management for hearing and hearing problems are discussed in this chapter. The purpose of all environmental and technological management strategies is to enhance the reception of clear and intact acoustic signals in order to access, develop, and organize the auditory centers of the brain. Without clear detection of the entire speech spectrum, higher levels of auditory processing are not possible. As Doidge (2007, p. 68) writes, "When we want to remember something we have heard, we must hear it clearly because memory can be only as clear as its original signal . . . muddy in, muddy out."

For Intervention, First Things First: Optimize Detection of the Complete Acoustic Spectrum

To facilitate the reception of clear and intact spoken language and environmental sounds, the following must occur: control and management of the listening environment; favorable positioning of talkers, whether parent, teacher, or clinician, so that they are always within earshot of the baby or child; and consistent use of the appropriate amplification—hearing aids, cochlear implants, and/or FM systems (Boothroyd, 2004).

Sounds reach the brain by traveling through the environment, the auditory system, and any technology worn by the child. An unmanaged hearing loss of any degree prevents certain sounds from having access to the brain, thereby interfering with the acquisition of language, literacy, and academic competencies.

Listening and Learning Environments

The integrity of the learning environment is the first item to be considered (Latham & Blumsack, 2008). In schools and in many other learning domains including the home and clinic, children often are placed in demanding, degraded, and constantly changing listening situations due to noise and distance from the talker (Crandell & Smaldino, 2002). The farther an infant or child is from the sound source, the greater the background noise, the poorer the speech-to-noise (S/N) ratio (Anderson, 2001).

Distance Hearing/Incidental Learning and S/N Ratio

Distance Hearing/Incidental Learning

Incidental learning through "overhearing" refers to times when the child listens to speech that is not directly addressed to him or her and learns from it. Akhtar, Jipson, and Callanan (2001) found that typical children as young as 2 years of age can acquire new words from overheard speech, showing the active role played by children in acquiring language. Furthermore, Knightly, Jun, Oh, and Au (2003) found that childhood overhearing helped improve speech perception and phonologic production of all languages heard. Unfortunately, children with hearing losses, even minimal ones, have reduced overhearing potential because they cannot receive intelligible speech well over distances. This reduction in distance hearing, also called *earshot*, can pose substantial problems for life and classroom performance because distance hearing is necessary for the passive/casual/incidental acquisition and use of spoken language. Therefore, a child's distance hearing needs to be extended as much as possible through the use of technology (Ling, 2002). Moeller, Donaghy, Beauchaine, Lewis, and Stelmachowicz (1996) found that more consistent auditory input can be obtained if FM systems are used in home as well as in school settings.

Signal-to-Noise Ratio, Also Called Speech-to-Noise Ratio (S/N Ratio)

S/N ratio is the relationship between a primary signal, such as the parent's speech, and background noise. Noise is everything that conflicts with the auditory signal of choice and may include other talkers, heating or cooling systems, classroom or hall noise, playground sounds, computer noise, and/or wind, among others. The quieter the room and the more favorable the S/N ratio, the clearer the auditory signal will be for the brain (Flexer & Rollow, 2009). The further the listener is from the desired sound source and the noisier the environment, the poorer the S/N ratio and the more garbled the signal will be for the brain. As stated previously, all children need a quieter environment and louder signals than adults do in order to learn (Anderson, 2004; Crandell, Smaldino, & Flexer, 2005).

Because overhearing conversations is such a critical way that children develop social/cognitive skills such as Theory of Mind and acquire and use spoken language, a child's distance hearing in various environmental settings must be known and extended. The Ling 6-7 Sound Test as a means of estimating distance hearing can assist in this regard. See Appendix 2 for directions about how to use the test. Further, FM systems should be fit at the same time that hearing aids are fit on babies/toddlers to extend earshot. Families require coaching in the effective use of the FM microphone as a means of promoting overhearing.

Adults with normal hearing and intact listening skills require a consistent S/N ratio of approximately +6 dB. This means that the desired signal needs to be about twice as loud as background noise for the reception of intelligible speech (Crandell, Kreisman, Smaldino, & Kreisman, 2004). Children, on the other hand, need a much more favorable S/N ratio because their neurological immaturity and lack of life and language experience reduce their ability to perform auditory/cognitive closure. They need the desired signal, including their own voice, to be about 10 times louder than competing sounds, which would be a S/N ratio of about +15 to +20 dB (remember that the decibel scale is logarithmic). Due to noise, reverberation, and variations in teacher position, the S/N ratio in a typical classroom is unstable and averages out to only about +4 dB and may be 0 dB—often less than ideal even for adults with normal hearing (Smaldino, 2004).

Acoustic access of the speech signal in a typical classroom environment is more problematic than initially thought. Leavitt and Flexer conducted a key study in 1991 to measure the effects of a classroom environment on a speechlike signal. They used the Brüel and Kjaer Rapid Speech Transmission Index (RASTI) which emits an amplitude-modulated broadband noise centered at 500 and 2000 Hz. This signal was transmitted from the RASTI transmitter to the RASTI receiver that was placed at 17 different locations around a typical occupied classroom. The RASTI score is a measure of the integrity of signals as they are propagated across the physical space. A perfect reproduction of the RASTI signal at the receiver has a score of 1.0.

Results showed that sound degradation occurred as the RASTI receiver was moved away from the RASTI transmitter, as reflected by a decrease in RASTI scores (Leavitt & Flexer, 1991). In the front row center seat, the most preferred seat, the RASTI score dropped to 0.83. In the back row, the RASTI score was only 0.55, reflecting a loss of 45% of equivalent speech intelligibility in a quiet, occupied classroom. Only at the 6-inch reference position could a perfect RASTI score of 1.0 be obtained. Note that the RASTI score represents only the loss of speech fidelity that might be expected at the student's ear or hearing aid microphone in a quiet classroom. The RASTI score does not measure the additional negative effects of a child's hearing loss, weak auditory or language base, or attention problems.

Even in a front-row center seat, the loss of critical speech information is noteworthy for a child who needs accurate data entry to learn. The most sophisticated of hearing aids or cochlear implants cannot recreate those components of the speech signal that have been lost in transmission across the physical space of the classroom.

ANSI S12.6-2002 Acoustical Guidelines

There is increasing awareness about the importance of managing classroom acoustics. In 2002, the American National Standards Institute issued a landmark document titled, *Acoustical Performance Criteria, Design Requirements, and Guidelines for Schools.* This is a 36-page booklet that defines the acoustic criteria for classrooms and provides a great deal of information about how to attain a favorable background noise level of 35 dBA and a reverberation time of 0.6 seconds. These minimally acceptable background noise levels are specified with the intent of producing a classroom S/N ratio of +15 dB; the desired speech signal ought to be 15 dB louder than background noise. This S/N ratio is believed to be necessary to provide children with access to intelligible classroom instruction. Note that acoustical measurements are taken in unoccupied facilities. Currently, compliance with the ANSI standard is voluntary and very few classrooms meet the criteria (Nixon, 2005).

Steps can be taken to influence the level of noise in a school classroom (Smaldino & Crandell, 2004). To begin with, the greatest source of noise in a room is the number of children in the room and the number of simultaneous auditory activities that are occurring in the room (Flexer & Rollow, 2009). Thus, classroom noise levels are largely determined by classroom activity; the more children and the more active learning centers, the noisier the room (Nelson, Smaldino, Erler, & Garstecki, 2008). In addition, note the construction of the floor and ceiling in the room. The floor and ceiling areas comprise 60% of the total area of a school classroom and have considerable impact on the noise levels in the room. Rooms with hard floors and high ceilings will be much more reverberant (echo) and noisy than a carpeted room with acoustical tile and lower ceilings (Adrian, 2009). Heating, ventilating, and cooling systems (HVAC) are also substantial sources of noise that need to be managed (ASHA, 2005).

Talker and Listener Physical Positioning

One strategy for improving the S/N ratio is to move closer to the infant's or child's ear so that the talker's voice will take precedence over all background sounds (Figure 5–1). Yelling from across the

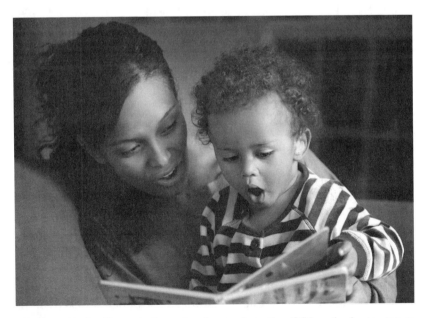

Figure 5–1. One strategy for improving the S/N ratio is to move closer to the infant's or child's ear so that the talker's voice will take precedence over all background sounds. This child is wearing hearing aids as he listens to his mother. (Photo courtesy of Oticon)

room promotes only audibility (hearing the presence of speech), not intelligibility (hearing differences among speech sounds), whereas an average loudness of speech very close to the ear facilitates intelligibility of the speech signal for the listener. Sitting across from a child does not produce as favorable a S/N ratio as sitting right next to a child, or holding a baby and speaking close to the ear or microphone.

A noisy room cannot possibly allow an effective S/N ratio. In fact, typical home and building noises (heating and cooling systems, televisions, computers, lawnmowers, hallway noise, Xerox machines, lawn sprinklers) can interfere with the child's ability to hear a clear speech signal.

If speech is being used as the primary communication vehicle, then educators and family members must be mindful of the potential intelligibility of the speech signal. The environment needs to be as quiet as possible. Turn off televisions, computers, videos, food processors, popcorn makers, electric mixers and blenders, lawnmowers, and radios. Close a window next to a noisy area such as a busy street. Position yourself close to the child's ear. The acoustic characteristics of the learning environment, whether the environment is in the home, car, school, store, or zoo, is a learning variable that must be managed to provide the child access to clear "data input."

Amplification

Hearing Aids /Hearing Instruments

Hearing aids (also called hearing instruments) usually are the initial technologies used to access sound for a baby or child who experiences a hearing loss. Hearing aids do not actually correct the hearing loss. Rather, they function to amplify and shape the incoming sounds to make them audible to the child without being uncomfortably loud. The hearing aid fit needs to be evaluated functionally (speech perception) as well as electroacoustically (real-ear measurements).

There are many excellent resources for detailed descriptions and discussions of both fitting and management strategies for hearing aids, cochlear implants, and FM technologies, The reader is referred to Dillon, Ching, and Golding (2008), Madell and Flexer

(2008), Schaub (2009), and Wolfe and Schafer, (2010). Other first-rate resources are The *Pediatric Amplification Protocol* and the *Pediatric Amplification Guideline* (American Academy of Audiology, 2004), which address issues such as candidacy, preselection issues and procedures, hearing aid circuitry and signal processing, electroacoustic verification and functional validation of the hearing aid fitting, hearing instrument orientation and training, and follow-up and referral. Refer to the American Academy of Audiology Web site for continual updating of Pediatric protocols.

New Context for Hearing Instruments

There is a new context for hearing instruments in today's world. In the "olden days," hearing aids may have had a negative connotation; a visible declaration that something was wrong. The small size feature of the hearing instrument was emphasized with the subtext that the hearing loss should be concealed. Now, "earwear" or "ear gear" is very common, popular and highly visible everywhere.

Hearing Aid Styles and Use

Hearing aid styles include *behind-the-ear* (BTE) also called *ear level* (the most appropriate for children, Figure 5–2), in-the-ear (ITE), in-the-canal (ITC), and completely-in-the-canal (CIC). The last three usually are not suitable for children due in part to the inability of these styles to connect to personal FM systems (they are not "bootable"), and also to continual ear canal growth. A fourth style

> *In today's world, "earwear" is a common and popular sight. Children and adults are observed with cords, buttons, flashing blue devices, cell phones, IPODS, etc. dangling from their ears. Hearing aids and cochlear implants attached to ears and heads are no longer noteworthy—no longer a unique proclamation that "something is wrong." This is the electronic and technological age where gadgets and devices are the rule rather than the exception. Using electronic technology (such as hearing aids, FM systems, and cochlear implants) for information access makes a positive statement in this era.*

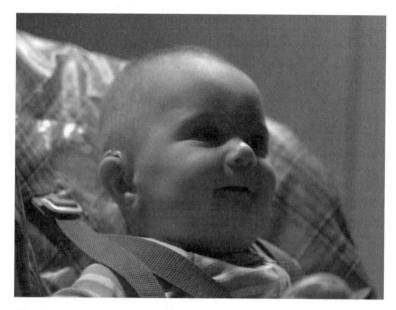

Figure 5–2. Ear-level hearing aids are the most appropriate style for infants and children.

is body-worn, once the rule for children, but now rarely used due to today's small and powerful BTE hearing aids. However, for infants, sometimes a body-style hearing aid can best accommodate the usual infant behaviors of lying down and drooling, as well as their small and soft ears and small ear canals.

Once sounds are made audible by the hearing aid, the baby or child must then have rich, meaningful listening experiences to learn to make sense of the new incoming signals. Sounds must be detected before higher level auditory skills and development can occur. Therefore, amplification is an initial step in the educational management of hearing loss, but it is not the only step, and it certainly is not the last step (Estabrooks, 2006; Ling, 2002; Sininger et al, 2009).

Hearing aids can and must be fitted on infants of any age who have hearing loss. The earlier that an infant's auditory brain centers are accessed the better, because of the need to take advantage of the time of maximal neural plasticity; therefore, every effort should be made to obtain a good fitting on very young children. However, obtaining a successful hearing aid fitting on infants less than 6 months of age is far from easy. Following are some practical challenges that need to be considered when fitting hearing aids on infants: (Kuk & Marcoux, 2002; Powers, 2010).

■ Parental acceptance of their infant's hearing loss (Moeller, Hoover, Peterson & Stelmachowicz, 2009; Sjoblad, Harrison, & Roush, 2004), and their commitment to keeping the hearing aids on the baby all waking hours,

> *Infant temperament, developmental stage, and life situations all influence the ease or difficulty of keeping hearing aids on the infant.*

■ Small ear canal and small overall ear size that can cause the earmold fit to be difficult—we have yet to obtain ergonomically appropriate earmolds and hearing aids for infants (Wolfe & Scholl, 2009),

> *For infants who may need earmolds made every two weeks due to ear canal growth, wrapping a Comply strip around standard size #13 tubing can create a functional earmold for a temporary fix.*

■ Soft, pliable infant ears can make it difficult to keep the hearing aids from "flopping,"
■ Acoustic feedback; infants tend to be lying down or held close to the parent's body, resulting all to commonly in feedback from the hearing aid (Kolpe, 2003), although feedback cancellation in digital hearing aids does help in some instances,
■ Money issues and funding availability; hearing aid loaner banks must be established to allow rapid access to appropriate technology,
■ Additional child health concerns, and
■ A conductive component to the hearing loss that can change and add to the degree of the child's overall hearing loss on a daily basis.

Loaner hearing aids, FM systems with a remote microphone, and specialized devices to help with hearing aid retention such as kiddy earhooks, double-sided tape, headbands, and bonnets can be used to address some of these practical issues.

Digital Hearing Instruments: Description and Terminology

There is much discussion about digital equipment for children. The advantage of digital instruments is their flexibility and more precise fit. Digital hearing instruments have a computer controlled sound processor inside the hearing aid. Traditional analog hearing instruments, which are mostly unavailable today, have a limited number of control options or the options are preset and not available for manipulation.

The following terms often are used when discussing and describing digital hearing aids.

- First is *advanced signal processing.* Advanced signal processing automatically adjusts the amount of amplification (gain) provided by the hearing aid according to the loudness of the sound reaching its microphone. So, softer sounds are amplified more than louder sounds and the *compression component* constantly adjusts the amount of gain available so that softer sounds can be heard more easily, while avoiding discomfort from louder sounds. Different signal processing configurations can vary the amount of compression, as well as the loudness level at which compression is activated, providing some benefit in noisy situations. Wide dynamic range compression (WDRC) may help children hear conversations at different listening distances.
- The amount of gain (amplification) a hearing instrument provides at each frequency is called its *frequency response.* Digital hearing instruments with *multichannel capability* divide the frequency response into two or more channels of control. Each channel can be adjusted independently so that different advanced signal processing schemes can be applied to each frequency region.

■ Many digital hearing instruments have memory, allowing them to store more than one frequency response or program, called *multimemory capability*. Multiple memories allow the child/parent/teacher/therapist to choose from different frequency responses and signal processing options with a remote control, or by pressing a button on the hearing instrument—or the hearing aid may have the ability to switch programs automatically. Multiple memories can be useful for children who communicate in many different listening situations or have fluctuating hearing losses. For example, for a child who often has otitis media (fluid in the middle ear), one program in the hearing aid might have added gain (amplification) to allow the child better access to sound when her hearing loss has been made worse by the addition of middle ear fluid.

■ Some digital hearing instruments have separate microphone settings (*multimicrophone capability*) that allow the child to pick up sound either from a broad area (omnidirectional) or from a narrower listening range (directional microphone), analogous to a camera having a wide angle and zoom lens. In noisy listening situations, the directional microphone can somewhat suppress sounds that come from behind (usually competing noise), which may improve the child's ability to hear speech that comes from the front. The assumption is that the most desirable speech comes from the front and the child likely will look at the intended auditory source, but such is not always the case. Some instruments will automatically switch between microphone modes depending on the listening environment.

> *Infants and children need to be able to overhear social conversations that occur around them. This overhearing/distance hearing is essential for learning the social cognitive skill of Theory of Mind (see Chapter 7) The most important acoustic information may not be in front of the child—it might be to the side or behind. Therefore, if a directional microphone setting is used, it is important that some access remains to sounds from the side and back.*

- Some digital instruments are designed to identify noise and automatically reduce the amplification in the frequency regions where it is detected. This *noise reduction capability* may provide the child with some improved ease of listening in background noise but the remote microphone of an FM system is still necessary.
- *Real-ear measurement* is a term used to describe electroacoustic verification of the hearing aid fit; it is a measurement of amplified sound in the ear canal through the use of a probe microphone. Real-ear measurements must be obtained as part of a valid hearing aid fitting for all infants and children (Figure 5–3).
- *Cortical Auditory Evoked Potential (CAEP)* can be used as a measure of aided functional performance by presenting speech stimuli through loudspeakers, and recording an electrophysiological response from the cortical region of the child's brain through electrodes placed on the infant's head. The infant is awake, positioned on the parent's lap,

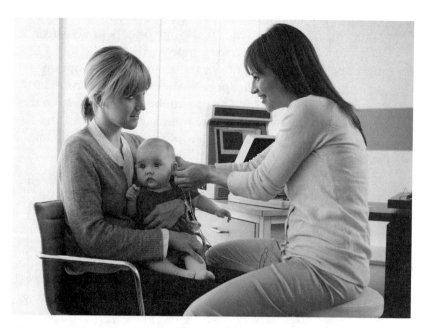

Figure 5–3. Real-ear measurements are an essential part of every hearing aid fitting. (Photo courtesy of Oticon)

and distracted by quiet toys. Research suggests that the recording of CAEPs can assist in verifying the hearing aid fitting in infants and young children who cannot respond behaviorally (Dillon, Ching, & Golding, 2008). Families often are overjoyed to view the recorded CAEPs to speech stimuli in their aided infant because they now have visible evidence that the stimuli are detected at the cortex, showing that conversational speech is indeed audible to the infant through his or her amplification technology.

■ *Articulation Index (AI)* is an expression of the proportion of the average speech signal that is audible to a person with hearing loss. Typically, the AI is compared in the unaided and then in the aided condition as one way of determining the extent of hearing aid benefit in making the speech spectrum audible (Killion & Mueller, 2010). The AI is calculated by dividing the average speech signal into several bands and obtaining an importance weighting for each band; a process first described by French and Steinberg (1947). Two ways to compute the articulation index include: (a) a "count the dots" audiogram (Killion & Mueller, 2010) that represents the weighted speech spectrum depicted as 100 dots, representing 100% of the speech spectrum, on an audiogram (Figure 5–4), and (b) accessing a Web site that will automatically compute the AI once the person's thresholds are entered into the formula (http://www.audiologyinfo .com/ai/). Note that not all speech sounds carry equal audibility importance. High frequencies carry more importance for speech intelligibility. However, please note that children must also have low frequency access for the critical vowel sounds that underlie the phonological process of reading (Robertson, 2009).

> *An audiologist can plot the child's unaided and aided (or cochlear implant) thresholds on a count-the-dots audiogram and use that graph as a counseling tool to explain to the family the proportion of the speech signal that is audible with and without technology. Viewing and counting the dots provides evidence that their child with a mild to moderate*

hearing loss, who seems to hear so well unamplified, is really missing a great deal when not wearing his hearing aid as shown in Figure 5–4. The AI is a very important tool to use in determining the effectiveness of a hearing aid, cochlear implant and FM system in making the speech signal audible.

The SII-Based Method for Estimating the Articulation Index

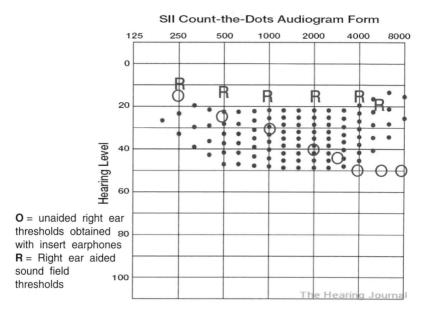

Figure 5–4. Plotting the child's unaided (*O*) and aided (*R*) right ear thresholds and counting the dots on this audiogram clearly displays the necessity of wearing the hearing aid during all waking hours. Without the hearing aid, this child has access to only 55% of the speech spectrum (AI = 55%). Whereas, when wearing his hearing aid, he has access to almost all of the speech information (AI = 97%). Of course, distance from the sound source and noise in the environment will still cause difficulty and will necessitate the added use of the remote microphone of an FM system. (Count the Dots Audiogram is printed with permission of the *Hearing Journal*).

■ *Frequency Lowering* is a general term that describes current technologies that take high-frequency input signals, usually consonant speech sounds, and shifts these sounds to a lower frequency region where the person has more residual hearing (Bentler, 2010). The idea is that this processing scheme will allow better speech understanding by making high frequencies audible. The concept of frequency lowering has been around for a long time, but better outcomes are now obtainable due to the digital-processing chip that is part of most current hearing aids; that chip allows real-time manipulation of the input signal. The two methods currently available that control input frequencies are called *frequency transposition* and *frequency compression* (Glista et al., 2009). Some children with moderate to profound high-frequency hearing losses benefit from this fitting protocol. The effective programming of frequency-lowering technologies can be very tricky, not all children benefit, and real-ear measurements must be made to verify the appropriateness of the fitting. Positive outcomes are possible; however, more evidence is needed for establishing best-practice guidelines.

■ Some hearing aids offer a feature called *data logging.* Data logging allows the hearing aid to retain relevant usage data that lets the audiologist know exactly how long the hearing

The degree of success that a child experiences from a hearing aid results from several interactive factors such as the child's residual or remaining hearing, the quality of the hearing aid fitting, the amount of time each day that the hearing aids are worn, the baby's age at amplification, the quality and quantity of auditory-based therapy, the ability of family, therapists, and teachers to create an "auditory world" for the child, and the use of necessary additional technologies such as an FM system with a remote microphone to facilitate distance learning.

aid has been worn, and sometimes, the types of signals received.

■ An additional feature to consider for hearing aids is their *compatibility with FM devices.* All hearing instruments that are fitted on children ought to be "bootable." Bootable means they have direct audio input capability for attachment of FM receivers directly to the hearing aid.

Hearing Aids for Infants and Children: Points to Ponder

Following are some issues about hearing aids that parents, early interventionists, clinicians, and teachers should consider.

The hearing aid fit needs to be *evaluated functionally* as well as electroacoustically (real ear measurements). That is, one needs to know how the hearing aid actually functions to access the speech spectrum for the baby or child (Madell, 2008). Comparisons should be made between amplified and unamplified speech perception capabilities, and also between unaided and aided audiograms for detection data. Although initially it was believed that aided thresholds were useful only for linear hearing aids, aided thresholds can still be very effective for estimating potential hearing for soft sounds, even with wide dynamic range compression hearing aids (Cox, 2009). Please refer to the efficacy discussion at the end of this chapter for more information about how to obtain functional speech perception information.

Children require more gain (amplification) for their hearing loss than do adults, and hearing aid prescriptions should reflect that fact. That is, different hearing aid prescriptions need to be used for children and adults (Dillon, 2006).

Hearing aids fitted on infants require vigilant audiologic monitoring. For infants birth to 3 months of age, weekly audiologic hearing aid checks are necessary. From ages 3 to 6 months, audiologic hearing aid checks should occur every 2 to 4 weeks. Hearing losses can change (typically the change is a progression) as will ear canal size.

If a hearing loss exists in both ears, *two hearing aids should be fitted*, one for each ear. Binaural fitting is the rule, not the exception.

Hearing aids should be *worn during all waking hours* within several days of fitting, augmented by the necessary assistive listening devices. It is important to access the brain during the early months and years of maximum brain neuroplasticity.

Hearing aids should have a strong *telecoil and capability of coupling to an FM receiver boot*. A telecoil is an internal hearing aid component that is activated by an external switch, labeled "T," or by a remote control to access the telecoil program. The telecoil picks up magnetic leakage from a telephone or an assistive listening device. All of a child's listening, learning and communicative environments must be considered when fitting hearing instruments.

Hearing aids should be *programmable for flexibility* regarding frequency response and power requirements. Sometimes initial fittings need to be adjusted as the child becomes a more reliable test-taker and listener. It also is possible that a child's hearing loss could change over time. In addition, fluctuating hearing losses demand adjustable hearing aids.

There are *water-resistant hearing aids* on the market that can be useful at the beach and pool. They can be worn during surface swimming, but not for underwater swimming or diving. In addition, there are hearing aid socks or sleeves made out of absorbent cotton or rubber that can assist in absorbing or repelling moisture. Some children wear these during hot, strenuous activities when they perspire a great deal (Figure 5-5).

A listening check must be performed on hearing instruments at least once a day by parents and/or teachers who have normal hearing (Estabrooks, 2006). A hearing aid stethoscope should be readily available for this purpose. Hearing aids break, and a malfunctioning hearing aid is of no value to anyone, especially to a baby with a hearing loss. Over the years, about 50% of amplification devices checked in school programs are found to be malfunctioning at any given time (Edwards & Feun, 2005; Sjoblad, Harrison, & Roush, 2004). Families and teachers need to be coached in performing this daily *troubleshooting* of hearing aids and other technologies. Troubleshooting means performing various visual and listening inspections to determine whether an amplification unit is malfunctioning and, if so, evaluating the nature and severity of the malfunction.

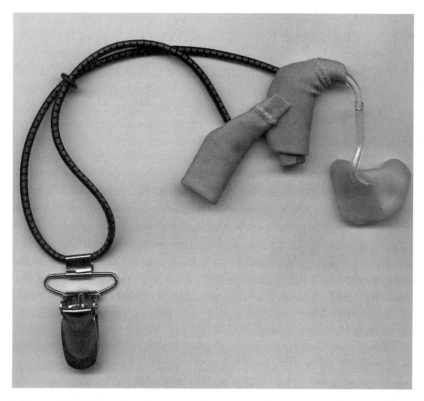

Figure 5–5. Hearing aid socks/sleeves made out of absorbent cotton, spandex, or rubber in many colors can assist in absorbing or repelling moisture. The cord and clip provide a safety feature by attaching the hearing aids to the child's clothing. (Photo provided courtesy of Ear Gear at http://www.gearforears.com)

Hearing aids are electronic devices, so moisture can cause a hearing aid to malfunction. Therefore, hearing aids need to be kept as dry as possible. *Dehumidifiers are airtight containers* that contain chemical compounds to remove moisture from hearing instruments; they must be used to store hearing aids whenever they are not on the child's ear.

Parents should order a *hearing aid care kit* when they order their child's first hearing aids. This kit contains earmold and hearing aid cleaning tools, a hearing aid stethoscope to listen to the hearing aid, a battery tester, OtoFirm (a cream to put on the ear-mold that can help seal it in the ear canal and prevent feedback), and a dehumidifier. The audiologist should provide information, literature, and demonstration of all items in the kit.

Battery problems cause many hearing aid malfunctions. Unlike watch batteries, the tiny hearing aid batteries last only a few days to a week in a high-power hearing aid. Battery life depends on the power output of the hearing aid, the added battery drain of coupling the hearing aid to an FM receiver boot, and how often the hearing aid actually is worn.

Earmolds are custom-made earpieces that direct the sound from the hearing aid into the ear canal. They are a crucial aspect of an appropriate hearing aid fit (Oliveira et al., 2006). Not only must they be comfortable (usually made of soft material for children), but they can be modified to allow better sound transmission to the ear canal because the earmold shapes the sound coming from the hearing aid (Pirzanski, 2006). For example, a horn-shaped earmold will enhance high-frequency transmission. An "open" earmold or a vented ear mold allows some of the low frequencies to filter back out of the ear canal as well as letting air in, an important consideration if the child has ear infections or ventilating tubes in her ears. If earmolds do not fit well, feedback can occur. Feedback is that high-pitched annoying squeal that comes from hearing aids. Finally, children's earmolds may need to be remade often to accommodate growing ears and to obtain a comfortable fit.

Amplification typically should *emphasize the high frequencies* if the child has any high frequency residual (remaining) hearing. The higher frequencies carry the acoustic energy necessary for discrimination of consonant sounds, and consonants are necessary for intelligibility of speech. Low frequencies, however, are also important for suprasegmentals and vowels, and should not be deleted. The relationship between low- and high-frequency amplification needs to be evaluated carefully in the applied hearing aid fitting formula (Dillon, Ching, & Golding, 2008; Killion & Mueller, 2010; Ling, 2002).

Visual deviancy and stigma issues should be considered when fitting amplification devices (Sjoblad, Harrison, & Roush, 2004). Equipment can be fitted in an attractive, colorful, and interesting manner. Technology should facilitate, not intimidate, communicative interactions.

If a baby or child resists wearing her hearing aids, it may be because the child has somehow sensed that the parent is not yet committed to having the child wear the hearing aids as they are a clear and constant reminder of the child's hearing loss. Professionals need to know that the parents' ability to cope effectively with the technology may be affected by the parents' raw emotional state. Sometimes parent groups or professional counseling are helpful—but sometimes just getting the hearing aids on, and having the child begin to respond is the best therapy possible. However, sometimes the problem is an audiologically correctable one. The first step is to investigate the following issues and then work with the audiologist to rectify any identified problems:

■ *Earmold fit. The earmold could be too small, too large, or it could rub and irritate specific parts of the ear or ear canal.*

■ *Hearing aid fit. The hearing aid could rub or irritate the child's ear or flop around annoyingly when the child moves.*

■ *Hearing sensitivity change. The child's hearing loss may have progressed so that current hearing aid settings no longer provide sufficient amplification;*

■ *Ear canal or middle ear infection. The child may have an infection that hurts when the hearing aid is put on. Medical evaluation and treatment then would be necessary.*

■ *Hearing aid settings. The hearing aid could be shorting out, it may present sound that is too loud, too soft, or too distorted, or it may provide inappropriate amplification of the speech spectrum. For example, a 3-year-old with a mild to moderately severe hearing loss did not want to wear his newly fitted hearing aids. He cried and ripped them off his ears about 10 minutes after they were put on. The parents were afraid that the hearing aids were too loud. However, a second opinion revealed that the hearing-aid settings were too soft, so that, when inserted, the earmolds and hearing aids functioned like ear plugs! The child heard better without the hearing aids than he did with them because he was underamplified. When the hearing aids were adjusted to allow more amplification, he not only kept his hearing aids on, he was reluctant to take them off.*

Bone Anchored Hearing Aid (Baha)

The bone anchored hearing aid (Baha), also called a bone-anchored hearing system (BAHS), an alternative to a traditional bone conduction hearing aid, is suitable for children with conductive or mixed hearing losses or single-sided deafness (complete sensorineural hearing loss in one ear; Figure 5-6). The conductive hearing loss could have been caused by a congenital middle or external ear malformation, or occur as part of a syndrome such as Treacher Collins syndrome.

The traditional bone conduction hearing aid is held on the head with a steel spring headband, and may be uncomfortable due to the constant pressure of the headband. The Baha is different. The Baha's sound processor is attached to a small titanium fixture that is surgically inserted in the bone behind the ear (Tjellstrom, 2005). A titanium sleeve connects the fixture through the skin; therefore, thorough daily hygiene using a special cleaning brush and soap and

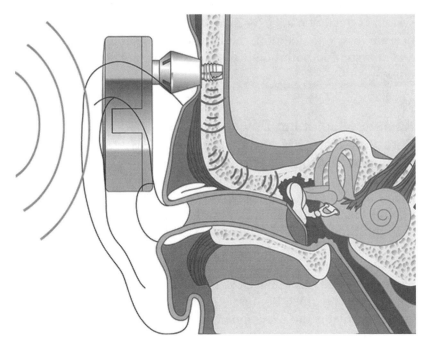

Figure 5–6. The Baha's sound processor is attached to a small titanium fixture that is surgically inserted in the bone behind the ear. (Schematic provided courtesy of Cochlear Americas.)

water is necessary. Through a process called osseointegration, taking 10 to 12 weeks, the fixture bonds with the surrounding tissue. Osseointegration is a direct structural and functional connection between living bone and the titanium surface of the implant that provides secure retention of the sound processor (Tjellstrom, 2005). Sounds therefore bypass the outer and middle ear, and stimulate the inner ear directly, a process known as direct bone conduction. At this point in time, the minimum age for Baha implantation is 5 years; however, some children receive the Baha at 2–3 years of age. For infants, the Baha Softband can be used until the child is old enough for the surgery. The Softband is an elastic headband with a Baha sound processor connected to a plastic snap disk sewn into the headband (Beck, 2010).

The verification procedure for bone-conduction devices is the attainment of aided sound field thresholds, and comparing unaided to aided results. Christensen et al. (2010) demonstrated the benefits of both the Baha Softband and implanted systems over traditional bone-conduction hearing aids and recommended the Baha system as the first choice for intervention of inoperable conductive hearing losses. In addition, the Baha can and should be used with an FM system in both home and school learning situations (Christensen, 2009).

Assistive Listening Devices (ALDs): Personal-Worn FM and Sound Field FM and IR (Classroom Amplification) Systems

Even though hearing instruments are the initial form of amplification for infants and children, hearing aids are not designed to deal with all listening needs. Their biggest limitation is their inability to make the details of spoken communication available under the following conditions: when there is competing noise, when the listener cannot be physically close to the speaker, or when both conditions exist together. Because a clear and complete speech signal greatly facilitates the development of oral expressive language and reading skills, some means of improving the speech-to-noise ratio (S/N ratio) must be provided in all of a child's learning domains (Anderson, 2004; Estabrooks, 2006; Ling, 2002).

Assistive listening device (ALD) is a term used to describe a range of products designed to solve the problems of noise, distance from the speaker, and room reverberation or echo that cannot be solved with a hearing aid alone (Boothroyd, 2002). ALDs enhance the S/N ratio to improve the intelligibility of speech and expand the baby's or child's distance hearing and incidental learning.

There are many categories of ALDs ranging from listening devices (which are discussed in this section) to telephone devices and alert/alarm devices. The types of ALDs most relevant to the population addressed in this book include personal-worn FM systems and sound field IR and FM (classroom) amplification systems. All ALDs enhance the S/N ratio by improving the audibility and intelligibility of the speaker's voice. Note that a pediatric audiologist must be involved in the recommendation and fitting of all hearing aids and assistive listening devices.

Wireless Connectivity

Wireless connectivity to the environment and to electronic devices is an evolving horizon for hearing aid wearers (Schum, 2010). Indeed, Bluetooth technologies are having a significant impact on developments of wireless assistive devices (Levitt, 2004). Bluetooth technologies use very high-frequency wireless signals to link computers and other digital devices together, offering flexibility and increased access to multiple technologies. Even though Bluetooth is the primary wireless technology used in cell phones and other electronics, Bluetooth wireless transmission poses a problem for hearing aids because the size of the transmitters and receivers is large compared to the components of hearing aids. In addition, Bluetooth transmission has high power requirements that exceed the capabilities of hearing aid size batteries. The current solution is to use a body-worn gateway device that accepts signals from various formats such as Bluetooth, direct audio input, and FM; converts the input signal to a digital magnetic signal; and then sends the signal to a digital magnetic receiver that is integrated in the electronics of the hearing aid (Nyffeler & Dechant, 2010). Wireless reception directly in the body of a hearing aid, although highly desirable, likely will not occur for years because a newer wireless technology would need to be developed to replace the current generation of Bluetooth. Nevertheless, wireless connectivity allows access to technologies for children with hearing loss in exciting and ever expanding ways.

Personal-Worn FM Unit

A personal-worn FM unit is a wireless personal listening device that includes a remote microphone placed near the desired sound source (usually the speaker's mouth, but it could also be a tape recorder or TV) and a receiver for the listener who can be situated anywhere within approximately 50 feet of the talker. No wires are required to connect the talker and listener because the unit is really a small FM radio that transmits and receives on a single frequency (Figure 5-7). Because the talker wears the remote microphone within 6 inches of her mouth, the personal FM unit creates a listening situation that is comparable to a parent or teacher being within 6 inches of the child's ear at all times, thereby allowing a positive and constant S/N ratio (Sexton, 2003). Personal FM systems, therefore, offer a direct communication connection between the talker and listener in any communication situation (ASHA, 2000; Launer, 2003).

Personal FM units are essential for a child with any type and degree of hearing loss, from minimal to profound, who is in any classroom or group learning situation (Anderson, Goldstein, Colodzin, & Inglehart, 2005; ASHA, 2000; T. S. Flynn, M. C. Flynn, & Gregory, 2005). Several models of FM equipment are available, costing approximately $2,500 per unit. The most common styles currently used include one where the FM receiver is built into the ear-level hearing aid case and another where a small FM receiver boot is attached directly to the bottom of the ear-level hearing aid, as seen in Figure 5-7, or to a cochlear implant speech processor. This small, attachable FM receiver has the advantages of a clear signal and small size. Obviously, care needs to be exercised in avoiding loss, especially when used by a small child. Fitting an FM system is not without its challenges and substantial audiological expertise is called for in selection, adjustment, implementation, monitoring, and maintenance of the device. Hearing assistance technology (HAT) fitting procedures are detailed in the AAA Clinical Practice Guidelines (2008). These procedures include a combination of electroacoustic,

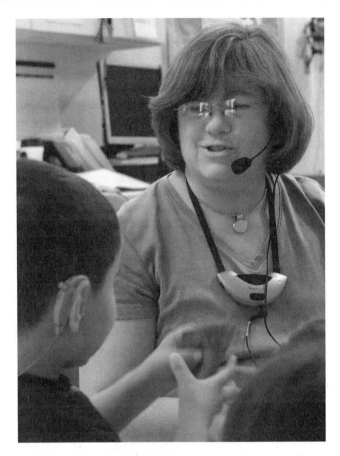

Figure 5–7. Personal FM receiver and remote microphone in the classroom.

real-ear, and behavioral measures to ensure compatability and transparency of the HAT with the needs of the child's personal technology. See a sample of Web sites—Phonak (MicroLink), Lexis (Oticon and Phonic Ear), Sonovation, Comtek, Widex (SCOLA), Audio Enhancement, and Lightspeed—for product information about their wireless personal FM systems.

Home Use

Traditionally, personal FM systems coupled to hearing aids have been used for school-aged children in the classroom setting, but

growing evidence suggests that infants and toddlers also can benefit from personal FM systems used at home. Moeller, Donaghy,
Beauchaine, Lewis, and Stelmachowicz (1996) compared two groups
of children, with one group who was encouraged to use an FM system at home, and another group who used hearing aids alone. The
families who wore the FM systems at home were provided with
training regarding how to operate the units. Subjective reports
from parents suggested that appropriate use of the FM at home
facilitated effective communication in a variety of listening situations. Another reported advantage was that two of the children felt
an increased sense of security when they could hear their parents
from a distance.

In another study about home FM use, Gabbard (2003) reported
preliminary information that was gathered from the Colorado
Loaner FM Project. The project utilized the FM Listening Evaluation
for Children as a way to gain an understanding of the use and benefit of hearing aids and FM systems with children. Parents were
asked to complete the evaluation form at least 3 to 6 months following FM fitting and then again at quarterly intervals. Some of the
parents' comments regarding perceived benefit of the FM included
"being mobile while continuing to hear," "consistent sound whether
noisy or not," "provides the best amplification to help auditory
skills," and "keeps him focused on the speaker." T. S. Flynn et al.

*In light of the advantages of FM technology use in home
environments, and because babies and children require distance hearing for incidental learning, personal FM systems
ought to be attached to hearing aids soon after the initial
hearing aid fitting. Families do require coaching about
when and how to use the personal FM unit outside of school
environments. Most families use the FM system about 60 to
70% of the baby's/toddler's day; the hearing aids are worn
every waking moment. The wearer of the FM transmitter
could be the mother, father, grandmother, sibling, playmate,
caretaker, etc. Typical FM use situations include the car,
playground, store, dance class, Sunday school, soccer field
(baseball, etc.), kitchen, dining room, etc. Think of the FM
microphone as the baby's "third ear."*

(2005) concurred that FM use at home improved speech understanding as measured by functional auditory assessment tools.

Multiple Wireless Microphone Use

There are many family and small-group situations where the use of several wireless microphones at the same time would be very beneficial for the educational, linguistic, and cognitive growth of the child with hearing loss. The Companion Mics Noise Reduction System from Etymotic offers one possible way to fill this need (see Figure 5-8). Based on a variation of Bluetooth wireless technology, the Companion Mic System offers three wireless (talker) microphone units and one wireless (listener) receiver unit; all can be used at the same time. The receiver unit can be coupled to a hearing aid or a cochlear implant using a neck loop or direct audio input cord, or the receiver can be worn with headphones. The system is reasonably priced and can allow the child with hearing

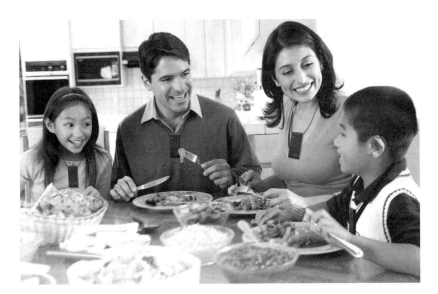

Figure 5-8. Companion Mic System can be used by a family around a dinner table. Three wireless (talker) microphones are capable of being used at the same time, allowing the child wearing the receiver unit (with a neck loop) easy access to the comments of all family members. (Photo courtesy of Etymotic Research, Inc.)

loss in noisy and dynamic situations (such as at a family dinner, in a small group learning situation, at the museum, in the car with both parents in the front seat and the child secured in the back seat) to converse with up to three people at the same time with an enhanced signal-to-noise ratio.

Auditory Feedback Loop: A Concept Facilitated by Using a Remote Microphone

The auditory feedback loop is the process of self-monitoring (input) and correcting one's own speech (output). Auditory feedback is crucial for the attainment of auditory goals and fluent speech (Perkell, 2008). That is, a child must be able to hear his or her own speech clearly in order to produce clear speech sounds (Laugesen et al., 2009). Improving the signal-to-noise ratio of the child's own speech can boost the salience of the speech signal.

To facilitate development of the child's auditory feedback loop, place the microphone of the FM system within 6 inches of the child's mouth when she is speaking or reading aloud. Because speaking and reading are interrelated, speaking into the FM microphone will highlight the child's speech, thus allowing her to monitor and control her speaking and reading fluency. The lapel microphone of a cochlear implant can be used in the same way.

Sound Field FM and IR Systems (Also Called Classroom Amplification Systems)

Sound field technology is an exciting educational tool that allows control of the acoustic environment in a classroom, thereby facilitating acoustic accessibility of teacher instruction for all children in the room (Crandell et al., 2005). A sound field system looks like a wireless public address system, but it is designed specifically to ensure that the entire speech signal, including the weak high frequency consonants, reaches every child in the room (Figure 5–9). By using this technology, an entire classroom can be amplified through the use of one, two, three, or four wall- or ceiling-mounted loudspeakers.

The teacher wears a wireless microphone transmitter, and her voice is sent via radio waves (FM) or light waves (infrared—IR) to an amplifier that is connected to the loudspeakers. There are no

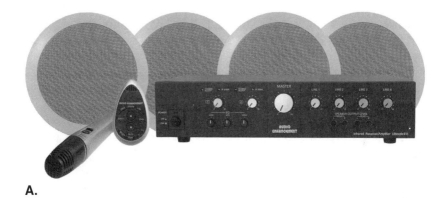

A.

B.

Figure 5–9. A. A classroom sound field system has a wireless teacher-worn microphone, a pass-around microphone for students, an amplifier, and evenly dispersed ceiling-mounted loudspeakers. **B.** Infrared is the most commonly used mode of transmission where the infrared signal is sent (emitted) from the teacher microphone to the diode in the center of the ceiling, to the amplifier on the wall, and then to the four loudspeakers in the ceiling. (Photo and schematic, courtesy of Audio Enhancement.)

wires connecting the teacher with the equipment. The radio or light wave link allows the teacher to move about freely, unrestricted by wires.

Why Is *Sound Field Distribution System* a More Descriptive Term?

Sound field distribution system is more accurately descriptive of sound field function. To explain, some teachers, parents, and acoustical engineers interpret the labels *sound field amplification* or *classroom amplification* to mean that all sounds in the classroom are made louder. This misunderstanding may give the impression that sound is blasted into a room causing rising noise levels, interfering with instruction in adjacent rooms, and provoking anxiety in pupils. In actuality, when the equipment is installed and used appropriately, the reverse is true. The amplified teacher's voice can sound soothing as it is evenly distributed throughout the room, easily reaching every child. The room quiets as students attend to spoken instruction. In fact, the listener is aware of the sound distribution and ease of listening only when the equipment is turned off. The overall purpose of the equipment is to improve detection by having the details of spoken instruction continually reach the brains of all pupils (Flexer, 2004a).

Who Might Benefit from Sound Field Distribution Systems?

It could be argued that virtually all children could benefit from sound field distribution systems because the improved S/N ratio creates a more favorable learning environment. If children could hear better, clearer, and more consistently, they would have an opportunity to learn more efficiently (Edwards & Feun, 2005; Flexer & Rollow, 2009; Rosenberg et al., 1999). Some school systems have as a goal the amplification of every classroom in their districts (Knittel, Myott, & McClain, 2002).

No one disputes the necessity of creating a favorable visual field in a classroom. A school building never would be constructed without lights in every classroom. However, because hearing is invisible and ambiguous, the necessity of creating a favorable auditory field may be questioned by school personnel. Nevertheless, studies continue to show that sound distribution systems facilitate opportunities for improved academic performance (Crandell et al., 2005; Flexer & Long, 2003; Mendel, Roberts, & Walton, 2003).

The populations that seem to be especially in need of S/N ratio enhancing technology include children with fluctuating conductive hearing losses (ear infections), unilateral hearing losses, "minimal" permanent hearing losses, auditory processing problems, cochlear implants, cognitive disorders, learning disabilities, attention problems, articulation (speech) disorders, and behavior problems.

Teachers who use sound field technology report that they also benefit. Many state that they need to use less energy projecting their voices; they have less vocal abuse, and are less tired by the end of the school day (Blair, 2006). Teachers also report that the unit increases their efficiency as teachers, requiring fewer repetitions, thus allowing for more actual teaching time.

With more and more schools incorporating principles of inclusion where children who would have been in self-contained placements are in the mainstream classroom, sound field distribution systems offer a way of enhancing the classroom learning environment for the benefit of all children. It is a win-win situation.

Keep in mind that about 90% of today's population of children who are identified at birth with hearing loss likely will go directly into general education classrooms by 5 years of age. Those classrooms must be acoustically ready for them.

To summarize, classroom amplification facilitates the reception of consistently more intact signals than those received in an unamplified classroom, but signals are not as complete as those provided by using a personal FM unit (Crandell et al., 2005). In addition, the equipment, especially the loudspeakers, must be installed appropriately, and teachers must be in-serviced about the rationale and effective use of the technology.

A primary value of sound field is that it can focus the pupils and facilitate attention to relevant information. To that end, the effective use of the sound system's microphone can be a powerful teaching tool. Teachers need to be in-serviced about how to use the microphone to create a listening attitude in the room; the purpose of the microphone is to quiet and focus the room, not to excite or distract the children.

Choosing a System

Should an audiologist recommend a personal FM system or a sound field system or both for a given child? Once it is determined that a child has a hearing problem that interferes with acoustic accessibility, the next step involves recommending, fitting, and using some type of S/N ratio enhancing technology. One thing is certain: we cannot manage hearing by not managing hearing. Preferential seating does *not* control the background noise and reverberation in the classroom, stabilize teacher or pupil position, or provide for an even and consistent S/N ratio everywhere in the room.

In many instances the best listening and learning environment can be created by using both a sound field IR and a personal-worn FM system at the same time. The sound field IR unit, appropriately installed and used in a mainstreamed classroom, improves acoustic access for all pupils and creates a "listening" in the room. The individual personal-worn FM system allows the particular child with hearing loss to have the most favorable S/N ratio.

In several parts of the country, many general education classrooms already have infrared sound field distribution systems in them with two microphones: a teacher-worn microphone and a pass-around microphone for pupils. Teachers have been in-serviced about how to use the classroom system as a teaching tool in order to manage the class, create an auditory focus, and deliver direct and incidental instructional information.

Of course, children with hearing loss must use a personal FM system for a superior signal-to-noise ratio. Most of the time, the child's personal FM transmitter can be carefully attached to the audio-out port of the sound field system, using an appropriate patch cord. The child with hearing loss greatly benefits from having access to the two microphones of the sound field system. She also benefits from having a quiet environment in the classroom and a specific auditory focus. Teachers do require in-servicing about both technologies, including how to troubleshoot and use them together.

Small, Portable Desktop Sound Field Systems

One type of sound field FM system is called a personal sound field unit or desktop system (Figure 5–10). This is a small, lightweight,

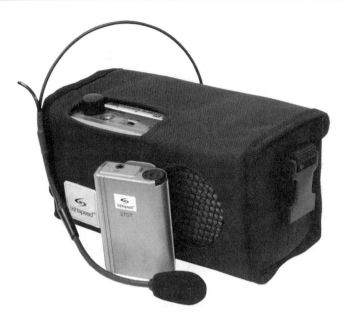

Figure 5–10. This small desktop sound field system, placed on a desk, provides close-up sound and can be carried easily from class to class. (Photo courtesy of LightSPEED Technologies, LES 391 Desktop SoundPak.)

battery powered, portable loudspeaker that can be carried from class to class and that delivers a clear, close-up sound right at the student's desk. Anderson et al. (2005) found either the personal FM system or the small, portable desktop sound field FM to be particularly useful for children with cochlear implants.

Following recognition and resolution of the equipment-related issues mentioned above comes the realization that, at best, *technology is simply a tool, a means to an end.* The purpose of classroom amplification, or any S/N ratio enhancing technology, is to facilitate the reception of the primary speech signal. Once children can detect word-sound differences clearly, they will have an opportunity to develop and improve their language skills and to acquire knowledge of the world. A 34-minute videotape, *Classroom Amplification and the Brain,* can be useful in conveying these concepts to parents, teachers, and therapists (Flexer, 2004b).

Whichever type of ALD is selected, personal-worn, sound field, or both, the following common-sense tips could facilitate use and function of the technologies:

- Try the equipment. *People must experience ALDs for themselves; they cannot speculate about benefit.*
- Be mindful of appropriate wearing and placement of the remote microphone on the teacher or parent. *Microphone placement dramatically affects the output speech spectrum. Specifically, high frequencies are weaker in off-axis positions. A head-worn boom microphone provides the best, most complete, and most consistent signal. A collar microphone, worn around the teacher's neck, also allows some level of control of microphone distance. If a lapel or lavaliere microphone is worn, it should be situated midline on the chest about 6 inches from the mouth.*
- Check the batteries first if any malfunction occurs. *Weak battery charge can cause interference, static, and intermittent signals in all FM or IR technologies.*
- Audiologists should write clear recommendations *for FM and/or IR equipment, specifying the rationale, type or types of S/N ratio enhancing technology needed, equipment characteristics, coupling arrangement chosen, parent and teacher in-service needed, and follow-up visits.*

Cochlear Implants

A cochlear implant is a surgically inserted biomedical device designed to provide sound information to children and adults who experience severe to profound hearing loss (ASHA 2004b). The cochlear implant is very different from a hearing aid. Hearing aids amplify sound, but cochlear implants compensate for damaged or nonworking parts of the inner ear (Niparko, 2004). In fact, the cochlear implant bypasses some of the damaged parts (typically the hair cells) of the inner ear; coded electrical signals stimulate different hearing nerve fibers which then send information to the brain. Hearing through an implant might sound different than typical hearing, but a properly inserted and programmed cochlear implant can allow many children to develop complete spoken communication skills if they receive appropriate early intervention (Geers et al., 2009).

The main components of a cochlear implant are the surgically implanted electrode array and the external speech processor that either can be body-worn or worn behind the ear like a hearing aid (Clark, 2003; Figure 5–11). Speech and sounds in the wearer's environment are processed by the components as follows. First, at the level of the speech processor, the microphone picks up sounds

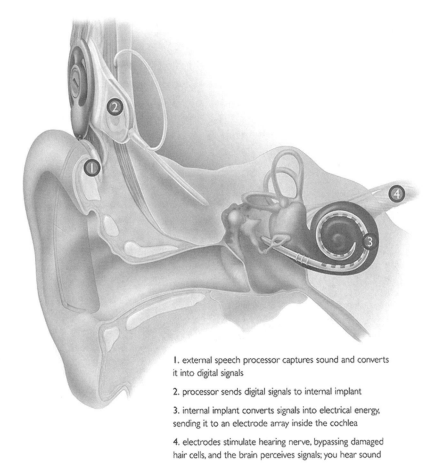

1. external speech processor captures sound and converts it into digital signals

2. processor sends digital signals to internal implant

3. internal implant converts signals into electrical energy, sending it to an electrode array inside the cochlea

4. electrodes stimulate hearing nerve, bypassing damaged hair cells, and the brain perceives signals; you hear sound

Figure 5–11. Schematic of a cochlear implant. (Provided courtesy of Cochlear Americas.)

from the environment and transmits them to the circuitry inside the speech processor. The circuitry in the speech processor then changes the input from the microphone into an electrical signal that is sent to the transmitter. The signal from the processor's transmitter is then sent, via an FM signal, through the skin behind the ear to the internal electrode array that has been surgically inserted into the cochlea. The internal electrode array stimulates auditory nerve fibers and the signal is sent to the brain. Finally, with auditory experience and learning, the signal is interpreted by the brain as sound and the person is able to hear. See the following company Web sites for more specific and updated product information: http://www.cochlear.com; http://www.cochlearimplant.com; http://www.medel.com.

Once implanted, the speech processor is linked to a computer and custom programmed for the individual child over several months (Zeng, Popper, & Fay, 2004; Figure 5–12). All current devices on the market have multiple program capacities that facilitate the mapping process and reduce the amount of time spent for mapping at the implant center. Please note that if a child is not progressing as

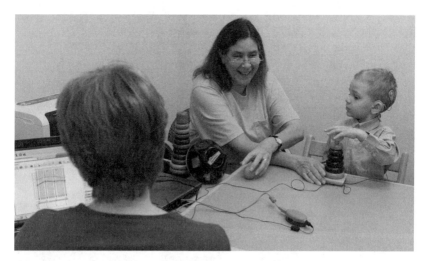

Figure 5–12. Once implanted, the child's speech processor is linked to a computer, either at a cochlear implant center, school, or in the home, and custom programmed. Multiple and repeated programming sessions need to be conducted to obtain and maintain an optimal program, also called a map, for the child.

expected or behavior and performance alter in a negative direction, contact your implant center and check the integrity of the device's map/program immediately (Wolfe & Schafer, 2010).

Implant Candidacy

As cochlear implant technology improves and as more outcome data are available, candidacy criteria are changing and becoming more liberal (Tobey, 2010). General trends are that children are being implanted at increasingly younger ages and they have more residual hearing (Fitzpatrick et al., 2009; Waltzman, 2005). Why? Because data continue to show that the younger a child is when implanted, the better are the desired outcomes of meaningful spoken language and literacy development due to stimulation of critical auditory brain centers during the early years of neural plasticity (Geers, 2002; Geers et al., 2009; Nicholas & Geers, 2006; Robbins, Koch, Osberger, Zimmerman-Philips, & Kishon-Rabin, 2004).

Identifying a baby or child as a candidate for a cochlear implant means that she should obtain significantly better hearing ability from a cochlear implant than she would from the most optimally fitted hearing aids. Following are generally accepted candidate criteria. There might be some variability between implant centers—and it is the implant team that ultimately determines who is or is not a candidate (ASHA, 2004b).

- Age 12 months and older; although more children are being implanted even younger than 12 months.
- Severe to profound bilateral sensorineural hearing loss.
- Intact auditory nerve.
- Little benefit from hearing aids—although the term *benefit* is subject to interpretation.
- Prior to approval for cochlear implantation, a 3- to 6-month trial with well-fitted hearing aids typically is recommended in conjunction with intensive auditory therapy. These criteria may be waived under certain circumstances, such as a history of meningitis with subsequent cochlear ossification.
- No medical contraindications to undergoing surgery. The surgery is typically performed on an outpatient basis, and takes 2 to 3 hours.
- No active middle ear disease.

> *View the cochlear implant as a value-added technology rather than as a "failed with hearing aids" technology. Even if the child is doing okay with hearing aids, can the implant add to the child's auditory access and distance hearing? Can the implant facilitate the child's exposure to conversations and information, both directly and indirectly conveyed?" Obtain audiological evidence to answer these questions.*

- An educational setting that emphasizes auditory therapy and communication.
- The family and, if old enough, the child should be highly motivated and have realistic expectations.

The following criteria often are added to the above in determining who to refer to an implant center for evaluation:

- A desired outcome for the baby or child of spoken language and reading skills consistent with hearing peers.
- Mainstream classroom placement.
- When wearing well-fitted hearing aids, the child is unable to understand speech at normal conversational levels without lipreading. The child can score up to 30% on open-set single syllable words and still be referred to an implant center. A child with a severe to profound hearing loss who demonstrates some benefit from hearing aids typically makes rapid and substantial progress with a cochlear implant. Why? Some benefit from hearing aids means that the auditory centers of the brain have been stimulated so that when the superior "keyboard" of the cochlear implant is provided, the child already has a neurological network in place for sound utilization.
- Unaided thresholds of 70 to 90 dB HL or worse from 1000 Hz through 8000 Hz.
- An aided speech recognition threshold (the softest level that known speech material can just barely be recognized using a closed-set task; this task focuses on vowels) of 35 dB HL or worse. There is a distinction between hearing aid gain and sound-quality benefit.

In this era of constant refinement of medical technologies and treatments, consumers expect the most current advice and interventions. One doesn't want the hip replacement that the mother had 10 years ago, or the cardiac treatment that the uncle had 5 years ago, or the knee surgery that a sister had just last year. Up-to-date information, recommendations, and interventions are required.

■ Aided distance hearing less than 10 feet for /s/ and less than 20 feet for *sh*. Distance hearing with a cochlear implant often can exceed 40 feet in a quiet environment, even for /s/. The greater the distance hearing, the better opportunity the baby or child will have for incidental learning.

Therefore, if a family previously was told (even in the recent past) that their child was not a candidate at that time—because he or she had too much residual hearing, or was getting too much gain from the hearing aid, or had some open-set discrimination, or was too young or too old—they should ask the implant center for an updated opinion (Allegretti, 2002; Tobey, 2010). Neither medicine nor technology is static. As we learn more about this wonderful device and about the possibilities it holds, different decisions will be made about candidacy.

Benefit of Cochlear Implants

Data are very exciting and show that children with multichannel cochlear implants demonstrate significant improvements in all areas of speech perception and production as compared to their preoperative performance with vibrotactile or conventional hearing aids (Geers et al., 2009; Moog & Geers, 2003; Waltzman, 2005; Zwolan et al., 2004). Benefits range from improved detection of sounds to understanding speech without lipreading and often include easy telephone use. In general, children who benefit the most from cochlear implantation are younger and/or have received the implant after a shorter duration of deafness. They are in good auditory-based training programs and have families who are firmly committed to the training process. An additional key factor is the length of time the child has used the implant. Even children who have used their device all day every day for more than 3 years continue to show substantial improvement in listening abilities.

Like the hearing aid and ALD technologies discussed previously in this chapter, a cochlear implant is only a tool, analogous to a computer keyboard that improves "data entry" to the brain. The ultimate effectiveness of the tool, however, is determined largely by the type and degree of aural rehabilitation and education that follow implantation (Geers et al., 2009; Moog & Geers, 2003; Tobey, 2010; Waltzman, 2005; Zwolan et al., 2004). Is the child placed in an environment that emphasizes spoken communication? Are listening skills systematically developed? What are the expectations for the child's ultimate use of the cochlear implant? Nicholas and Geers (2006) found that a key variable is the age of the baby/child at implantation. Those children who were implanted at the youngest ages when the brain has the most neuroplasticity developed the highest skills if they received appropriate auditory-based intervention.

Data entry and auditory-linguistic skill building take time, often years. The child who has an implant needs to be taught to interpret and derive meaning from the sounds that now enter his or her brain via the cochlear implant. The child who has access to an appropriate, auditory-based program has the best opportunity to benefit from a cochlear implant. The remainder of this book details the necessary intervention strategies to attain a listening and spoken language outcome.

> *There is now enough evidence that every month of access to sound makes a difference. Because of that, the decision to implant should be made by the time the infant is 9 months of age so that implantation can occur no later than 12 months of age.*

Bilateral Implants

Just as with bilateral hearing aids, bilateral cochlear implantation may offer assistance in difficult listening situations and subsequently can optimize speech, language, educational, and psychosocial development. Research has shown that bilateral cochlear implantation offers substantial benefits to the child. However, it also presents challenges (Tyler et al., 2002; Figure 5–13).

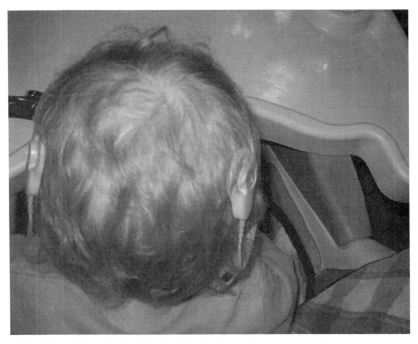

Figure 5–13. This baby is wearing bilateral cochlear implants with ear-level speech processors.

The value of bilateral implants is based on the value of bilateral hearing in general. To date, research on bilateral implants has shown advantages for many children in the following areas (Litovsky, 2010; Litovsky et al., 2006; Litovsky et al., 2009): improved speech recognition in noise through the binaural squelch; improved localization of speech and environmental sounds (also called spatial hearing); better access to sound originating from second CI side; access to binaural summation; and opportunities to capture the better ear. Team collaboration is critical in determining candidacy for a second implant and in arranging for the appropriate follow-up to maximize functional outcomes for each child.

The wear-time schedule for first and second cochlear implants, therapy activities, and therapy structure are dependent upon a number of individual variables, some of which include:

- Age of the child
- Auditory skill development with first CI or with hearing aids
- Time elapsed between the first and second implant

■ Family commitment to structured wear-time and activities for the second implant

Following are some observations about binaural implants that have been made so far. The better the child's auditory abilities (with either hearing aid or first cochlear implant) prior to implantation, the faster the child will learn to utilize the new electroacoustic input. It must be that the central cortex that is accustomed to dealing with auditory information more quickly recognizes and makes sense of the new source of auditorily coded input. The older the child is at the second implantation, the longer the adjustment might be and the longer that therapy tasks must be used focusing on the second implant alone. It appears that the younger the child is at the time of the first and second implant, the shorter the time needed for the second device to "catch up" (Litovsky, 2010). In addition, the shorter the time between implants, the less structured therapy is needed in the second implant-only condition. The degree to which children tolerate wearing the second implant alone varies, and parents should encourage that activity at home.

Bimodal Fittings

Bimodal hearing means that the child is wearing a cochlear implant in one ear and a hearing aid in the other. The hearing aid provides acoustic stimulation, and the cochlear implant provides electrical stimulation, hence the term "bimodal." The cochlear implant offers the advantage of high frequency audibility, and the hearing aid provides low frequency access because residual hearing typically occurs in the low frequencies.

When cochlear implants were first approved for children age 2 years and older in 1998, most candidates had very profound hearing losses and received virtually no benefit from continuing to wear a hearing aid in the unimplanted ear (Tobey, 2010). Subsequently, children with more residual hearing have been implanted and questions arose as to the value of wearing a hearing aid in the unimplanted ear. That is, for children who are not using bilateral implants and who have more residual hearing, is there benefit to wearing a hearing aid? Research has demonstrated that there can be substantial value to wearing a hearing aid in the ear contralateral to an implant if that ear has some low frequency residual hearing and such use should be encouraged (Cullington & Zeng, 2010). It seems that the low-frequency acoustic information below 250 Hz can provide speech perception benefit, assist when listening to multiple talkers, and add value to music appreciation (Cullington & Zeng, 2010; Zhang et al., 2010)

There also is continuing interest in combining electric and acoustic hearing in the same ear, called hybrid stimulation (Fabry, 2008). More research is needed about this fitting in children.

Cochlear Implants and FM Systems

Cochlear implants, like hearing aids, perform better in quiet than in noise. In fact, real-world listening environments (typically noisy) may slow language processing in young children with cochlear implants (Grieco-Calub, Saffran, & Litovsky, 2009). Because children must have access to soft speech at a distance in less than ideal environments, some sort of FM arrangement with remote microphone must be used. Schafer and Thibodeau (2003) and Anderson et al. (2005) evaluated the benefit of FM use with cochlear implants. They found that either a personal-worn FM coupled (attached) to the implant receiver, or a desktop sound field system, resulted in significantly improved performance in noise when compared to the implant-alone condition (Figure 5–14). The personal-worn FM must be programmed to the CI speech processor by the implant audiologist to avoid electrical interference, and to verify the relationship between the level of the FM signal and the environmental signal.

Accurately fitting a personal-worn FM to a cochlear implant depends on the child's ability to respond to the integrity of the sound. Only the child knows what she is actually hearing through the cochlear implant. Even though today's generation of FM/CI coupling is quite advanced, we recommend using a small desktop loudspeaker with a child who is too young or whose listening skills are not yet developed enough to provide good feedback regarding signal clarity.

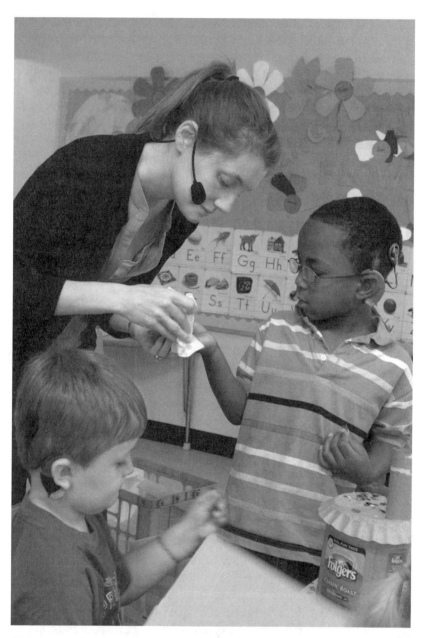

Figure 5–14. Both boys have an FM receiver boot coupled to their cochlear implants, and their teacher is wearing an FM transmitter to improve the signal-to-noise ratio in a classroom environment.

Measuring Efficacy of Fitting and Use of Technology

Efficacy can be defined as the extrinsic and intrinsic value of a treatment (Crandell et al., 2005). Even though technological treatments for hearing loss clearly have value, some measurement needs to be made to show that the individual baby or child in question is obtaining benefit. Benefit may be measured through educational performance, behavioral speech perception tests, direct measures of changes in brain development, or functional assessments.

Assessing cochlear implant benefit (as well as hearing aid and FM/IR benefit) in infants and young children has been challenging because this population has limited communication skills, limited attention span, and immature behaviors. Functional auditory assessments, therefore, are the most common and easily administered efficacy measure (Tharpe, 2004).

See Table 5–1 for an overview of functional auditory assessment tools.

Equipment Efficacy for the School System

The key to securing technology from the school system is to obtain data documenting need (Ackerhalt & Wright, 2003). A multifactored comprehensive evaluation, which is a thorough evaluation by a multidisciplinary team, is necessary to document the need for a child to receive special services. The last category on most multifactored comprehensive evaluation forms is Assistive Technology Needs. In order for assistive technology to be recommended within any legislative framework, some type of evaluation must be conducted. That is, can we document that the child in question cannot obtain an appropriate education unless a personal-worn FM system or an FM or IR sound field distribution system is utilized? Can the child's access to and performance in the general education environment be linked to hearing difficulties in the classroom? What tests can be administered to document acoustic access and listening difficulties in the classroom?

Table 5–1. Functional Auditory Assessment Tools for Infants and Young Children

Measurement Tool	Authors	Age Range	Purpose
Auditory Behavior in Everyday Life (ABEL) (2002)	Purdy et al.	Children 2–12 years	Twenty-four-item questionnaire with three subscales (aural-oral, auditory awareness, social/conversational skills) which evaluates auditory behavior in everyday life
Children's Home Inventory for Listening Difficulties (CHILD) (2000)	Anderson & Smaldino	Children 3–12 years	Parent and self-report versions that assess listening skills in 15 natural situations
Children's Outcome Worksheet (COW) (2003)	Whitelaw, Wynne, & Williams	Children 4–12 years	Teacher, parent, and child rating scales of classroom and home listening situations with amplification device; to specify five situations where improved hearing is desired
Early Listening Function (ELF) (2000)	Anderson	Infants and toddlers; 5 months–3 years	Parent observational rating scale of structured listening activities conducted over time to record distance learning
Functional Auditory Performance Indicators (FAPI) (2003)	Stredler-Brown & Johnson	Infants through school age	Parent or interventionist assessment of functional auditory skills over time
Infant-Toddler Meaningful Auditory Integration Scale (IT-MAIS) (1997)	Robbins, Renshaw, & Berry	Infant-toddler and older child versions	Structured parent interview scale designed to assess spontaneous auditory behaviors in everyday listening situations
Listening Inventories for Education (LIFE) (1998)	Anderson & Smaldino	6 years and above	Student and teacher rating scales designed to assess listening difficulty in the classroom

Measurement Tool	Authors	Age Range	Purpose
Little Ears (2003)	Kuhn-Inacker et al.	Birth and up	Questionnaire for the parent with 35 age-dependent questions that assess auditory development
Meaningful Auditory Integration Scale (MAIS) (1991)	Robbins et al.	Children 3 to 4 years and up	Parental interview with 10 questions that evaluates meaningful use of sound in everyday situations; attachment with hearing instrument, ability to alert to sound, ability to attach meaning to sound
Parent's Evaluation of Aural/Oral Performance of Children (PEACH) (2000)	Ching et al.	Preschool to 7 years	Interview with parent with 15 questions targeting the child's everyday environment; includes scoring for five subscales (use, quiet, noise, telephone, environment)
Preschool Screening Instrument for Targeting Educational Risk (Preschool SIFTER) (1996)	Anderson & Matkin	3 to 6 years	Questionnaire with 15 items completed by the teacher that identifies children at risk for educational failure; has five subscales (academics, attention, communication, class participation, behavior)
Screening Inventory for Targeting Educational Risk (SIFTER) (1989)	Anderson	6 years through secondary school	Teacher questionnaire designed to target academic risk behaviors in children with hearing problems; has five subscales (academics, attention, communication, class participation, behavior)
Teacher's Evaluation of Aural/Oral Performance of Children (TEACH) (2000)	Ching et al.	Preschool to 7 years	Interview with teacher having 13 questions targeting the child's everyday environment; includes scoring for five subscales: use, quiet, noise, telephone, environment

One way that an audiologist can document the need for technology and also measure efficacy of technology fitting is to perform speech-in-noise testing in the clinical sound room. Typically, audiologists test children's speech perception in quiet at advantageous intensity levels. If phonetically balanced (PB) words are presented only at 40 dB sensation level (SL) under earphones, functional information is not provided about accessibility to typical classroom instruction. Words presented at a loud level in perfect quiet always overestimate a child's real life auditory discrimination ability. By adding two speech assessments to the basic audiologic test battery, an audiologist in a school or clinical setting can document efficacy by providing functional information about the child's acoustic accessibility to the speech spectrum. Using appropriate speech material, such as the WIPI, word identification testing should be performed in the sound field in the unaided condition. Then, while wearing hearing aids or cochlear implant(s), these same tests also should be performed in the aided condition, in quiet and in noise. Appropriate speech stimuli for the language level of the child should be presented at the average loudness level that a child in a favorable classroom environment—50 dB HL—receives speech. Because the child also must hear soft speech, another list of words should be presented at 35 dB HL.

Conclusion

The purpose of technology is to efficiently, effectively, and consistently channel sounds to the brain. The purpose of intervention is to use the technology to provide the child with redundant and meaningful auditory-linguistic communicative experiences to allow the brain to develop a substantial auditory neurolinguistic infrastructure. The development and programming of the baby's/child's auditory neural centers serve as the basis for spoken language, literacy, and academic and social-emotional growth. Therefore, the fitting and use of hearing aids, cochlear implants, and FM/IR technologies is a critical first step in attaining the desired outcome of listening and talking.

6

Intervention Issues

Key Points Presented in the Chapter

■ The framework for intervention presented in this book is based on the premise that the most effective ingredients of intervention for young children who have hearing loss include beginning intervention (both technological and instructional) when the child is very young, following a normal developmental sequence, and having parents be the primary teachers of their children.

■ Educational programs for children who have hearing loss differ on several important dimensions. Parents and professionals need to know what those dimensions are so that they can ask questions to find out where each program stands on each of the dimensions.

■ For a child with a hearing loss, challenges to the process of learning spoken language can arise from late wearing of hearing aids or cochlear implants, from disabilities in addition to the hearing loss, or from the child living in a multilingual environment.

■ Preschoolers with hearing loss have widely varying abilities and needs, and their educational programs need to be carefully and individually planned. A full continuum of options needs to be available in order to determine the program that most appropriately fits the child's needs.

Basic Premises

The goal of this text is to provide a framework for professionals and families who want to help promote spoken language development in their young children who have hearing loss. Ideas about intervention in this book are grounded on the following four premises:

- The first premise is that it makes sense to begin intervention with children who have hearing loss when they are *very young* because of the research on particular sensitivity of the brain's neural pathways to auditory input prior to the age of 3 (Sharma, Dorman, & Spahr, 2002; Sharma et al., 2004; Sharma, Dorman, & Kral, 2005; Sharma, Martin, et al., 2005) as well as because of the verbal and academic deficits often seen in children whose audiological and educational management begin later (Geers & Moog, 1989; Nicholas & Geers, 2006; see Chapters 1 and 2).
- The second premise is that it makes sense to help these children learn to *listen and talk* in order to keep as much of the world open and available to them as possible (see Chapter 7).
- The third premise is that it makes the most sense to help the *parent* help the young child learn spoken language through listening. The idea is to maximize the child's development through optimizing the family's capacity to address the child's needs. Working in partnership should result in the most effective intervention with very young children (Bromwich, 1981; Girolometto & Weitzman, 2006; Law, Garrett, & Nye, 2004; Rini & Hindenlang, 2006; Tannock & Girolometto, 1992; Yoder & Warren, 1998, 2002; see Chapters 9 and 10).
- The fourth premise is that in acquiring spoken language through listening, a child with a hearing loss will generally follow a normal developmental path. The pace may be somewhat slower (or not!), and there may be some asynchronies in learning related to difficulty in hearing particular aspects of language (Ertmer, Strong, & Sadogopan, 2003; Estabrooks, 2006; L. Kretschmer & R. Kretschmer, 2001; Uchanski & Geers, 2003; Schauwers, Gillis, & Govaerts, 2005; Tye-Murray, 2003). Much of the intervention described in this book is based upon the child following the normal developmental

sequence of spoken language learning. However, carefully preplanned and structured teacher- or parent-directed strategies will need to be used to address asynchronies as they are uncovered. The longer the child is without hearing, the more the need for structured, adult-directed instruction (see Chapters 7 and 10).

The primary focus of much of this book is on work by *parents* who are helping their children learn *spoken language through listening*. Certainly, by the age of 3 years, when parents and school districts may be thinking of preschool, each child presents unique educational needs to be met. No one single method or educational setting can meet the needs of all children who have hearing loss. The section in this chapter entitled "Educational Options for Children with Hearing Loss, Ages 3 to 6" discusses some of the possible educational choices that could be considered by parents and school districts as they are trying to make decisions. Much of the information in this book could be applied to work in small group preschool settings, where the teacher of the hearing-impaired has knowledge and experience in helping children with hearing loss learn spoken language through listening. Appendix 5 lists needs that are common to all children with hearing loss who are learning in group settings. What will be different for each child will be the amount of intensive individual therapy required. That amount should be based on what is needed in order to get (or keep) the child's auditory and spoken language learning at an appropriate level for realizing the child's potential for cognitive, social, and academic development.

Not every child with severe or profound hearing loss does learn to talk, sometimes in spite of the best efforts of parents and professionals. Reasons for a lack of satisfactory progress in spoken language can include late diagnosis, poorly fitting and/or poorly maintained hearing aids, an impoverished educational program, lack of appropriate sensory aids for those with no measurable hearing, insufficient or ineffective parental involvement, additional disabilities, or additional problems in learning (either general or specific in nature). None of these factors by itself precludes the possibility of the child learning to talk, but a combination of several of them can mitigate against it. The section in this chapter entitled "Challenges to the Process of Learning Spoken Language" provides more detail on this issue.

Differentiating Dimensions Among Intervention Programs

There are hundreds of programs, both publicly and privately supported, that provide services based on spoken language development for children who have hearing loss in the birth to 6-year-old age range. These programs may describe themselves as "oral," "auditory-oral," or "auditory-verbal." Professionals in these programs may have certification by the A. G. Bell Academy as Listening and Spoken Language Specialists (either LSLS Educators or LSLS Therapists).

Although the primary aim of all these early intervention programs and individuals is to help children who have hearing loss learn to talk, close inspection reveals that such programs can vary on several theoretical and methodological dimensions. Parents need to be aware of these distinctions in order to understand the nature of the program in which their child is enrolled. Additional information for parents who need to make decisions about group placement for their children at age 3 or older can be found in Appendix 5.

1. **The nature and manner of parent involvement in the child's learning can be different in different programs.** This can be reflected in details such as the number of sessions per week; whether or not the parent is in the therapy room or observing from outside; whether it is primarily the parent or the therapist who interacts with the child during the sessions; the locale of the sessions (center-based, home-based, or a flexible combination of the two); the existence of parent group meetings and activities outside of the sessions; and the nature and amount of information supplied to the parent about how to help the child outside of the intervention sessions. If the program truly is providing intervention aimed at having the parent become the child's primary language teacher, then there are likely to be one or two parent guidance sessions per week. The parent is expected to be integrating auditory strategies into all that they do with the child, during all the rest of the week, all of the child's waking hours. It is not the hour spent with the teacher or therapist that causes the child to learn to listen and talk! It is all of the work that the parents and family do in the remaining 83 or so hours of the week that the child is awake and alert.

2. **Programs vary in the emphasis placed on normal everyday interactive events as the context within which the**

child will learn language, versus an emphasis on the child learning language from participating in adult-directed teaching activities. The contrast is between a normal developmental approach and a remedial approach. Helping very young children who have hearing loss learn to listen and talk can be accomplished primarily through a normal developmental process, with "embellishments" that include hearing aids and cochlear implants, and parents employing strategies to help children integrate listening and talking into their way of interacting with the world. However, if the child's hearing loss is detected late and/or if there are other interfering problems that have resulted in the child being very far behind, then the approach will need to include more adult-directed and preplanned activities. Programs differ on the extent to which they employ either approach, both in general and with regard to their work with individual children at different points in their development.

3. **Programs and interventionists also vary in their use of sense modalities in providing spoken language input, both in normal everyday conversations and in more adult-directed activities.** There are three likely avenues of sensory input for spoken language: auditory, visual, and tactile:

   a. A program that emphasizes *audition* will treat the child's need for stimulation of the auditory centers of the brain as a neurological emergency. They will have the parent and child come in to fit hearing aids within 2 weeks of an initial contact, they will teach the parent how to manage the equipment, and they will provide guidance on how to keep the equipment on the child all waking hours from the very beginning. Professionals in an auditory program will also be talking with the parents about ways in which they can help the child learn to listen in the course of everyday interactions, right from the beginning. For example, audition can be maximized in normal interactions by speaking at a relatively close distance to the child, by sitting behind or beside him, or by having the child's visual focus on the toys or activity at hand, rather than on the speaker's face.

   b. The *visual* sense modality in this context refers to whether or not the child is frequently encouraged to watch the speaker's face for cues provided by speech-reading—that is, for example, to watch the speaker's lips and facial expressions when the speaker is talking. In addition, although it is now only rarely done with young children, it is also possible to consciously teach differentiations among or between particular lip positions and their associated sounds (e.g., the difference in lip position and movement of a /fa/ versus a /ba/).

c. The *tactile* sense modality can be employed in a global way through the use of vibrotactile devices that are intended to be worn by the child to aid in perception of speech in normal conversational situations. Vibrotactile devices are also sometimes used in a more limited way for speech and auditory training exercises. With or without a vibrotactile device, touch can be employed in demonstrating features of particular speech sounds where tactile sensation is salient such as the breathstream of fricatives and plosives.

Some of the possible permutations of the use of sense modalities include programs that advocate the use of audition only; programs that include the use of vision and touch as supplements to audition, when needed; programs that always encourage the child to watch the face when someone is speaking (and are thus purposely presenting the input through audition and vision at the same time), with the use of touch also, as needed; and programs which might do any of the above, depending upon the needs and abilities of a particular child.

To the uninitiated, these differences may seem to be insignificant, but within the field of education of children who are deaf or hard of hearing, they have, with some justification, been hotly contested issues. There are strong research- and logic-based reasons to rely primarily on audition as the major means of helping a young child with a hearing loss learn spoken language. The key program elements seem to rest most squarely on the knowledge, persistence, and enthusiasm of the teacher and the parents.

Challenges to the Process of Learning Spoken Language

Providing the conditions for a young child with hearing loss to acquire spoken language through listening requires knowledge-driven effort on the part of all the adults in the child's life. Necessary conditions (whether the child is at home, at daycare, or in a preschool setting) include:

■ **Consistent, appropriately excellent auditory access to speech all waking hours from a very young age.** The child needs auditory access (by means of appropriately fit and maintained technology, e.g., hearing aids, cochlear implants, and FM systems) all waking hours. That access needs to be verified through constant adult vigilance about the functioning of the child's equipment, and about the acoustic conditions of the child's environment, as well as through appropriate use of personal FM technology in any situation where noise or distance from the speaker is likely to reduce the child's access to the speaker's message.

■ **Multiple and varied repetitions of linguistic input and linguistic practice in meaningful, everyday interactions with fluent speakers of the target language.** We do not have research that tells us exactly how much talking and interacting is enough. However, there is research on children with normal hearing who experienced widely varying amounts of verbal interacting with their caregivers, which clearly demonstrates the advantages to the child's own language and literacy growth from being exposed to a rich quantity and variety of adult talk and interaction in at least the first 3 or 4 years of life (Hart & Risley, 2003). For the child with hearing loss, access to the verbal messages to and around him is necessarily at least somewhat limited by the very presence of the hearing loss. How much more important must it be to have adults in his or her life who consistently go out of their way to play and interact verbally, providing a rich and varied linguistic experience for the child?

The following circumstances can present additional challenges for the child with hearing loss as he or she learns spoken language:

1. Child is late to full-time wearing of appropriate amplification.
2. Child has disabilities in addition to the hearing loss.
3. Child's family does not speak the language used by the aural habilitationist, by teachers and students in the child's school, and by the "mainstream" community.

Each will be addressed in turn.

Late to Full-Time Wearing of Appropriate Amplification or Cochlear Implant(s)

Research has not yet told us a precise age after which the child is too old to acquire spoken language. However, we do know that the earlier the child begins wearing appropriate audiological technology, the better the child's progress will be (Nicholas & Geers, 2006, 2007; Sharma, Dorman, & Kral, 2005; Yoshinaga-Itano, 2004). Time before the child is wearing hearing aids is lost listening time, and delays the child's immersion in listening, which is a necessary first step for the child's brain to begin sorting out all of the auditory "noise" into meaning. A child who is 18 months old before his hearing loss is identified, and hearing aids are worn full time, has lost 18 months of listening time, and has missed the time period during which all of his hearing peers were listening and learning spoken language. Now, to begin at 18 months, the child is out of synchrony, out of sequence—his nonverbal cognitive abilities may be those of an 18-month-old, but his ability to understand and express himself using words is not.

In addition, in order to catch up to his hearing peers before kindergarten, the child has to learn at a faster-than-normal rate. The normally hearing 18-month-old child will proceed to do 3½ years of learning before age 5, whereas the newly aided 18-month-old will have to do 5 years of learning in those 3½ years in order to be on an equal footing with his normal-hearing peers. Children with hearing loss have caught up with their normally hearing peers, but it does take consistent effort on the part of all involved. Unfortunately, the child wearing hearing aids often is working at the further disadvantage of not being able hear well in even low-level noise, or at a distance of more than about 12 feet from the speaker, which makes normal overhearing of others' language difficult or impossible. (*Note:* (1) Noise and distance problems can be addressed by parent use of FM and (2) children with cochlear implants are likely to have better distance hearing than this, on programs set for distance listening.)

Children with hearing loss *are* able to learn at amazing rates, once they wear amplification technology on a full-time basis, and once all of the adults in the child's life are providing appropriate, meaningful spoken language in interactions with the child. Achieving 18 months to 2 years progress in 1 year on standardized language measures is not uncommon for preschoolers with hearing loss who have appropriate amplification and input.

Even children with mild or unilateral hearing loss are known to have speech and language-learning problems with greater incidence than children with normal hearing (Delage & Tuller, 2007; Lieu, 2004; Tharpe, 2008). Because today's technology can nearly always bring the speech signal to the child more intensely and with great fidelity, it is imperative that parents explore the audiological technology that may be of help to their child. Parents (and all family members) then need to insist that the child wear the amplification all waking hours as soon as it is prescribed and fit. There can be challenges in keeping hearing aids on a child's head at any age, but the greatest challenge has been surmounted when the child's parents are convinced that the child needs to wear the equipment in order to learn to listen and talk.

The challenges to keeping hearing aids or cochlear implants on young children vary, depending on the age at which the child is just beginning to wear the technology. Unlike some adults, children do not need gradual acclimation to having access to sound—they need it as soon as possible, all waking hours. The parents' job is to make the technology the first thing they do with the child in the

Parental belief that the audiological equipment is helping the child has key importance to this process. If at all possible, the audiologist and aural habilitationist need to demonstrate the child's improved hearing when the child is wearing the equipment at the first appointment. But it is one thing to know intellectually that the technology helps your child, and another to be able to be "happy" about having your child wear it all of the time. That is, it is important to remember that most new parents are likely to be much less enthusiastic about the wonders of today's technology than the professionals! Hearing loss and hearing equipment are new to the parents, and in fact when the child is wearing the equipment, it is proof that their child has a hearing problem. The equipment is likely to bring on questions from family members and from strangers that the parent may only be beginning to be able to answer for herself or himself.

morning, which goes on as soon as the child wakes up, and only comes off when the child is sleeping (although some children like to wear their technology when they are sleeping, too). Just as they would not allow the child to go around without a diaper, or to run in the street, they make sure that the child is not running around without his or her "ears," without the technology that will provide the child with auditory access to develop the auditory centers of the brain, during all of the experiences of childhood.

With tiny babies, the problems usually are those of large fingers (adults') getting used to putting earmolds into tiny ears, and knowing that the pinna (external ear) is pliable and can be pulled a bit without causing any harm to the child. The audiologist and/ or aural habilitationist will demonstrate techniques for identifying which earmold is which (right versus left), holding the earmold in a certain way, and then inserting it while gently and firmly pulling the pinna back and up and then making sure that the earmold is seated properly. It is awkward at first, but with practice, inserting an earmold becomes second nature. Another challenge can arise from the fact that the child frequently is held close to the body (e.g., during feeding), and one ear and earmold can be covered or can emit feedback, simply from the positioning. Sometimes shifting position slightly can take care of the problem. In addition, most current digital hearing aids have feedback suppression circuits that help reduce feedback. (See Chapter 5 for additional information about putting hearing aids on very young babies.)

With children who have the dexterity to able to take off hearing aids or cochlear implants, parents may need to cheerfully keep putting them back on time after time for the first week or so. Distracting the child with toys or with another child or adult interacting with them, as well as putting something else into the child's hands are additional strategies that often help. However, if the child learns that taking off the equipment brings an upset mommy or daddy running and upset, it may increase the frequency with which the child takes off the equipment. For that reason, simply saying, "Uh-oh. We need to put this back on! Here you go," and smiling calmly is likely to be a better strategy. That may be easier said than done, the 900th time, so be easy on yourself. It is better to leave the hearing aids off for an hour, and give yourself a break until you can *be* that cheery mom or dad and have someone else distract the child while the equipment is being put back on.

With children who are 18 months or older, the ease with which the child adjusts to the equipment is likely to be similar to the ease with which he or she adjusts to any change in daily routines. Parental strategies for managing the child's behavior also will come into play. Again, maintaining a cheerful, matter-of-fact demeanor is likely to be helpful, as is distracting the child's attention with favorite toys or videos. The stipulation may need to be that the toys or videos only get played with (or only work) when the equipment is on the child's head.

Nearly all parents will want their children to have "alligator clips" with one end looped around the child's earhook and the other clipped to the back of the child's shirt. If and when the child removes the equipment, it will dangle, rather than fall and be lost. Dental floss and safety pins can provide the same function. In addition, there are other means of keeping hearing aids in small ears, which may be helpful, including "huggies" (small plastic tubing that goes around the child's ear to provide more stability), head bands, and hats. The following Web sites may be helpful: http://www.gear forears.com and http://www.silkawear.com.

Disabilities in Addition to the Child's Hearing Loss

A child with a hearing loss may have the hearing loss alone, or may have disabilities in addition to the hearing loss. According to data reported from Gallaudet's 2005–2006 Annual Survey of Deaf and Hard of Hearing Children and Youth, the approximate incidence of deafness with no other additional condition 51%. In contrast, approximately 47% of the children with deafness in their survey were reported to have at least one additional condition. The other conditions include problems such as cerebral palsy, visual problems (including blindness), learning disabilities, developmental delays, cognitive problems, orthopedic disabilities, ADD/ADHD, traumatic brain injury, behavioral problems, problems with the heart, kidney, or liver or other conditions.

The data from Gallaudet do not indicate the severity of the additional conditions, which can vary widely from mild to very severe. Having clear auditory access to speech, and having all of the adults in the child's life providing appropriately enriched linguistic input, is a positive situation for any child. For a child with multiple, very severe disabilities, having access to sound may play a pivotal role in connecting the child to the environment. The child may begin to alert to some of the sounds that surround him, and may begin to smile or be more animated when adults talk with him—which further connects the adults with the child, and creates a cycle of positive interactions for both the child and others in the child's life. Sometimes the child's hearing and talking abilities become strengths relative to the other disabilities.

The aural habilitationist and audiologist will need to work closely with the other professionals involved in the child's life and intervention. Each of the professionals needs to bring his or her information and expertise to the table, and to collaborate in providing a cohesive program for the child and family. Aural habilitationists have much to offer with regard to ways of promoting an optimal auditory environment for the child, auditory strategies to integrate into any other intervention that is being carried out, and appropriate spoken language to use in particular situations. This means, for example, that the occupational therapist and physical therapist need to wear the FM, and need to be comfortable in reinserting the child's hearing aids, and they need to know that it is incredibly important to talk to the child about what they are doing, and about what the materials or toys are that they are using, and to pause for the child's responses. Similarly, the aural habilitationist needs to be aware of positioning the child appropriately for play and interacting, understand the importance of a sensory diet for some children, and needs to have snipping scissors and pencil grips for activities where they are needed by other children. Protecting perceived professional turf is unlikely to be productive, whereas respectful collaboration is likely to result in a more cohesive picture for the family of what needs to be done and how.

The presence of other disabilities may create additional challenges to practicalities such as keeping the hearing aids on in the presence of other equipment, the existence of ever present noise from other life-saving equipment, the difficulty of continuing to persist with encouraging listening and spoken language when progress is very slow. Aural habilitationists need to be especially sensitive to these issues, and to be ready to address them creatively and with compassion, along with other members of the child's team. Regular co-treating with other professionals is an excellent way for cross-fertilization of ideas and techniques which enrich the practice of all of the adults working with the child and family, and keep everyone using similar language and similar strategies, which is much less confusing for everyone involved.

Multilingual Environment

Being multilingual in today's world can be an important asset, and in some families is essential for communication with all of the members of the family. Individuals with hearing loss certainly are capable of becoming fluent in more than one spoken language. (Robbins, Green, & Waltzman, 2004; Thomas, El-Kashlan,& Zwolan, 2008). Not surprisingly, ***consistent auditory access*** to both languages from a young age seems to be a key factor. With today's technology, early consistent auditory access is a reachable goal for all children with hearing loss, so bilingualism also is a possibility.

However, learning two languages simultaneously may be less advisable if the child's hearing loss is identified late, or if there are multiple disabilities or other challenges. When the goal is for the child to learn a first language, it is logical that first language-learning is going to be faster and more efficient if all energies are devoted toward helping the child learn one language to a complex level, before introducing a second one. There are only about 12 to 14 waking hours in most young children's lives, and most hearing children are using all of those hours to learn only one spoken language. When the quality and quantity of listening are reduced because of the child's hearing loss, it would seem to become even more important for that reduced input to the child to be consistently in one language. The situation may be analogous to a situation where a child is being taught to play both the flute and the guitar at the same time. It is possible to do, of course, but the amount of practice time for each will be reduced by the simple fact that there are only 12 to 14 waking hours in the child's daily life, with many other activities also occurring during that time.

The choice of *which* language will be the child's first language should be entirely up to the child's parents. Factors that can weigh into the decision include:

- ■ Fluency of the adults in the child's home in the languages being considered;

■ Comfort of the adults in using each of the languages being considered (this is important for adult-child bonding, as language is such an integral part of the bonding process);

■ Language of instruction in the child's school environment.

None of the challenges mentioned here is insurmountable, but the process of learning spoken language is likely to require additional time and sustained effort on the part of the child and all the adults in the child's life.

Educational Options for Children with Hearing Loss, Ages 3 to 6

In the United States,[1] each state now has early intervention programs under Part C of IDEA that provide services to children with hearing loss and their families from birth until the age of 3. Starting at age 3, children with special education needs become the financial responsibility of the school district for the town in which the child resides. This change in funding agency, causes the necessity of a transition process from one agency (Birth to Three or early intervention) to another (the school system). Early intervention programs are set up to educate and support families in their efforts to address their children's developmental needs. For children with hearing loss, early intervention programs address the child's hearing needs and the child's language-learning needs, in addition to other needs as they are identified. Many of the sessions occur in the child's home.

In contrast, school systems are set up to educate children in classrooms in schools, and with very few exceptions, are set up to do that without much involvement from parents in the actual daytime educational process. In school, teachers teach the children rather than instruct the parents in how to address their child's developmental needs, as is done in Birth to Three early intervention programs. School systems generally are not equipped, nor are

---

[1]Readers in other countries may not have to deal with this transition from one agency to the other when the child turns 3 years old, but they are very likely to have similar issues to consider when trying to develop an appropriate educational program for a preschool-aged child with hearing loss.

they funded, to provide educational services in ways other than through classroom instruction. Not surprisingly, the expectation often is that most children with special education needs will be educated in the district's existing special education preschool classes, which may have some typical peers, but are primarily classes for all preschool children with special needs, regardless of disability.

However, according to the U.S. Department of Education, children with hearing loss have unique communication needs (United States Department of Education, 1992, 2004). Those unique communication needs are to be central to decision making regarding each child's educational placement, and central to the determination of what constitutes the least restrictive educational environment for a child who has hearing loss. For a child with hearing loss who is learning spoken language, the fundamental needs at school age (age 3 years and older) are related to the child's need for auditory access to spoken language, as well as to the child's need for individualized spoken language stimulation. The preschooler with hearing loss needs a professional with the appropriate knowledge to and experience to provide appropriate auditory/linguistic stimulation as well as to guide the parents in providing appropriate auditory/linguistic stimulation all waking hours outside school. Even by the age of 3, children with hearing loss vary widely in factors such as the age of identification of the hearing loss, the degree of hearing loss, the age at which they began full-time wearing of appropriate hearing technology, and in the quantity and quality of spoken language exposure. Consequently, at the age of 3 years, children with hearing loss have widely varying profiles with regard to hearing loss and communication needs. The decision to provide intensive specialized support for a child whose language lags far behind age peers may be easier to make than determining the level of support for a child whose language scores on standardized tests appear to be within the normal range (which is occurring with increasing frequency, due to infant hearing screening and the availability of excellent audiological technology and improved pedagogy). However, for children who appear to be doing very well, it must be considered that the reason that the child's language scores are within the normal range may well be because of all of the professional and parent work that has taken place during the birth-to-three period. For the child to continue to make the same gains in the two remaining years before kindergarten, it is crucially important that appropriate supports continue to be provided, because language learning is exponential between age 3 and 6 for children with normal access to sound 24 hours of the day. Relative to their normally hearing peers, 3-year-old children with any degree of hearing loss continue to be at a marked disadvantage for spoken language learning because their access to auditory/linguistic input in the environment is significantly reduced in both quantity and quality. Removing all supports until the language of the child with hearing loss shows statistically significant deficits follows a failure-based model. It cannot be justified in terms of the ongoing effects of the permanent sensory deficit on the child's learning. Each child's ongoing educational needs must be individually considered in determining services, as dictated by federal law. Clearly, there needs to be an array of options available, not just the existing special education preschool.

Some of the educational options that may be appropriate for individual children with hearing loss at age three include the following:

- **Child and family receive Auditory-Verbal Therapy (which includes audiological support services), with the parent deciding whether or not to send the child to a regular nursery or preschool for socialization purposes.** If the child goes to regular nursery or preschool, classroom educational audiology support services are needed.

- **Child with appropriately aided hearing, excellent listening abilities, and language abilities apparently on age level attends regular nursery or preschool setting**, with FM equipment provided and regularly monitored by an educational audiologist, and with the regular preschool staff receiving regular consultation from knowledgeable professionals regarding the equipment, and the child's listening and language-learning needs. That same professional will monitor the child's language learning throughout the year to be certain that the child's language learning is progressing normally.

- **Child attends a specialized inclusive listening and spoken language preschool for children with hearing loss**, which has small groups of both other children with hearing loss and at least an equal number of typically developing peers, with a Teacher of the Hearing-Impaired all day long, as well as an Early Childhood Instructor, weekly parent guidance sessions, and audiological support services. When parents cannot or do not choose to engage in Auditory-Verbal Therapy, this may be the most appropriate option for children with hearing loss whose spoken language abilities at age 3 are more than a year behind those of their typically developing peers. This inclusive preschool preschool offers intensive instruction specialized for children with hearing loss, that focuses on helping the child learn to listen, and on helping the child increase his or her rate of spoken language learning. It constitutes the Least Restrictive Environment for these children, because the specialized instruction makes the curriculum available to the child, and because play and other regular preschool activities are carried out with typically developing peers and facilitated by the teacher of the hearing impaired and other staff.

■ **Child with appropriately aided hearing, excellent listening abilities, and language abilities apparently on age level attends a preschool class for children who are learning English as a Second Language, with full educational audiological support services.** The advantage to this class is that it is entirely devoted to language stimulation; the disadvantage is that there may not be peers who are fluent speakers of English. The child will need full educational audiological support services in this setting, as well as ongoing direct service and consultation from a teacher of the hearing-impaired or speech-language pathologist who is knowledgeable and experienced in promoting listening and spoken language development in children who have hearing loss.

■ **Child with severe multiple disabilities including hearing loss attends special education preschool class where there are typical peers, class size is small, and the disabilities of the other children do not compromise the child's auditory access.** Full educational audiological support services need to be provided in this setting, as well as frequent consultation and/or direct service from a teacher of the hearing-impaired or speech-language pathologist who is knowledgeable and experienced in promoting listening and spoken language development in young children who have hearing loss. The advantage to this setting is that the child's needs in addition to hearing loss will be addressed by professionals with expertise in those areas. The disadvantages of these settings can include:

- Noise levels that are excessive, due to the number of professionals and paraprofessionals required to attend to all of the varying needs of the children in the classroom and/or due to other children who vocalize nonstop;
- Special educators, paraprofessionals, and administrators whose expectations for children with hearing loss may be similar to expectations for children with intellectual disabilities;
- Special educators, paraprofessionals, and administrators who are resistant or unable to achieve the levels of vigilance about noise that are needed to provide appropriate auditory access for the child with hearing loss.
- Lack of at least a 1:1 ratio of children with disabilities and typically developing children to provide sufficient models of normal sociolinguistic behavior.

Appendix 5 contains a Checklist for Evaluating Preschool Group Settings for Children with Hearing Loss, with items listed according to the child's needs. These items could apply to any preschool group setting that parents and educators may be considering for the child. What would vary according to the child's language abilities, would be the level of support needed from a teacher of the hearing-impaired, Auditory-Verbal Therapist/Educator, or other professional with appropriate expertise in order for the child's language to continue to grow exponentially at ages 3, 4, and 5.

It is difficult to imagine a more effective language teacher for a 3-year-old than a parent who is home with the child all day, who loves everyday play and interacting with a baby or young child, and who thoroughly understands the importance of integrating auditory strategies throughout the child's day. Much of this book is intended to provide information for professionals in supporting parents who are doing exactly that, throughout the preschool (birth to six) years. However, by the time the child is 3 years old, not every parent can or wants to continue to take on that role. In addition, many parents believe that young children need to be exposed

As a result of incredible advances in technology for children with hearing loss, in addition to early identification of hearing loss through newborn hearing screening programs, the needs of 3-year-old children with hearing loss are very different now from what they were even 8 or 10 years ago. Expectations of the general public and of many school systems have not necessarily kept up with those advances. Today, because of technological and pedagogical advances, there is no limit to what a child with early identified hearing loss can achieve —other than the limits we create by denying them auditory access or by denying them (and their parents) the specialized support that will help the children learn to listen, talk, and achieve. Given appropriate auditory access and appropriate specialized early educational experiences, there is every reason to expect that the children will learn spoken language well enough to achieve on grade level, go to college or other postsecondary education if they so choose, and eventually lead independent productive, tax-paying lives.

This expectation is what drives the field today, beginning with viewing the infant's hearing loss as a neurological emergency, which requires speedy provision of appropriate hearing technology to provide auditory access from as young an age as possible, so that the child's brain loses as little time as possible without auditory and linguistic stimulation. Unfortunately, this expectation is also what can drive parents into conflict with school personnel who are unaware of the new world of opportunities for children with hearing loss, and of what it takes from the school system to permit the child to access those opportunities.

to group activities with their age peers for social-emotional development and/or for "getting ready for school."

Second only to being toilet-trained, probably *the* most important aspect of "getting ready for school" for any child is acquiring as much spoken language ability as possible (Hart & Risley, 2003). The child who is staying home with the parent described above may be in an optimal situation for language-learning. A child with very low language abilities due to hearing loss is likely to learn the most language from adults in his environment who keep the environment relatively quiet, and who take the time to try to help him understand and to help him make himself understood. Even though he may learn other important things from a preschool group experience, the child with low language abilities and hearing loss is unlikely to learn much *language* from his preschool peers as the language level and the pace of teacher talk and instruction is likely to be well above his or her zone of proximal development (Vygotsky, 1978). Of course, he may learn language from the adults in the preschool, particularly if those adults are vigilant in providing auditory access and in interacting in language-promoting ways. However, it should be noted that, even with an excellent teacher-to-child ratio, that ratio cannot compete with a ratio of one parent to a child or two.

So why should preschoolers with hearing loss go to preschool? What children learn from preschool is, above all, how to feel comfortable away from family, how to play and learn in a group, and how to conform to school expectations for group social behavior. Children also may be exposed to readiness skills (colors, shapes, letters, numbers), but they could easily also be exposed to that information at home. However, because children are likely to be taught in groups in kindergarten, there may be a rationale for exposing them to group learning situations before that time.

When should a child with hearing loss go to preschool, and for how much of the child's day? Ultimately, that should be a parental decision. Considerations that could be part of that decision include the parents' ability and desire to be at home with the child for language stimulation, and other practical factors. What is appropriate can range from no preschool experience to full-time 5-days-a-week preschool experience. Whatever decision the parents make, they should remember that even a full-time preschool experience is only for about 25% of the child's waking hours, and they (the parents) remain their child's primary sources of language stimulation and his or her primary advocates for maintaining their child's auditory access to spoken language for the other 75% of the child's waking hours outside of school.

Preschool special educators are often wonderful, dedicated teachers and human beings. They love young children, and they want to help. However, preschool special education classes are almost never appropriate settings for children with hearing loss.

A 3-year-old child with hearing loss, even when his or her language scores suggest normal receptive and expressive language, is at a very vulnerable stage. For typically developing children, the period between 2 to 5 years of age corresponds to Brown's Stages II through V, when the Mean Length of Utterance goes from 2 words per utterance to 5 words per utterance. This is "the most explosive stage of language development," the period in which children move from telegraphic utterances to the mastery of basic sentence structures. (Paul, 2007, p. 318). Normally hearing children make this progress as a result of a combination of their own innate abilities with 20,000 hours of "relentless auditory attention" (English, 2010), to copious spoken language input from the people in their environment—input which is almost entirely auditorily based! Children with hearing loss, even with the most current, appropriate audiological technology, still miss chunks of spoken language input, particularly if they cannot (or have not yet learned to) overhear (listen to language that is not directly addressed to them), and particularly if they are in noisy environments where the noise blocks out (masks) the spoken language around them.

Due to the decreased quantity and quality of access and exposure imposed by the hearing loss, even the most "successful" 3-year-old with hearing loss, still needs more guided experience in two areas:

- *Learning to over-hear, to auditorily scan the environment for spoken language that is not addressed to them, and to learn from it.*
- *Continuing to learn all of the pragmatic, semantic, syntactic, and phonological elements and items that typically developing children are learning during this early time of exponential learning.*

Providing the supports and resources in these early years offers the best chance of reducing the levels of support needed for all of the child's academic learning to come.

As noted above, the reasons are related to the preschool special educators' lack of experience and knowledge of hearing loss, the noise level in a classroom that has children with all kinds of disabilities with attending paraprofessionals, and the ratios of children with disabilities to children without disabilities. Many children in special education classes are children with developmental and/or cognitive delays. The child with hearing loss (who has a cochlear problem, not an intellectual deficit) is likely to "look great"—and the teacher is unlikely to have appropriately high expectations for the child's auditory and linguistic learning. This creates a less than optimal situation for the child with hearing loss, for whom the potential—given an appropriate setting—is unlimited.

Securing an appropriate educational setting for a preschooler with hearing loss is sometimes complicated. Even with the best intentions, some school systems have a tendency to think in terms of placing children in the classes that they have, rather than considering the individual child's needs first, and creating a program that is appropriate for that individual child (as was the intent of the U.S. federal legislation entitled IDEA). Another complication is school districts often do not have a teacher of the deaf and hard of hearing on their staff—or if they do, it is quite likely to be a teacher of the deaf and hard of hearing who does not have background or expertise in helping children with hearing loss learn to listen and talk.

Wherever they live, it is essential for parents to become informed about the rights and responsibilities guaranteed under special education law, as well as to become informed about what services are available in their town and region long before their child will need them. For families in the United States, parent advocacy groups and Web sites exist to assist with that endeavor (e.g., http://www.wrightslaw.com). In 1992, the U. S. Department of Education published a specific guidance on how IDEA is to be interpreted with regard to children with hearing loss (United States Department of Education, 1992). This document can be used to assist decision-makers in educational placement team meetings in focusing attention on the unique needs of the child who has hearing loss.

7

Auditory "Work"

Key Points Presented in the Chapter

- Hearing is the only sense that can perceive acoustic subtleties. Since spoken language is acoustically based, the ear is the most useful and efficient sensory receptor for speech.
- Speech characteristics can be described in terms of the three primary acoustic dimensions: intensity, pitch, and duration.
- Advances in technology such as miniaturization of powerful hearing aids, improvements in fidelity of signal transmission, digital hearing aids, small personal FM receiver boots, classroom sound field amplification, and of course cochlear implants have all contributed to making learning spoken language through listening a strong and viable option for the vast majority of children with hearing loss.
- Early auditory stimulation causes measurable differences in brain organization and neural activity.
- Auditory skills are the components of theoretical models that researchers have developed to explain how language is processed auditorily. The auditory skills overlap and interrelate, and are not necessarily hierarchical.
- In essence, auditory/linguistic learning consists of the child becoming aware of sound, then connecting sound with meaning, and then understanding more and more complex language—first in quiet circumstances, and then in a variety of more difficult listening conditions.

■ Children with hearing loss can learn to listen in ordinary, everyday ways with the adults being vigilant about the viability of the child's amplification, the listening conditions, the distance between speaker and the child's microphone, and the use of auditory strategies.

Introduction

This chapter begins with a rationale for teaching spoken communication auditorily, including specific examples of the acoustic dimensions of speech, and how these acoustic dimensions relate to major aspects of language. The concept of Listening Age is introduced, followed by discussion of auditory development, auditory "skills," and auditory processing models as well as discussion of the importance of the child being able to overhear for his or her development of Theory of Mind and Executive Functions. These sections are then followed by two explicated scenarios. The scenarios illustrate how normal everyday interactions between caregivers and children with hearing loss can be slightly altered or "embellished" to emphasize and make more salient particular acoustic aspects. Consistent use of auditory "embellishments" and auditory strategies by caregivers in varied contexts throughout the child's waking hours is one of the central keys to helping the young child who has hearing loss learn to listen and talk through natural play interactions.

Let us begin with a discussion of the reasons behind using audition as the primary sense modality for helping a baby and child learn spoken language.

The Primacy of Audition

The easiest way to understand the primacy of audition for speech reception is to consider what happens every time you turn on the radio or use the telephone. If you have normal hearing, you are able to understand the speaker based on listening alone, without using

> *Who is doing the "work"? For babies and young children, the auditory "work" is primarily done by the parent, who consciously employs strategies to help the child learn to have confidence in his or her ability to understand based on listening alone. This is in contrast to the situation that starts at about age 3, for children whose auditory abilities may need to be improved through the same all day-everyday adult auditory strategies, but who also benefit from short periods of more adult-directed and planned practice to fill in gaps in the child's knowledge. Having a hearing loss means that the individual misses or hears only partially some auditory events. The parts of spoken language that are missed will need to be brought directly to the child's attention through preplanned activities that will become part of the child's auditory work. In any case, since the responsibility for hearing, listening, and learning will ultimately be the responsibility of the individual with the hearing loss, whatever responsibility for the auditory "work" that the child is able to assume, he or she should.*

any other sense modality. This is because talking, or spoken language, is primarily an acoustic event (Chermak, Bellis, & Musiek, 2007; Erber, 1982; Fry, 1978; Ling, 2002). The other senses (smell, taste, touch, vision) are of very limited use in understanding others' spoken messages. Consider each of the other sense modalities in turn.

- **Smell.** The sense of smell has no use for speech reception.
- **Taste.** The sense of taste has no use for speech reception.
- **Touch.** The sense of touch has some limited use for the reception of individual speech sounds. For example, one can feel the vibration or breathiness of sounds. Specifically, you can feel breathy sounds on your hand, or feel the difference in the temperature of the air for the /s/ vs. /sh/ sounds when produced next to a wet hand, or feel vibrations in the bones of your face when producing nasal sounds. However, those tactile cues cannot be used by themselves to identify the sounds. The tactile sense is useful only for speech reception (or teaching) when the sounds are produced in isolation, not in running speech.

There also are tactile devices that can be worn on the body that can supply gross information about the duration and loudness of spoken language that reaches the microphone. (See Chapter 5 for more information about tactile devices.) But again, the prosodic features in normal conversational speech occur too rapidly and in such complexity that tactile devices cannot adequately capture them in such a way that they can be used by themselves with a child learning a first language. An additional problem with tactile devices is that they respond to nonspeech noise as well as speech, further muddying the signal that the child receives.

■ **Vision.** Vision has limited use for speech reception in that the listener can watch the speaker's lips (lip-rounding, spreading, closure), frontal tongue movements, teeth positioning, larynx movements regarding sounds. If you turn off the sound when you are watching the news, you will see how little information is available from simply watching a person talk. Vision has very little use for speech reception in running speech, but can be useful in discriminating between speech sounds produced in isolation. However, about 70% of sounds in English are sounds that look like other sounds on the lips (i.e., they are homophonous, such as *ba, pa,* and *ma*), so vision is only potentially useful for about 30% of speech. However, when you are already listening, being able to see the speaker's face often does make it easier to understand because the visual cues provide redundancy with the auditory cues, as a kind of underlining.

■ **Hearing.** None of the other senses can provide clear information about the speaker's prosodic features (intensity, pitch/intonation, rhythm/duration) or about specific speech sounds in the way that the ear can. Much of speech perception is based on perception and discrimination of timing-related events in the speech signal. Only the ear has the ability to respond to the speed of the temporal events that occur in speech, and the ability to discriminate fine differences among them.

In that hearing is the sense that can most effectively perceive the subtleties of acoustic events, it seems that the ear was "built" for being able to receive and deal with speech! Clearly, some parts of a spoken message have redundant representation in the visual and tactile modalities that may need to be used by some children with hearing loss as a supplement to audition. But since spoken language is acoustically based, the ear provides the most useful and efficient sense receptors for speech.

The Acoustics-Speech Connection

This section provides explicated examples describing how each of the three primary acoustic dimensions (intensity/loudness, pitch/frequency, and duration) is realized in speech. The section is based on information from Cole (1994), Kent and Read (2001), Ling (1989, 2002), and Pickett (1998).

Intensity/Loudness

- The average intensity of normal conversational speech is used as a general guideline in fitting hearing aids and in mapping cochlear implants, which is not surprising as the goal of wearing primary amplification devices such as hearing aids and cochlear implants is to be able to hear speech. The term *speech banana* was coined by Dr. Daniel Ling as a means of describing the area on the audiogram that includes the essential intensity and frequency characteristics of speech (Figure 7-1). Generally speaking, audiologists try to program hearing aids and cochlear implants so that the child's thresholds fall near the top or just above the speech banana on the audiogram.
- Differences in typical loudness can assist the listener in identifying who the speaker is.
- Loudness differences are used by speakers to express particular emotional states. A very loud voice can often be an angry one, whereas a soft and quiet voice is often used to express affection or soothing.
- Differences in the loudness of particular words in sentences are used to emphasize the important information in the sentence (It's *mine*!), or to mark phrase boundaries or accompany intonational changes to enhance the listener's understanding.

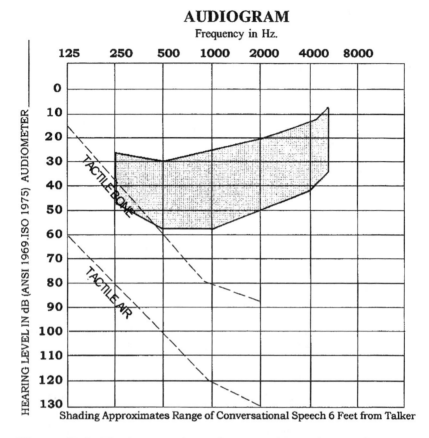

AUDIOGRAM

Figure 7–1. The banana shape drawn on this audiogram illustrates the approximate area (intensity range and frequency range) within which speech would fall if it were drawn on an audiogram.

■ Differences in the loudness of particular syllables occur within words, and using typical syllable stress will assist the listener's comprehension. Syllable stress can also signal differences in meaning such as the meanings intended by *ob*ject versus ob*ject*, or by *pres*ent versus pre*sent*.

Frequency/Pitch

■ The pitch of a speaker's voice varies with the speaker's age and sex, and is a very important characteristic of an individual's speech. Men's voices tend to be the lowest in pitch, children's the highest, and women's in the middle. Most children with hearing loss can easily learn to discriminate pitch differences among male, female, and child voices.

■ Every language has its own intonational melody that goes up and down in pitch. Intonational changes can signal whether the utterance is a question or a statement, the speaker's emotional state, or the end of a thought group. These intonational cues are within acoustic reach of nearly all children with hearing loss, although they may need to be brought to their attention. Emphasizing intonational cues with very young children is a normal part of the way that most adults talk with young children, and is probably one of the cues that babies use to know that they are being spoken to.

■ Each speech sound has particular frequencies associated with its production that listeners automatically use to know immediately that sound has been produced. For example, the words *father* and *feather* are heard as different words because of the acoustic differences between the two initial vowels. The vowel /a/ as in *father* has strong energy produced at about 800 and 1200 Hertz (Hz) (a term used to describe frequencies); and the vowel /ɛ/ as in *feather* has strong energy produced at about 600 and 2200 Hz. Using knowledge of the typical characteristics of speech sounds, it should be possible to predict which speech sounds a child with a particular aided audiogram is likely to be able to learn to detect and produce using hearing alone. A child with no usable hearing at about 2000 Hz could not be expected to imitate the /ɛ/ sound based on listening alone, but he would certainly be able to imitate the /a/ based on listening alone.

Knowledge of the formants of speech sounds can also be used by audiologists in setting hearing aids or mapping cochlear implants, based on the fact that a child talks the way that he or she hears. If a child is not producing an /s/ sound, for example, the audiologist may well believe that the child is not hearing its band of energy that spreads from about 4000 Hz upward, and make adjustments in the child's equipment to provide access to the /s/.

Duration

■ Durational differences are usually one of the first cues that children with hearing loss learn to listen for and produce. For example, if the parent says a long "Mmmmmmmm." sound in connection with eating or taking bites, it will not be long before the child will be repeating or imitating a similarly prolonged sound. If the parent says, "Hop! Hop! Hop!" in short staccato syllables in making a bunny hop, then the child is likely to make a similarly short sound in play with the bunny. Approximating the length of the speech segment in imitation is highly desirable listening and producing behavior! Precision in the young child's speech can come later, but imitating the correct number of syllables is clear evidence that the child is listening carefully, and is an enormously important early listening milestone. This is one of the reasons that adults need to speak to children who have hearing loss using complete phrases and sentences of a length and content consistent with what they would use for any young child. Modeling for the child with a non-normal durational pattern such as "I . . . want . . . juice" is highly inappropriate from an acoustic point of view, not to mention a linguistic one!

■ The overall rate of speaking is another duration-related item. Obviously, very fast speech is difficult for anyone to understand, but what is to be avoided in speech to children with hearing loss is speech that is abnormally slow and consequently *over*articulated. This kind of extraordinary slowing down (as in "I . . . want . . . juice." or in saying the word *bell* very slowly) distorts both the auditory and visual cues to the message. Abnormally slow speech makes the message harder to understand, rather than easier. Because most people do not talk that way, the child runs the risk of being able to understand only when spoken to in that same slow and overarticulated manner. In the old days, it was often possible to spot teachers of the deaf because of their overarticulated speech, mistakenly used to "help" the children.

■ Individual speech sounds have characteristic durational features (as well as the intensity and frequency characteristics mentioned above). Sounds can be short or long in their usual duration, such as a /k/ versus a /ʃ/ at the end of "walk" versus "wash." They can have gradual or sudden onset, such as an /r/ versus a /g/ as in "run" versus "gun," and they can stay relatively stable throughout their production, such as an /s/, or can change throughout their production, such as a /w/. These differences in speech sound durations are only milliseconds of difference, so short that they can only be perceived by hearing, not by any of the other senses.

■ Individual speech sounds can have variations in timing as one of their primary features. For example, the unvoiced and voiced sound pairs such as /p/ and /b/ are differentiated by the presence or absence (respectively) of a 20 millisecond "airy space" (silence) between the production of the consonant and the following vowel. A grossly simplified drawing of the sounds is in Figure 7–2. It is this timing difference between the consonant and vowel that makes these two sounds different. Interestingly, even though this is only a 20 millisecond difference, it is usually fairly easy for children with hearing loss to learn to hear as well as to produce.

In summary, the human ear is the most efficient sense organ for perceiving and analyzing the central aspects of speech, which are acoustic. Information provided by the tactile or visual senses offers only secondary correlates of the speech sounds.

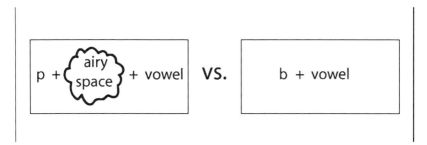

Figure 7–2. This is a theoretical drawing of the difference between the syllables /ba/ and /pa/, which are identical except for the initial voiced or unvoiced bilabial. The unvoiced /p/ is followed by 20 milliseconds of aspiration (the "airy space") before the vowel, whereas that aspiration is absent in the /ba/ syllable.

The Effect of Hearing Loss on the Reception of Speech

The effect of hearing loss is to reduce the amount and quality of acoustic information or speech that is available to the listener. Depending upon its severity, hearing loss will distort, reduce, or eliminate a number of acoustic cues. However, hearing loss is rarely total. At least since the 1960s and 1970s, it has been technologically possible to provide amplification with the potential of permitting the majority of children with hearing loss to learn to use their residual hearing.

With recent advances in cochlear implants, in the power and clarity of digital hearing aids, and in the precision of instrument fitting, the use of audition in the reception of spoken language is within reach of the vast majority of children, even those with profound hearing loss. Naturally, the more hearing the child has, the more acoustic cues are available when amplified. Even with minimal residual hearing (e.g., aided hearing within the speech range at only 250 and 500 Hz), the child can learn to perceive and monitor durational, rhythmic, and intonation cues. The result can be improved understanding by the child, as well as improved intelligibility and predictability in the child's own speech, even when cochlear implants are not used. However, current best practice would dictate that the parents of a child with such minimal residual hearing be encouraged to consider a cochlear implant, which could provide the child with access to all of the acoustic aspects of speech at close to normal intensity levels.

A Historical Look at the Use of Residual Hearing

Markides (1986) has eloquently described the history of the use of residual hearing for educating individuals with hearing loss. The first recorded (and as Markides says, rather drastic) attempts were those of Archigene (98–117 A.D.) who tried to stimulate residual hearing by blowing a trumpet in the deaf person's ear. However, publications concerned with utilization of residual hearing in very young children with hearing loss are a rather more recent phenomenon, beginning with authors such as Fry, 1966; Griffiths, 1964; Horton, 1974; Pollack, 1970; Tervoort, 1964; and Whetnall, 1958. There has long been supportive evidence for the importance of early auditory stimulation in studies of sensory deprivation using animals (Riesen, 1974; Tees, 1967). One of the first attempts to explore systematically the effects of early auditory stimulation for children with hearing loss was that of Griffiths (1955). This study compared the speech of a group of children aided at a mean age of 3 years, 8 months with a group aided at a mean age of 5 years, 3 months. The speech of the earlier-aided children was rated as more normal and more intelligible by four separate panels of judges. Of course even the earlier-aided children in this study would be considered very late-aided by today's standards.

Since Griffiths' study in 1955, a great deal of other research has been done which strongly supports the contention that early auditory stimulation has long-term beneficial effects on speech reception, speech intelligibility, language development, and academic achievement. Recent work includes that by Kirk et al., 2002; Moog, 2002; Moog and Geers, 2003; Nicholas and Geers, 2006; Niparko, 2004; Robbins, Koch, Osberger, Zimmerman-Philips, and Kishon-Rabin, 2004; Sharma, Dorman, et al., 2005.

But studies of the efficacy of particular educational approaches (such an auditory one) with very young human subjects with hearing loss are methodologically difficult to design and implement. One relatively minor problem is that of trying to assemble large enough groups of very young subjects with hearing loss who are similar with regard to relevant variables (e.g., age, degree of hearing loss, age at detection, age when full-time wearing of amplification was begun, degree and nature of parental involvement). Then there is the problem of gaining consensus in an experimental sense regarding exactly what an auditory emphasis or auditory stimulation is. Related to that is the problem of attempting to standardize how the work is implemented and measured in a rigorous, as well as educationally meaningful, manner. All of these problems contribute to the ultimate difficulty of separating the effects of early *auditorily-based* intervention from the effects of early intervention of any kind.

Recent very exciting research by Sharma and colleagues (Sharma et al., 2004; Sharma, Dorman, et al., 2005; Sharma, Martin, et al., 2005) and Nicholas and Geers (2006) all resoundingly supports the contention that early auditory stimulation is essential for normal development of the auditory system at the cortical level. Children who are deprived of sound, due to unidentified hearing loss or to very profound hearing loss that does not respond to traditional amplification, demonstrate clear differences in brain waves. Refer to Chapter 1 for more information.

A number of these studies suggest that if the children begin wearing hearing aids or cochlear implants by 3½ years of age, then their brain waves (specifically, the P1 cortical auditory evoked potential) begin to reflect a normal response to sound within 3 to 6 months of the child having access to sound. In one study (Sharma et al., 2004) of two children who received cochlear implants at 13 months and 14 months of age, the latency of their P1 waves was within normal limits by 3 months post-implant. The two children also demonstrated significant increases in the proportion of more mature vocalizing (reduplicated babbling) by 3 months post-implant.

Although the Sharma et al. (2004) study examined the development of only two children, the results parallel other studies reporting significantly higher speech perception and language skills in children who had access to sound through cochlear implants from a young age (by age 3 or 4 years), compared with those who were deprived of appropriate and consistent access to sound until 6 to 7 years of age (Kirk et al., 2002; Nicholas & Geers, 2006). The evidence clearly supports the concept that auditory stimulation from as young an age as possible provides the easiest route to spoken language development.

The Concept of *Listening Age*

A child with normal hearing generally listens to spoken language for at least 10 to 12 months before he or she starts to produce a few single words, and it is not until another 10 to 12 months later that the child begins combining those words into two-word phrases. A child with hearing loss is likely to need a similar length of time to listen to spoken language before he or she can be expected to use words singly, or in combinations. Whether or not the child can do that, and do it intelligibly (so that others can understand him or her), will depend on whether or not the child's technology provides access to all of the frequencies of speech (particularly the high frequencies), and allows the child to hear soft or quiet speech. It also depends on whether or not the child is wearing the technology all waking hours.

The day that the child begins wearing appropriately selected and fit technology all waking hours is Day Zero for the child's *listening age*. The child who begins full-time wearing of appropriate technology at 3 months of age has lost only 3 months of listening time, and will have a listening age of 9 months at her first birthday. Chances are excellent that this child will make up for those lost 3 months, and have language development that closely parallels her hearing peers at least by the time she is 2 years old, if not before. However, a child with hearing loss who only begins full-time wearing of technology at 2 years of age has lost 2 years of listening time, and will have a listening age of 2 years, when the child's chronological age is 4 years. Closing that two-year gap in listening time and spoken language learning is not impossible, but is much more difficult than closing the three-month gap for the previous child.

This is not a new concept. Pollack (1970) and Northcott (1972) both discussed the concept, calling it the child's *hearing age*, and used it to help parents have an idea of what to expect regarding the child's progress after the child began wearing hearing aids. Calculating the child's listening age can be complicated by periods of time when the child's access to spoken language is compromised by events such as chronic otitis media, behavioral issues, poorly fitting earmolds, equipment malfunction, or progression of the child's hearing loss. Any time the child does not have appropriate access to quiet speech, he or she is not able to listen to spoken language in the manner that is needed for language development. Consequently, that time cannot be counted as part of the child's listening age. Patton, Hackett, and Rodriguez of Sunshine Cottage School for the Deaf (2004) developed a formula for taking a number of those issues into account in an attempt to determine a more accurate listening age.

Whether or not an actual formula is used for calculating the child's listening age, the concept of *listening age* is a good one to use in understanding the crucial impact of a child's auditory access to speech through his technology, and about reasonable expectations to have for the child's spoken language development. Flexer and Madell (2009) identified the following factors that may advance or delay children's auditory function and, consequently, the interpretation of their *listening age*.

■ Age at which hearing technology was acquired
■ The audibility of the speech signal made available by the technology (including high frequencies and soft speech)
■ The amount of time each day that the child actually wears the technology (e.g., 2 hrs/day; 4 hrs/day; 12 hrs/day; all waking hours). (**Reminder: typically hearing persons have auditory access to their brain, 24 hours per day.**)
■ The impact and skill of the family and therapist in providing auditory language enrichment.

The *Listening Age* concept is based on the fact that high-integrity auditory brain access of the speech spectrum is absolutely essential for the child's listening and spoken language development.

Auditory "Skills" and Auditory Processing Models

All of the informed auditory training work done with children with hearing loss to develop auditory skills is based on theoretical models and constructs. We are still far from comprehensive knowledge of the complicated process of human communication, including the exact role of audition in communication.

For example, we really do not have certain knowledge of exactly how humans formulate ideas, encode them in language, perceive and analyze acoustic signals, and process linguistic messages produced by others. However, based on research, empirical data, and reasoning, hypothetical models have been developed that integrate existing pieces of knowledge and thinking. The researcher's intention is that the models' integrity and usefulness will then be experimentally tested and accordingly revised—not that the component units are necessarily ready to be treated as realities upon which to base intervention practice. However, the teacher or therapist cannot wait for scientific knowledge to be complete, and sometimes the practitioner's zeal for certainty embues the theoretical constructs with more reality than they deserve. Perhaps the essential thought to bear in mind is that the auditory processing "whole" is greater than the sum of current knowledge of its hypothesized parts.

Auditory processing models are presented and explained in Bellis (2003), Kuhl (1987), and Musiek and Chermak (2006). Some of the presumed components of commonly agreed-upon stages will be mentioned, and then implications illustrated for children with hearing loss. What follows is, of necessity, overly simplistic in an attempt to describe the exquisitely complex process of listening and understanding.

For an overview of the sequence, let us assume that the child's peripheral ear has received a bit of speech/acoustic information and that the child was *motivated to attend* to it (or to *detect* it). According to the auditory processing models cited above, there is first some sort of frequency, intensity, and time analysis done by the peripheral ear, with transformation of the input into representative neural patterns. Brief sensory memory storage must be occurring at this stage in order for the analysis and transformation to take place.

Next, it is known that some preliminary auditory processing occurs in the brainstem related to *localization,* and separation of competing messages (i.e., selective listening or selective attention). And finally, when the auditory cortex receives the input, higher levels of analysis occur about which we have the least certain knowledge and, consequently, the most theorizing. This processing presumably includes phonetic, phonological, syntactic, semantic, and pragmatic/contextual processing. It may very well require hypothesized cortical activities such as the following: *discriminating* from close cognates, *identifying (categorizing* or *associating)* with other similar items, and *comprehending (integrating* or *interpreting)* as meaning is derived. And clearly, both short-term and long-term *memory and retrieval* are essential to this higher level processing of auditory/linguistic messages.

The preceding discussion has highlighted a number of items that are featured in most texts and curricula as the content or goals of auditory work with children who have hearing loss (e.g., Cole, Carroll, Coyne, Gill, & Paterson, 2005; Erber, 1982; Estabrooks, 2006; Hirsch, 1970; Northcott, 1978; Pollack, 1985; Pollack, Goldberg, & Caleffe-Schenk, 1997; Rossi, 2003; Sindrey, 2002) as well as in online resources such as "The Listening Room" sponsored by Advanced

Bionics (http://www.hearingjourney.com) and Cochlear's HOPE materials and courses (http://www.cochlearamericas.com/Support).

Particularly in view of the additional concurrence of scholarly opinion in including these items in their models, it seems reasonable to assume that each of these components is involved in some manner or at some level in processing spoken language. And it is certainly beneficial (with a particular child, or at given points in time, or as part of a specific game or activity) to focus on one auditory dimension alone. *But these auditory components overlap and interrelate in both natural and structured activities to such a degree that they cannot seriously be considered to be discrete or necessarily hierarchical* (Bellis, 2003; Ling, 1986). Curricula that attempt to train these as isolated auditory skills may play a useful role for the teacher of older children because the curricula systematize instructional objectives and activities related to improving the child's use of residual hearing. But isolated rote training on hypothetical auditory subskills is generally inappropriate—and unnecessary for children with hearing loss under 3 years of age. With young children, the auditory subskill will be in the adult's mind, but in most cases, the child will be interacting, playing, or solving a problem (in a way that just happens to require that auditory subskill).

For the young child, the ability to demonstrate capability concerning any of the highlighted auditory components is inextricably linked to the child's cognitive and spoken language growth. That is, for the toddler to be motivated to attend selectively; to localize; to discriminate; to identify, categorize, associate; to integrate, interpret, comprehend—for all of these, there must be meaning attached to the event. And, to paraphrase Winnie-the-Pooh (Milne, 1926), the main place that meaning in acoustic input comes from is from Gradual Acquisition of Spoken Language. And the main place spoken language comes from is from Normal, Everyday Interacting and Play with Caregivers Using Spoken Language.

Informality does not mean that there is a lack of planning and structure in the intervention and interacting processes. For example, simply being aware of the importance of consistently noticing relevant sounds or remarking on the child's noticing them could be viewed as introducing a "structured" or contrived element into a conversational interaction between caregiver and child. Certainly, parents of normally hearing children also notice sounds and notice their children's reactions to them. But parents of children who have hearing loss become especially conscious of the importance of these particular events for encouraging the child's use of his or her residual hearing, and consequently they attempt to do both kinds of noticing consistently, and perhaps with a bit more deliberate interest and enthusiasm.

Theory of Mind and Executive Functions

Special note needs to be made of the importance of being able to overhear the conversation of others. This ability requires appropriate settings on audiologic equipment so that the child has access to listening to quiet speech at a distance, and may not be technologically possible for every child. Overhearing also requires motivation and practice in having one's attention primarily focused in one direction or on an activity, but still being aware of quiet conversation going on in the vicinity, without being directly addressed. Overhearing is essential for natural learning of particular grammatical items, such as first and second person pronouns (e.g., I, me, you) and deictic terms (e.g., here, there). As we know, a child's language development depends on exposure to both direct and overheard spoken conversations and on development of the auditory centers of the brain. However, overhearing has crucial importance for stimulating development of the higher level social and cognitive abilities and knowledge that comprise Executive Functions and Theory of Mind, both of which are essential for becoming a competent and socially appropriate member of society.

A *"Theory of Mind"* (often abbreviated in ToM) is a specific cognitive ability that enables the understanding of others as independent, intentional agents; essentially, it means understanding that other people have minds that can be perceiving and thinking in ways that are totally different from one's own mind. It means that one is able to maintain, simultaneously, different representations of the world, and know that there are many ways of looking at things. An example of a child who has acquired Theory of Mind would be a child who, looking at the 12 inches of snow that fell during the night would know that he and his teenage sister would be happy about it (because of making a snowman and going skiing), but that his parents might be unhappy about it because they would have to shovel the driveway and drive in slow traffic because of it. This child would know that others could have different feelings, perceptions, or beliefs about the same event. Not surprisingly, the development of ToM is dependent on one's language abilities, and one's ability to overhear conversations that are not necessarily directly experienced.

ToM seems to be an innate cognitive potential in humans, one that requires social/linguistic experiences over many years for full development. With social experience and conversations, both direct and overheard, a child learns to gauge others' beliefs, desires, perspectives, and intentions, and then to predict their behavior (Moeller, 2007).

Having a ToM is critical for understanding many aspects of human social life such as surprises, secrets, tricks, mistakes, and lies. As children age and achieve more social and language skills, ToM forms the basis for inference, perspective taking, social reasoning, and empathy. Having a ToM is critical for academic development, especially in collaborative educational and work environments where listening to and understanding other points of view and engaging in joint mental activity is not only essential to the process of working together, but actually is the basis of the creative problem-solving process. "Language provides us with a means for *thinking together,* for jointly creating knowledge and understanding" (Mercer, 2000, p. 15).

A working ToM does not develop before the age of 4 years. By that age, a child should be able to distinguish between what is so and what people believe is so. One of the most important milestones in ToM development is gaining the ability to attribute *false belief;* that is, to recognize that others can have beliefs about the world that are wrong (Sabbagh & Moses, 2006).

The language skills in children with hearing loss are directly related to their ToM skills. The child needs to be at a fairly complex syntactic level. For example, the child could demonstrate ToM knowledge through being able to combine two clauses (ideas) in one sentence using coordinating or subordinating conjunctions (e.g., I am happy about the snow, and/but Mommy is sad about the snow); or through using "that" to combine clauses (e.g., She believes that snow is a big bother.) ; or both (e.g., I know that the cake is in the cupboard, but he thinks that the cake is still in the refrigerator). Theory of Mind also requires rather specific vocabulary skills, such as knowing words for describing internal processes like thinking,

> *Siblings in the home facilitate the development of ToM because there tend to be discussions of mental and emotional states that lead to differences in behaviors. Those discussions must be made available acoustically (through technology) to be overheard by the child with hearing loss, and the child needs to communicate in the same language as others in his or her environment. Therefore, wearing hearing aids and/or cochlear implants at home, and also using remote microphones (FM and Bluetooth technologies) in home environments are critical for the development and maturation of social/emotional skills.*

feeling, imagining, knowing, and believing. That is, if a child can understand and also produce sentences such as, "He *thought* his cake was in the refrigerator," he is more likely to understand and predict behavior that stems from a false belief.

The child learns these linguistic structures and the vocabulary to describe mental activities (thoughts and feelings) after multiple exposures in varied contexts, just as he or she learns any language. Overhearing "self-talk" (of parents, or others in the environment) such as, "where are those car keys," or "I forgot the doctor's name," also contribute to the child understanding that others have a state of mind that is different from their own.

One important way that children gain an understanding of others' thoughts is by attending to the back and forth viewpoint exchange of family members. Therefore, the child must be able to track multitalker conversations, a skill that demands the maximum possible auditory access to speech at a distance, and in the same language as other talkers in the environment.

Executive Functions are a collection of processes that are responsible for guiding, directing, and managing cognitive, emotional, and behavioral functions, especially for novel problem solving (Sabbagh & Moses, 2006). The primary behaviors that comprise this collection of regulatory and management functions include the ability to initiate behavior while inhibiting competing actions, choosing relevant tasks and goals, planning and organizing problem-solving strategies, shifting attention, behaving flexibly, and monitoring and evaluating behavior (Meltzer, 2007). A very important feature for preschoolers is the inhibition of ineffective behaviors.

> *Even for normally hearing children, noise in the environment disrupts the child's ability to access Executive Functions because their auditory focus is fragmented. The detrimental effects of noise on the speech perception of a child with hearing loss are known to be even greater than for a child with normal hearing. Thus, the consequences of noise for the child's cognitive development (including Theory of Mind and Executive Functions) can be even more detrimental. Acoustic management of the classroom and use of personal FM technologies are a crucial necessity.*

Many executive functions continue to mature well into the third decade of life, a process that parallels the prolonged neurodevelopmental growth of the prefrontal regions of the brain.

According to Schneider et al. (2005, p. 2), "An interesting question is whether executive functions represent a precursor of ToM, or whether ToM understanding predicts the development of executive functions. It is reasonable to assume that individual differences in vocabulary and verbal understanding are particularly important for predicting performance on executive functioning and ToM tasks in samples of young children (e.g., 3-4 years old). For older children, individual differences in working memory and executive functioning, rather than verbal abilities, may be better predictors of ToM performance." In any case, though, it seems clear that in the early years, developing a Theory of Mind and developing rudimentary executive functions both depend on the child's language development, which in turn depends on the child's auditory access.

How to Help a Child Learn to Listen in Ordinary, Everyday Ways

In essence, auditory/linguistic learning consists of the child becoming aware of sound, then connecting sound with meaning, and then understanding more and more complex language—first in quiet circumstances, and then in a variety of more difficult listening conditions. Each of the parts of this process will be fully discussed in

Chapter 10. However, there are several steps that need to be taken in order to provide a facilitative auditory environment for the child to learn to listen and talk (Figure 7–3).

Step 1. The most important step that parents can do to help the process along is to be sure that the child is wearing appropriate, well-maintained amplification [hearing aids and/or cochlear implant(s)] all waking hours. The importance of keeping the hearing aids or cochlear implant on the child all waking hours cannot be overemphasized. The child's access to appropriate, consistent sound is, quite simply, fundamental to learning to listen and talk.

Accessing sound means that the child must be wearing the equipment, and it must be functioning well. With young children, it is the parents' responsibility to learn what they need to know to be sure that the child's technology is functioning in topnotch condition every day through daily listening checks, troubleshooting, having back-up accessories on hand, and keeping the audiologist's phone number on speed dial!

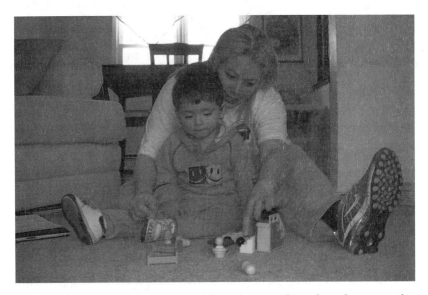

Figure 7–3. This mom is speaking close to the microphone on the child's hearing aid while his visual attention is focused on the toys in front of them. Through her actions in this ordinary play situation, the mother is providing an environment which is highly facilitative of auditory and linguistic growth.

Step 2. The next step that parents can take is to be very conscious of the listening conditions around the child in all communication situations. These conditions include the amount of background noise in the environment, and how far away the child is from the person speaking.

Background noise includes any noise that could interfere with the child's being able to hear a person speaking to him or her, or being able to hear him- or herself vocalizing or talking. Background noise includes TV, radio, cars or trucks going by outside, fan noise, or other people talking—any of those absolutely normal noises can mask over a message that the child was supposed to hear. Unfortunately, noise is amplified and processed by the hearing aid or cochlear implant right along with the speech signal. Current digital hearing aids and speech processors do attempt to pull the speech signal out of the surrounding nonspeech noise, but are far from perfect. It is important to note that the auditory centers of the brain are being stimulated 24 hours of the day for children with normal hearing. For children with hearing loss, it is essential that we optimize the daily 14 hours or so that the child is awake and alert because it is valuable listening and learning time. Background noise needs to be absent or minimal to provide the child with the best chance to hear, and/or an FM system should be used to improve the signal-to-noise ratio (see Chapter 5).

Step 3. The other part of the listening environment that needs to be managed is the distance between the speaker and the child's microphone. Amplification is usually set so that the child can easily hear about two yards from a speaker. However, the best distance between the speaker and the microphone for a child wearing hearing aids is still within about six to eight inches, and for a child with a cochlear implant, about three feet.

Luckily, when they are intentionally interacting, adults are usually talking with babies and young children from very close by. Once the child is mobile, parents need to make sure that they move close to the child and get down on the child's level so that the child has optimal access to the sound of what the parent is saying. Speaking louder will not solve the problem, because although the speech may be louder, it will not be clearer.

FM technology (discussed in Chapter 5) can help overcome the negative effects of noise and distance by making the speaker's

All of this discussion has centered on creating optimal conditions for intentional interacting and communication. As just discussed in the Theory of Mind and Executive Function section, it also is important that the child is provided with the opportunity to learn from overhearing the conversations of others. That is, the child needs to be able to learn from conversations between other people, which are not intentionally directed toward him or her. This may require adjustments on the child's hearing aids or cochlear implants to provide the ability to hear quiet speech at a distance.

voice louder than the surrounding noise. FM can be used in the home, outside on the playground, or in the classroom. Personal-worn FM systems work like a small radio station where the speaker wears a microphone and transmitter that sends the signal directly into the receiver attached to the child's hearing aids or cochlear implant.

Step 4. And lastly, here are some strategies that parents can adopt to promote the child's listening abilities in the course of any communicative interaction:

- Hold the child on your lap facing away from you, or sit beside him or her, with the child's attention directed toward toys or activities that you are both engaged in playing with. Talk close to the child's microphone, without the child constantly looking at you.
- Expect the child to understand without watching your face. If the hearing aids or cochlear implants are properly set, the child will definitely be able to hear you. What the child needs is experience listening in the course of repeated, routine events and play with toys or activities that are of interest.
- If the child doesn't seem to understand an auditory-only message, try saying it again, closer to the child's microphone. If the child still doesn't understand, then help him or her to understand by watching or demonstrating, and then say it again, auditory-only. The idea is to help the child build up confidence in his or her ability to understand auditory-only messages.

Two Examples of Auditory Teaching and Learning

What follows are two scenes that illustrate how to create a good listening environment by utilizing auditory strategies. The scenes are each followed by explanations.

Scene I: Tony

The Context

A father and his 14-month-old son are building with blocks on the floor in the living room after supper. The child has a severe to profound sensorineural hearing loss, and has been wearing hearing aids consistently for 2 months. The mother has been in another room, but at the beginning of this scene appears in the doorway which is about 10 feet away from the child. The child is playing beside his father, with his back to the doorway where the mother is now standing.

The Action (which takes about 15 seconds)

Mother waits for a break in the conversation between father and son, and then calls, "Tony!"

The father ceases block-building, leans toward Tony, puts his head to one side as his face takes on an interested, curious sort of "listening" expression. He says, "Listen! Did you hear that? I heard something" (Figure 7-4). Tony has been looking at the father's face from the time the father stopped playing with the blocks and leaned forward. When his father continues to maintain the "listening" expression without saying or doing more, Tony looks back at the blocks and picks up one to start playing again.

The mother pauses a second or two, and then calls again, "Tony!'

Tony looks up, alertly, at the father.

The father says nothing, but still looks as if he is listening to something.

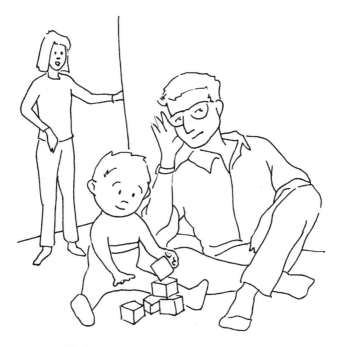

Figure 7–4.

His mother takes a step forward, and calls once more, "Tony! Time for your bath!"

This time Tony turns around and sees his mother She smiles and says, "Terrific! You heard me. It's time for your bath."

Tony smiles impishly, and toddles off, full speed, in the opposite direction.

The Explanation

Mother waits for a break in the conversation between father and son, and then calls, "Tony!"

The mother's voice is loud enough to be well within this particular child's range of hearing, so that it is reasonable for the child to *detect* it. Since the mother is 10 feet away, which is much further than a normal conversational distance, this could be viewed as an instance of a *distance listening* event. She has waited for a break in their conversation, partly because it is conversationally appropriate to do so, and partly because Tony stands a better chance of hearing her if her calling voice occurs in quiet. This is an effort to enhance the *figure* (signal) relative to the *ground* (noise). Some children, perhaps at a more advanced stage, may be expected to hear a calling voice in this sort of situation even when there is other talking going on. In fact, in any normal, everyday situation in the home, there is quite likely to be other noise in the room (e.g., from the toys at hand, from the street outside, from the dishwasher, from an older sibling turning pages in a book) which will be reaching the microphone of the child's hearing aid and being amplified. The signal, for example, the calling voice, must be louder than the surrounding noise in order for the child to detect it. The degree to which it is louder will be the degree to which it is easier for the child to hear. This simple fact is often easily forgotten in the course of normal activities where, for example, the radio or TV may be left on for long periods of time. In a sense, nearly all normal everyday listening involves *selective attention* or *selective listening* abilities.

The father ceases block-building, leans toward Tony, puts his head to one side as his face takes on an interested, curious sort of "listening" expression. He says, "Listen! Did you hear that? I heard something." Tony has been looking at the father's face from the time the father stopped playing with the blocks and leaned forward. When his father continues to maintain the "listening" expression without saying or doing more, Tony looks back at the blocks and picks up one to start playing again.

The father's behaviors are an attempt to *alert* Tony and *motivate* him to *attend*. Depending upon the degree of the child's hearing loss, his absorption in a task, and his or her backlog of positive experiences listening, he or she may respond immediately to a calling voice from 10 feet away. Others will need to be alerted to listen. As for the "listening" expression, it is impossible to actually present an appearance of listening that is unmistakable as listening. That is, one person cannot see another person hearing or listening. But it is possible to see the listener's reaction to sound, interest, or curiosity about it, which is what the father is demonstrating here.

The mother pauses a second, and then calls again, "Tony!"

In this particular instance, a certain number of repetitions of the mother's calling seems reasonable. However, the real goal is clearly for the child to respond after only one instance of the mother calling. If parents and professionals always quickly give the child multiple repetitions of messages or task demands, the child may come to expect that a second or third repetition is coming, and may not bother to respond initially. One simpleminded but vitally important strategy which may lead toward the child's responding after being called once (or after being asked to perform any kind of task, for that matter) is the one of being certain to provide ample time for the child to respond before calling again. (Of course, this is also important from a conversational, turn-taking perspective.) It is equally important to recognize that there are times when the child is not going to respond, and to stop repeating oneself long before it becomes a pointlessly frustrating exercise. Before that, however, there are several steps described below that one can take when it is necessary to enhance the audibility of the acoustic signal.

Tony looks up, alertly, at the father.

The father says nothing, but still looks as if he is listening to something.

This suggests that Tony *detected* a voice from the surrounding background noise *(selective attention),* but has incorrectly (but not surprisingly) assumed it was his father speaking to him. He has thus *localized* the sound incorrectly in that he thought it came from in front rather than in back of him. He is also not attending sufficiently to the higher fundamental frequency and harmonic cues which, one day, will tell him that it was his mother speaking and not his father. This could be viewed as a *discrimination* task, with the child being required to discriminate between his mother's and his father's voices. In situations where a large number of people could ostensibly be calling the child, the task may be more one of *identification.*

His mother takes a step forward, and calls once more, "Tony! Time for your bath."

This time, Tony turns around and sees his mother. She smiles and says, "Terrific! You heard me. It's time for your bath."

Tony smiles impishly, and toddles off, full speed, in the opposite direction.

The mother's behaviors are intended to make her acoustic input more salient (more easily *detected)* to the child. By stepping forward, she has somewhat decreased the distance from the sound source (her mouth) to the microphone on the child's hearing aid. This will make the sound a bit louder. By also adding the sentence, "Time for your bath!" she has provided a longer piece of acoustic input.

The child may not be able to *understand* this bit of information auditorally, but the mother's primary purpose here is simply to provide a lengthier clue to the child to help in his *localizing* (the source of the calling voice) and *associating* (that voice = mother) tasks. Naturally, it is important that she has used a contextually and prosodically appropriate, semantically meaningful, and syntactically correct sentence. These aspects of her input will eventually lead to Tony's *understanding.* And by doing all of these things in all of the hundreds of small events that occur in a day, the mother is building up Tony's belief that he is *expected* to understand spoken messages, with or (often) without looking at the speaker's face. In addition, Tony's mother has rewarded his turning by smiling and by using words which describe exactly what it was that he did that was pleasing. These parent responses are intended to be part of motivating Tony to want to listen the next time(s).

One interpretation of Tony's behavior in this scene could be that Tony soon detected the sound, localized it to a source behind him, identified the mother as the speaker, and comprehended the verbal message. Another interpretation could be that Tony detected the voice, saw that it was not his father speaking, began searching visually for the sound source, and happened to find his mother in the process. Then he saw the pajamas in her hand, and knowing what that meant, toddled off. In a research study, it might be important to try to determine which of these interpretations is correct. But in a real life situation, it doesn't much matter. The parents are not testing his ability to perform listening tasks. In this normal, everyday event, they are providing all the conditions which are likely to encourage and promote Tony's use of residual hearing. These include the provision of appropriate "input" in terms of the prosody, intensity, syntax, semantics, and conversational context. The conditions also include provision of motivation and social or circumstantial "rewards." If, this time, Tony saw his mother in the course of visual searching for "a voice—not father's," then this experience will simply be part of the learning process. If he did actually localize the source and identify the speaker auditorily, then this experience is an example of his having learned. Either way, at every future opportunity, the parents will continue to make the same effort to "set up" events in such a way as to allow, encourage, and expect Tony to listen.

Scene II: Tamara

This next scene is an example of a normal, everyday interactive event between a mother and her slightly older child. The mother smoothly and automatically employs a number of strategies to encourage the child to listen.

The Context

This child is 23 months of age, has a severe to profound sensorineural hearing loss, and has worn hearing aids consistently since 11 months of age. Consequently, she has a "listening age" of 12 months. The mother and child are playing on the kitchen floor with blocks, cars, and little people dolls. They have just built a very tall tower with the blocks. (The event took about 30 seconds in all.)

The Action

Tamara says, "Where block?" as she looks around for another block on the floor. She is standing as the tower they are building is so tall.

Guessing what Tamara meant, the mother says, "Where's another block?" Tamara is not watching the mother's face since she is still searching for blocks.

Tamara says, "'Nother block?"

Mother says, "Hmmm-well, let's see." Mother looks for more blocks; Tamara turns away. "Oh—here's one." Tamara turns back, and the mother hands her a block.

The mother then says, "Thank you."

Tamara says, "What?" and looks at her mother.

The mother rubs her nose, partially obscuring her mouth, and says, "You can say 'Thank you.'"

Tamara again says, "What?"

This time the mother lets Tamara look at her face as she says, "You're supposed to say 'Thank you.'"

Tamara repeats, "Thank you."

Tamara puts the block on the top of the teetering tower, which then topples. She steps back (right on the mother's finger), and says, "Uh oh!" looking at the blocks that fell.

The mother says, "Ouch! My finger!" (Figure 7–5)

Tamara looks at her mother who is shaking her finger.

The mother says, "You stepped on my finger! You gave Mommy a boo-boo."

Tamara looks stricken, and softly says, "Boo-boo" looking at the finger.

The mother says, "What are we going to do about it?" Tamara says, "Kiss boo-boo," and she does.

The mother hugs Tamara, and says "Oh thank you. It's all better now."

Tamara repeats, "All better now."

The Explanation

Tamara says, "Where block?" as she looks around for another block on the floor. She is standing since the tower they are building is so tall.

Guessing what Tamara meant, the mother says, "Where's another block?" Tamara is not watching the mother's face since she is still searching for blocks. Tamara says, "'Nother block?"

The mother is expanding Tamara's utterance in her question as she attempts to clarify her meaning and confirm her guess at what Tamara meant. This type of adult response/question is an especially important one to use in connection with expecting that the child will understand without having to look at the speaker's face. The child is likely to be motivated to attend to the mother's utterance since the mother is not introducing new concepts or topics. Instead she is using the child's topic, showing her interest in clarifying her

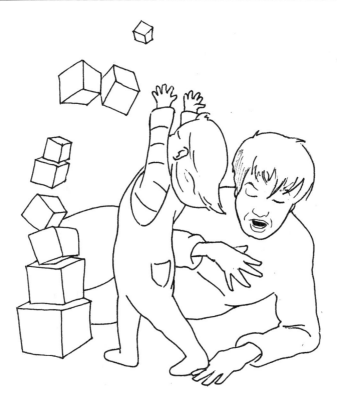

Figure 7–5. "Ouch! My finger!" says the mom as Tamara steps back onto it, oblivious in her glee about the tower toppling.

meaning, and adding only a small amount of relevant information to her original utterance. Clarification questions and expansions are strategies parents use that are likely to promote the child's language growth. They are also likely to promote the child's listening. In this instance, Tamara was not looking at the mother's face when the mother spoke. The fact that she then imitated the mother's question, employing the mother's word "another," suggests that Tamara did get the mother's message through listening alone.

Mother says, "Hmmm—well, let's see." Mother looks for more blocks; Tamara turns away. "Oh—here's one." Tamara turns back, and the mother hands her a block.

The mother actually contrived this listening opportunity. That is, she waited until Tamara had turned away to say, "Oh—here's one."

The mother then says, "Thank you."

Tamara says, "What?" and looks at her mother.

Here, Tamara detected the voice, but did not understand what was said.

The mother rubs her nose, partially obscuring her mouth, and says, "You can say 'Thank you.'"

Tamara again says, "What?"

This time the mother lets Tamara look at her face as she says, "You're supposed to say 'Thank you.'" Tamara repeats, "Thank you."

Tamara puts the block on the top of the teetering tower, which then topples. She steps back (right on the mother's finger), and says, "Uh oh!" looking at the blocks that fell.

In instances where it is desirable to insist on auditory-only input, and the child is looking directly at the adult, there are a number of strategies one can employ. The most obvious is for the speaker to cover his or her own mouth or to otherwise obscure the child's visual access to the mouth. Less obvious is directing the child's visual attention away from the face. Here the mother could have gestured to the block and said, "Look, Mommy gave you a block." When the child's gaze went to the block, she would then say, "You're supposed to say 'Thank you.'" In many instances, it is possible to simply sit behind or beside the child in such a way as to discourage the child from constantly watching the face. After two attempts to give the message auditorally only, the mother let Tamara look at her face as she spoke. There is controversy regarding how long one should "stay auditory," but in everyday situations, the most reasonable course may be to stay auditory as long as it is possible without destroying the conversational flow or unduly frustrating either adult or child.

The mother says, "Ouch! My finger!"

Tamara looks at her mother who is shaking her finger. The mother says, "You stepped on my finger! You gave Mommy a boo-boo."

Tamara looks stricken, and softly says, "Boo-boo," looking at the finger.

The mother says, "What are we going to do about it?"

Tamara says, "Kiss boo-boo," and she does.

The mother hugs Tamara, and says, "Oh thank you. It's all better now."

Tamara repeats, "All better now."

Tamara turned to the mother's loud "Ouch!" The mother shook her finger because it hurt, but that also meant Tamara looked at the finger while the mother said, "You gave Mommy a boo-boo." Thus Tamara's repeating of "boo-boo" is likely to be based on her having actually heard what her mother said. In hugging Tamara, the mother deprived her of visual access to her face. Tamara's imitation of "All better now" confirms that she heard and listened to her mother's utterance.

In a normal, everyday event such as the second one illustrated here, a general *motivation to listen* is assumed to have been established already, although every instance of listening and understanding is likely to build upon that motivation. *Selective attention* is operating because the child is listening in a normally noisy environment (block play); *localizing* is not much of an issue at the moment since the mother is the only other speaker. Each instance of the child's having understood when she was given access only to the auditory part of the message (through the techniques described above) is an instance of the child using her abilities to *discriminate, identify (categorize, associate),* as well as *integrate (interpret, comprehend).* This example will have been successful if it also illustrates why and how these higher level processes are all "of a piece" in real-life instances, as well as why and how they are inseparable from the child's overall cognitive and linguistic development and abilities.

Targets for Auditory/Linguistic Learning

Targets for Auditory/Linguistic Learning can be found in Appendix 3. The Targets are divided into four phases of auditory development:

Phase I: Being Aware of Sound

Phase II: Connecting Sound with Meaning

Phase III: Understanding Simple Language through Listening

Phase IV: Understanding Complex Language through Listening

Across the phases, the individual targets indicate abilities that the child demonstrates as he or she becomes aware of sound, then connects various sounds with meaning, and then gradually acquires the ability to understand more and more complex language. The chart can be used to understand the general progression of auditory/linguistic learning demonstrated by the child who is learning spoken language through listening. It also can be used as a record-keeping device, with dates noted for the child's increasing abilities as described in Appendix 3, and could be used as the basis for developing instructional objectives related to specific abilities.

The four phases represent sequential milestones in the spoken language development of the child who has hearing loss and is being taught spoken language through listening. However, individual items within each phase are not necessarily sequential, although some are logically so. This is not intended to be used as a rigid curriculum! Sometimes activities and abilities at higher levels are appropriate to try, even though the child may not have completed all of the targets at a lower level. In addition, an appropriate game or activity could easily tap multiple auditory/linguistic targets simultaneously.

Examples or indicators have been included as to clarify what is intended by particular targets, but the intention is that parents and interventionists will take advantage of all kinds of normal everyday events and routines where these targets will be easy to "fall over" in ordinary ways. When there is a need for more adult direction and focused structuring of preplanned activities, then the parent's or aural habilitationist's creativity will need to be used to develop activities that provide sufficient practice, while remaining playful.

A Last Word

The structure and knowledge of the importance of the child's ability to demonstrate the auditory abilities need to be more in the mind of the teacher or parent and generally not particularly obvious in the activities occurring with the child (Cole et al., 2005; Estabrooks,

2006). Pollack (1985) said that the child's auditory abilities develop "because emphasis is placed on listening throughout [all the child's] waking hours so that hearing becomes an integral part of [his or her] personality" (p. 159). Similarly, Ling (1986) said that "learning to listen occurs only when children seek to extract meaning from the acoustic events surrounding them all day and every day" (p. 24). At the same time, as mentioned above, for certain children with hearing loss, some structured practice on component parts may be useful as a supplement to the emphasis on audition in normal, everyday activities. With very young children this structured work will normally be done through games which, from the child's point of view, are meaningful and enjoyable. Excellent activities of this sort are detailed in a number of sources that the reader is strongly encouraged to consult, including both print materials (Estabrooks, 2006; Rossi, 2003; Sindrey, 2002) and online resources such as The Listening Room (http://www.hearingjourney.com) and the HOPE materials and courses (http://www.cochlearamericas.com/support). With regard to these more structured activities, however, it is important to close the chapter by reiterating two themes:

1. The skills and abilities being worked upon are theoretical constructs; consequently, the specific exercises may be somewhat arbitrarily derived; and,
2. Whenever the child learns to perform any task in a structured activity or game, the task must then be integrated into real-life situations in order to be functional for him or her. That is, provision must be made for allowing, encouraging, and expecting the child to demonstrate the same ability in the course of normal everyday events and activities. Clearly, the more similar to everyday life that an adult-planned activity is, the greater the likelihood that the child will automatically carry over what has been taught to everyday life events.

Spoken Language Learning

Key Points Presented in the Chapter

■ Communicative competence includes knowledge of pragmatics, semantics, syntax, morphology, and phonology.

■ By the age of 3, most typically developing children have basic communicative competencies in all areas; by the age of 6, sophisticated communicative competencies are well established.

■ There are a number of theories regarding how language develops, although we still don't know precisely what causes a child to move from one developmental stage to the next.

■ If appropriate auditory and linguistic experience is provided to most children who are deaf or hard of hearing from an early age, then cognitive and linguistic functioning can be expected to follow the normal course of development.

Introduction

Since this book is so centrally concerned with spoken language learning by infants and young children, it is appropriate to engage in a discussion of all that is involved in communicating verbally, and of how much of that learning is accomplished at a very young age. Theories about how children learn to talk are also addressed in this chapter, and are followed by consideration of the relevance of the nature/nurture controversy for intervention. The final section in this chapter concerns an overall perspective of spoken language intervention for children with hearing loss based on current informed views of the effects of hearing loss on psychological and cognitive processing.

What's Involved in "Talking"?

Above all else, language is a social tool. It is a shared code that lets people send and receive messages. That is its purpose. Hymes (1972) was the first to use the term "communicative competence" in talking about people effectively and appropriately exchanging messages. He describes communicative competence as the speaker's knowing not only what to say, but also how to say it, when to say it, where to say it, and to whom to say it. Knowledge of the interpersonal, cultural, and linguistic conventions that govern appropriate use of language is what is known as the area of pragmatics. In order to use language appropriately, the child eventually acquires three interwoven domains of communicative knowledge.

One of these levels of pragmatic knowledge is presuppositional knowledge. Presuppositional knowledge involves the speaker's automatic guesses about the general format or register that is appropriate, as well as the level of detail and explicitness that is needed for expressing oneself in a particular social context. For example, the decision that a bilingual individual makes about which language to use with a person who is new to him or her would be governed by presuppositional knowledge. In addition, the child must learn that it is important to attend to and interpret particular features of the listener (e.g., age, sex, social and educational status) and the setting, in order to determine the degrees of informativeness and politeness that are appropriate to a particular situation. This information contributes to the types of sentence structures used, the directness or indirectness of reference, and a host of other grammatical choices such as how much to use pronouns, subordinate clauses, and adjective embeddings.

Presuppositional knowledge influences decisions regarding the level of explicitness taken in a second pragmatic domain: the functions or intentions expressed by each utterance. As was said at the beginning of this section, the purpose of language is to send messages back and forth between two (or more) people. The speaker sends the message with the intention of expressing something. A newborn baby attends to and responds to stimuli, but probably does not communicate with intentionality for some time. By about 8 to 12 months of age, the baby does intentionally gesture and vocalize to demand, ask, label things, notice, and protest. By age 3, that number of functions has expanded at least 10-fold to include expression of even such subtle intentions as suggestions and hints (Dore, 1986).

The third of these interrelated domains of communicative knowledge concerns the conventions regarding the social organization of discourse—or the mostly unspoken rules for maintaining a dialogue with another person. These include conventional turn-taking, topic initiation and maintenance, and repair procedures to follow when there is a breakdown in the communication. All of these conventions need to be acquired by the child learning language.

In addition to pragmatics, other rule systems involved in learning to talk are the semantic, syntactic, morphologic, and phonologic systems. Semantics refers to knowledge of networks or hierarchies of meaning for individual vocabulary words (i.e., lexicon), as well as knowledge of meaning relationships of words in sentences (i.e., case grammar). The syntactic rule system is concerned with the permissible ways of ordering words within sentences in order to express particular meanings, and with ways of transforming basic sentences into more complex structures. Morphologic rules are concerned with the permissible combinations of free morphemes with affixes (such as *un* in *unhappy* or *ness* in *happiness*), and with inflectional morphemes which indicate grammatical features such as tense (The dog walk*ed*.), person (The dog walk*s*.), or number (The dog*s* walk.). The phonological system includes all of the sounds in the language, the permissible ways of combining those sounds into words, and the conventional ways in which the language uses prosodic features such as intonation, stress, and rhythm to express meaning. Rules for semantic, syntactic/morphological, and phonologic usage are all influenced by the pragmatic conditions of the communicative event, such as the speaker's guess about how explicit, detailed, or complex it is appropriate to be for a particular listener (Figure 8–1).

Clearly, the learning of all the conventions for the pragmatics, semantics, syntax, morphology, and phonology of a language is no small task. The wonder is that by the age of 3, most normally developing children have sophisticated knowledge in all of those areas It also is a fact that, given early and appropriate auditory and linguis-

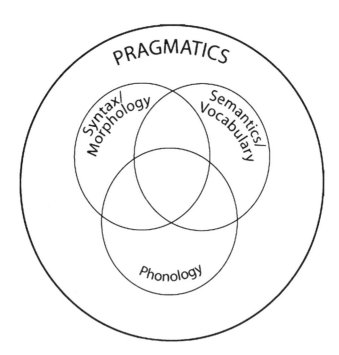

Figure 8–1. By the age of 3 years, typically developing children have a solid foundation in all of the interrelated areas of language.

tic experience, the language development of many children with hearing loss can be remarkably similar to that of their age peers (e.g., Geers & Moog, 1989; Geers, Moog, Biedenstein, Brenner, & Hayes, 2009; Hayes, Geers, Treiman, & Moog, 2009; Nicholas & Geers, 2006; Nittrouer & Burton, 2001; Nott, Cowan, Brown, & Wiggelsworth, 2009; Sininger, Grimes, & Christensen, 2010; Yoshinaga-Itano, Sedey, Coulter, & Mehl, 1998).

How Does a Child Learn to Talk?

The fact is that despite many theories and a great deal of research, we still do not really know just how and/or why language develops. Even though "development" implies change, present developmental research and theories seem to be best at describing what goes on within the "plateaus of non-change," as Snow and Gilbreath noted in 1983. In fact, we do not know how neurons in the brain represent human knowledge of any kind (Fodor, 1997). What is not known is how or why the child moves from one kind of knowing or one developmental stage to the next. This is not unlike the situation in other areas of human development, where the motivation or the mechanisms for the transitions from stage to stage are still basically unexplained through research findings.

Theoretical explanations of language development have traditionally fallen into either "nature" or "nurture" categories at opposite ends of a continuum. The nativist point of view is that language acquisition can be accounted for by innate, internally generated processes (a view usually attributed to nativists such as Chomsky [1993]). The extreme opposite point of view is that of behaviorism where all learning is considered to occur through externally controlled events [the perspective of behaviorists such as Skinner (1957)]. However, over the years, empirical evidence has not provided support for the extreme behaviorist explanations as a theory of language acquisition in typically developing children. An enduring alternative to the nature or nativist explanations are the interactionist (Braine, 1994) or constructivist explanations.

In essence, the interactionist perspective is that both innate and environmental factors determine development. Innate, internal, developmental abilities or propensities (some of which may or may not be specifically linguistic) interact with environmental factors and experiences in ultimately building up the child's knowledge of language. The environmental factors include all of the stable and changing features of the child's social, physical, linguistic, experiential environment: that is, the people and objects around the child throughout his everyday life. The child's social context interacts with his or her natural, genetic endowment in determining and promoting the acquisition of linguistic behaviors. Examples of the internal factors could include processing biases such as a capacity for symbolic representation, selective auditory and visual attention and processing, skill at "chunking" speech segments, skill at analyzing sequential information, categorical perception, a propensity for attempting to search for order and/or causality in events, and memory (Bates, Benigni, Bretherton, Camaioni, & Volterra, 1979; Braine, 1988). As Bates and Goodman (1999) put it, the question is no longer one of nature versus nurture, but one of exploring the "nature of nature" (p. 33). The debate concerning nature is now about whether language acquisition is based on language-specific abilities, or based on general-purpose cognitive abilities that apply to language learning as well as to other kinds of learning.

Consider for a moment the fascinating time when the child first begins to use words to communicate. In order to support the appearance of those first words, a number of hitherto apparently separate threads of development must converge. The Bloom (1983), Bloom and Lahey (1978), and Lahey (1988) division of language development into *form*, *content*, and *use* components is a useful construct for this brief discussion. *Form* development during the first 12 months of life includes multiple and dramatic changes occurring in the child's vocalizations as they gradually become more and more speechlike (Oller, 1995, 2000). *Content* development includes the child's gradual acquisition of differentiated repertoires of behaviors for using, pursuing, and/or dealing with objects and with people (Sugarman, 1984). Early *use* development includes the child's integration into the basic back-and-forth rhythm of human interaction (turn-taking), of being responsive and having others respond to him. Bloom (1983) suggests that the transition to the use of words comes about when these separate threads of development begin to intersect. That is, by about 12 months of age, the child knows how to behave interactionally with others, his vocal productions are speechlike, and he knows (for example) that a person can be used to get a hard-to-reach toy. Words will appear when all of these types of knowing begin to converge. Clearly, this is a very brief presentation of an extremely complex and multifaceted set of developments. However, there is intuitive validity to Bloom's concept of developmental transitions occurring when separately developing threads of abilities begin to converge.

To return to the nature/nurture issue, the foregoing discussion is an excellent example of the fact that we can describe what is acquired as the child develops, but we cannot account for why the changes in ability or behavior occur. Bloom's (1983) view is that the transitions to new levels of functioning require insight or intuitive understanding on the part of the child. Insight and intuitive understanding are unarguably internal to the child, as would be the child's propensity to even begin searching for understanding of the objects and people around him. But these innate abilities would have little value without the environment providing the objects upon which to act or the people with whom to interact. Both nature and nurture seem to be inextricably implicated as mediators in the acquisition of language.

Relevance for Intervention Decisions

Actually, for the educator or therapist with children and families needing immediate attention, the nature/nurture debate may be an interesting but immaterial one. With regard to the nature of the child, some aspects of the child's presenting repertoire undoubtedly are genetically endowed and/or internally generated. This may include aspects such as information processing rate, learning style (e.g., analytic, holistic, or some combination thereof), temperament, and the child's facility with language learning strategies such as the elicitation, entry, and expansion operations proposed by Shatz (1987). The child's genetic endowment clearly cannot be ignored. But for the interventionist, ethical practice demands that all of the child's abilities and inabilities must be considered amenable to influence or teaching until demonstrated otherwise.

With regard to the nurturing of the child, there is merit in the notion that language learning is a highly buffered or protected process, and that "the environment needs only to be sufficiently rich that the learner can at any point in time discover what [he] needs . . . " (Shatz, 1987, p. 4). At least, this may be so for normally developing and normally hearing children. But for children with language learning problems, there is evidence that differences in the environment can have considerable impact on the child's language development. And even for normally developing children, the defining characteristics of the "sufficiently rich" environment for language learning have yet to be unequivocally articulated. In any case, interventionists think more in terms of attempting to determine the components of an optimally *rich environment, rather than a* sufficiently *rich one. The environment, even with all of its individual and cultural variability, remains an extremely likely candidate for profitable examination and guidance toward becoming as language-facilitating as present scientific knowledge permits.*

How Should Intervention Be Organized?

The question that then arises for the interventionist is one of how to organize all of the kinds of learning and knowledge in order to assess the status of the child with hearing loss, and then implement a program intended to guide and promote the child's progress. In order to answer that question, one needs to consider two contrasting views regarding the effects of hearing loss on psychological and cognitive processing. Studies that have set out to define the effects of deafness on psychological and cognitive processing tend to be unavoidably fraught with weaknesses in experimental design. Sources of experimental weakness include the relatively low incidence of congenital sensorineural deafness which results in a small subject pool, complicated by the myriad of factors relating to individual differences that can affect the individual's use of residual hearing and learning of language. Research planning is often further limited by ethical questions regarding the withholding of habilitative treatment in order to establish control groups. The result is that for nearly every observation or research finding in this field, there is a counterfinding. Consequently, one is left with points of view, and many questions still open to research endeavor.

The traditional view is that, due to hearing loss, the child's psychological and cognitive abilities and strategies are somehow different, or at least reorganized. The result of this reorganization is language usage and understanding that are different from those of people with normal hearing (Furth, 1966; Myklebust, 1960). Proponents of this view tend to base their arguments on observations of people who are deaf and whose primary mode of communication is sign language. It seems quite logical that one's language usage and understanding would require a different sort of cognitive processing for a language whose semantic and grammatical subtleties are encoded visually, rather than acoustically. But these differences would seem to be more related to the modality or base (visual versus acoustic) through which the language is learned and used—rather than due to the sensorineural damage in the child's cochlea. In any case, espousing the view of cognitive and psychological difference resulting from deafness might logically lead one to the (circular) belief that visually based language is the "natural" language of the deaf.

A diametrically opposed view to the traditional one is that if adequate auditory and linguistic experience is provided to most children who are deaf or hard of hearing from an early age, then cognitive and linguistic functioning can be expected to follow the normal course of development (Geers, 2004; Geers et al., 2009; Geers, Nicholas, & Sedley, 2003; Hayes et al., 2009; L. Kretschmer & R. Kretschmer, 2001; Ling, 2002; Nittrouer & Burton, 2010; Nohara, McKay, & Trehub, 1995; Nott et al., 2009; Schauwers, Gillis, & Govaerts, 2005; Sininger, et al., 2010; Uchanski & Geers, 2003). Differences in the child's language ability are seen as due to lack of experience and exposure; as delay, rather than as deviance. The sequence of language learning is expected to include normal processes such as the intertwining of linguistic and cognitive activity. That is, assuming early and appropriate auditory, communicative, and linguistic stimulation, the early talking of the child with hearing loss is likely to mirror that of his or her hearing peers. For example, early semantic/syntactic performance will focus on objects and people in the immediate environment; the presence, recurrence, and/or disappearance of objects; actions related to the child; possession; basic characteristics of objects; locations in space; and cause and effect (Bloom, 1973; Nelson, 1973; Schauwers et al., 2005). The child is also likely to exhibit normal "errors" such as overgeneralizing or overrestricting syntactic and semantic rules during the learning process (L. Kretschmer & R. Kretschmer, 2001).

Assuming that audiologic and technological management is rigorous and appropriate, then providing enriched verbal interaction becomes the most important priority in order to promote the child's linguistic and cognitive development. The most reasonable course to follow in carrying out intervention for children with hearing loss is thus one of replicating (or re-establishing) the overall framework of a normal language learning environment. The child is expected to develop normal psychological and cognitive function and to follow the usual developmental sequences.

However, the provision of adequate auditory and linguistic stimulation requires *embellishments* of the normal situation which undeniably result in it being "non-normal" to some degree. One such embellishment would be the presence of the child's hearing aids, cochlear implant, and/or FM apparatus. Other embellishments would include the parent consciously employing specific techniques for helping the child learn to use his residual hearing, such as sitting close by (either behind or beside) the child when speaking to him, and using an interesting and animated voice when speaking. Another necessary embellishment might be to increase the frequency of caregiver-child interacting events throughout the day, specifically as an attempt to remedy the child's decreased exposure to spoken language. That is, the child who is deaf or hard of hearing may have a lessened ability to profit from each instance of interaction, as well as a lessened (or nonexistent) ability to overhear others' interactions with each other (Ling, 2002). Consequently, in order to achieve a desirable level of support, it may be necessary to establish an environment where interacting occurs more consistently and frequently than it otherwise might (Estabrooks, 2006; Snow, 1984).

The overall thrust of the parents and of the intervention program is to acknowledge and cope with the differences related to the hearing loss, while attempting to put them into perspective in a scene where most other aspects of interacting with their child will be normal.

Constructing
Meaningful
Communication

Key Points Presented in the Chapter

■ The essence of fluent communication between parent and child consists of sending and receiving linguistically encoded messages.

■ Language typically is acquired in the course of normal everyday routines and play.

■ The affective relationship between the caregiver and child has fundamental importance for the child's optimal acquisition of language.

■ Early learning about communication that the young child acquires includes knowledge about joint reference, turn-taking conventions, and the signaling of intentions.

■ Research on caregivers in mainstream middle class North American, British, Australian, and other cultures demonstrates the use of a number of characteristic behaviors in adult talk with young children. These characteristics include content, prosodic features, reductions in semantic and syntactic complexity, increased repetition of their own utterances and those of the child, employment of strategies to clarify meaning or to keep the child talking, and increased responsiveness to the child.

■ There are a number of theories about why caregivers engage in *motherese*, as well as about whether or not motherese actually is necessary or contributory to the child's language development. A child with no identified disabilities may develop language in the midst of a number of different language learning conditions. However, for a child with a hearing loss, it makes sense to strive for what research indicates is occurring in optimally supportive language learning environments. Professionals working with children and families from diverse cultures may find that some aspects are applicable to their own situations, and some are not.

Introduction

This chapter focuses on the communication and spoken language developments that occur for normally hearing children between birth and 6 years of age. This period begins with a time where the child is not actually using words—the time often referred to as *prelinguistic.* It continues to a time when the child is interacting in a broad variety of conversational contexts with different people, nearly always using complex, grammatically correct, mostly intelligible, multiple word utterances. The present discussion concerns the normal (presumably language facilitating) interactive environment whose basic features remain important throughout early childhood in mainstream English-speaking middle class families in North America, England, and Australia. This provides the theoretical background and rationale for the Framework for Maximizing Caregiver Effectiveness in Promoting Auditory/Linguistic Development in Children with Hearing Loss in Chapter 10. The information in this chapter is heavily based on research studies that are the foundation of theory and practice in the fields of speech-language pathology and deaf education today.

Let us begin by considering what happens when a parent and 3-year-old have a conversational exchange.

Language develops in the course of interactions between parent and child during routine, everyday play and caregiving activities. The essence of fluent communication between the parent and child consists of sending and receiving linguistically encoded messages. By the time the child is even 3 years of age, the caregiver or child can seek out the other in order to enjoy, share, request, assist, inform, and/or learn about the world (Dore et al., 1978). In order for any communicative attempt by either interactant to be successfully received, there are two necessary conditions: first, a shared focus must be established; and second, the message must be relevant to and interpretable by the listener (Bruner, 1975; Grice, 1967). That is, the parent and the child need to be jointly engaged in some activity or looking at each other or an object. Furthermore, the comment or question that is made needs to be of interest to the listener, as well as understandable. When the initiating attempt is successful, the receiver and sender quickly exchange roles, and a linked communicative chain ensues; the two are thus engaged in an intentional *communicative interaction*. The communicative aspect relates to the cycle of shared understanding (messages) sent and received, and then sent and received. The interactive aspect refers partly to the back-and-forth nature of the event (taking turns in a conversation), and partly to the fact that each partner actively derives meaning about the message from details of the participation of the other in the event.

But how do the parent and child arrive at this felicitous level of fluent conversation and interacting? This discussion of the development of communicative interacting will address three related areas: the affective relationship between parent and child, the child's development of interactional abilities; and features of caregiver talk that may be facilitative of the child's early development of verbal communication.

The Affective Relationship

The affective relationship between parent and child seems to have fundamental importance for the child's optimal acquisition of language from the very beginning. The question then arises regarding the nature of the affective relationship that would be most support-ive of language learning. It is interesting to note the adjectives scat-tered throughout one scholar's discussion of "personhood" and the interpersonal motivation for learning language. The environment provided by the parent during at least the early interactions was variously referred to as loving, rational, caring, thoughtful, caress-ing, joyous (Dore, 1986). This nurturing environment is not unlike the environment Clarke-Stewart's (1973) seminal research found to be most facilitative throughout infancy for social-emotional, intellec-tual, and linguistic development: an environment that was " . . . not only warm, loving, and nonrejecting, [but also] stimulating and enriching visually, verbally, and with appropriate materials . . . and . . . as well, immediately and contingently responsive" (p. 47). The socially competent infant gives clear, readable clues about what is wanted, is responsive when others approach him or her, and cap-tures the parent's ongoing attention by making the parent feel as if she is competent.

The results of Bromwich's longitudinal study (1981) demon-strated the importance and mutuality of influence of a positive rela-tionship between parent and child for all aspects of the child's development, including language. Interactions are a matter of "reciprocal reading and responding to each other's cues" which begins with bonding and attaching in the early months of life (p. 9). From a very young age, the normally developing infant's behaviors are seen as signals or cues by the parent who "reads" them and responds to them. The parent's behaviors eventually also become signals that the infant learns to read. It is through these early recip-rocal transactions that the emotional ties or bonds are established that are crucial to the child's social-emotional, intellectual, and lin-guistic development. Bromwich says that the child is developing a rudimentary level of trust in the predictability of the human and physical environment, and in his ability to have some influence on it. The parent, in turn, is being "captured" by the infant as a store-house of effective interactions is built up. For example, after the parent responds to the infant, the infant settles down, smiles, or babbles. These positive experiences can only serve to encourage both parent and infant to interact frequently, as both gain feelings of efficacy from it. As the infant develops socially and cognitively, the interactions become more complex. Eventually, the child is motivated to use verbal language as a more effective means of dealing with the complexity and sophistication of the interactions.

The success of the communicative process is entirely dependent upon the readability of each interactant's cues, as well as sensitivity to each other's cues (Figure 9–1). When the cues of either are not easily read, or one seems to be unresponsive to the other, it may begin a downward spiral in the affective and interactive relationship between parent and child. The parent becomes the focus of the intervention in this situation as it is the parent who has the potential of conscious control of his or her actions toward the child. The intention is to help the parent perceive the child's difficult-to-read cues and to modify parental responses in such a way that the child's cues become more predictable, and the likelihood is increased that the child will respond to the adult's behavior. Thus the downward spiral in the relationship would be reversed as the quality and mutuality of the interactions are enhanced—all of which favors optimal social-emotional, intellectual, and linguistic development of the child.

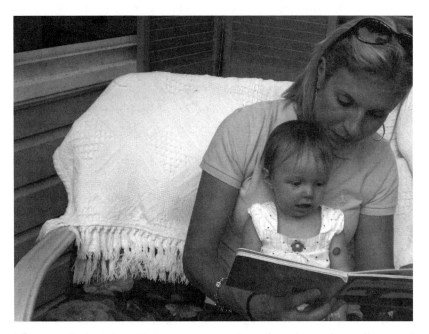

Figure 9–1. Interactions are a matter of reciprocal reading and responding to each other's cues. This child's cues may be expressed by direction of gaze, pointing, touching, and/or vocalizing.

The Child's Development of Interactional Abilities

Some of the issues regarding language development are whether or not there is a continuity between preverbal and verbal behaviors; whether or not preverbal behaviors are precursors, prerequisites, or simply antecedents for verbal behaviors; and once again, the degree of importance that should be attributed to biological development and caregiver/environmental influences. It seems likely that child behaviors that occur prior to the child's use of spoken language share at least some features in common with spoken language behaviors (Bloom, 1983). For example, the shared affective environment and timing of the "dance" of interactive behaviors in the very early months has features in common with the notion of reciprocal synchronization that occurs in verbal conversations. And the child's first words tend to be words about characteristics, movement, and locations of objects—the very concepts about which the prelinguistic child gradually acquires knowledge. But this relatedness or similarity should not be construed as implying that the linguistic behaviors necessarily develop out of the prelinguistic behaviors. For example, the child does not use speech *because* he has learned to babble; he does not talk about objects and their relationships *because* he has developed knowledge of them; and he does not communicate verbally *because* he can communicate nonverbally. On the other hand, as Sugarman (1984) says:

> Some preverbal experiences and acquisitions may nonetheless be critical to some aspects of language development. For example, it may be that unless children have learned something about communication prior to speaking they would have little motivation to look for a language to learn . . . (p. 136)

To the careful observer, early infant behavior and learning (birth to 12 months) seem to be "all of a piece." Attempts to describe it seem to impose artificial structure, uniformity, and order on what is actually a very complex, dynamic, and interwoven phenomenon. Added to that are the possible erroneous inferences resulting from the widespread application of linguistic terminology to preverbal behaviors. The reader should be aware that, lacking a better way, the following discussion is guilty on both counts: it divides early communication learning into three (untidy) areas for consideration, and it uses the same widely accepted terminology.

It appears that the preverbal learning having the clearest relationship to later verbal learning has to do primarily with the establishment of the social structure and communicative groundwork, rather than with semantic or syntactic groundwork (Kaye & Charney, 1980). Three essential features of discourse structure that are learned preverbally include joint reference to objects and events, turn-taking conventions, and the signaling of intention.

Joint Reference

One of the fundamental rules of fluent communication requires that the interactants share a focus or topic about which the message(s) is/are sent and received. For very young children, gaze and gesture are two of the means through which mutual attention is established and regulated. It generally is believed that it is through gaze and gesture that the child eventually acquires an understanding that part of communicating involves the establishment of topics and the means by which to establish them. Initially, a joint focus may be getting established, for example, as the mother and newborn engage in patterns of mutual gazing and mother vocalizing or talking to the baby. Then, as the child begins to notice objects, colors, and movement, the mother frequently follows the child's direction of regard and comments on what the child is presumably observing. By about 4 to 6 months of age, the child can follow the mother's gaze and will do so even more readily if the mother has just said something such as "Oh, look!" The consistency of a mother's encouragement of the child attending to a topic during the first 6 months of life correlates with later language development. Over time, as the child begins to understand more and more spoken language (albeit initially within much practiced routines), the mother can increasingly establish topics using verbal means alone.

Infant gestures are an important part of early communication development. At about 9 months of age, the child sometimes points at objects in the process of inspecting or examining them. This is not considered to be communicative. However, the child also now exhibits a "showing" gesture, whereby the child holds out an object for someone else to look at. This showing gesture is considered to be a step toward being communicative in that another person's involvement is essential, which is often signified by the child's looking toward the adult's face. This showing may or may not be accompanied by vocalizing. Soon after, the child not only shows the object to others, but actually allows the other to take it (i.e., the "giving" gesture). By about 11 months, the child points to objects in communicative fashion—not necessarily to obtain them, but just to point them out and presumably share the experience with another person. Similar to the previous gestures, the child's pointing is most likely to be effective in obtaining and maintaining the other person's attention if it is accompanied by vocalizing. Pointing out objects to have others look at them using vocalizing is an extremely important communicative achievement (Goldin-Meadow, 2007; Tomasello, 2008).

Turn-Taking Conventions

Fluent communicators know their culture's conventions regarding aspects of turn-taking such as when, in the flow of the other person's talk, it is and/or expected that one should take a turn. They also know how to signal that they are finished, and that it is the other person's turn to talk. This is acquired knowledge, presumably learned in the course of the multitudinous interactive exchanges that the child begins experiencing at birth. Even the "jiggle-suck" sequence that occurs as the infant is nursed may be an initial kind of turn-taking prototype. The adult orchestrates the turns, with clear indications to the child when it is time to take a turn. With the nursing infant, when the infant stops nursing, the mother jiggles the baby slightly, which seems to make the child begin nursing again for a time. When the infant stops nursing, the parent jiggles again—and so on, back and forth (Kaye & Wells, 1980). The clear openings for the child to take a turn continue in early childhood. In fact, Snow (1977) observed that, in conversations with a young child, the adult's primary purpose seems to be to try to get the child to take a turn, unlike the situation in adult-to-adult conversation where the purpose often seems to be to get to take as many turns as possible.

There are a number of characteristics in adult interactions with young children that could be interpreted as part of an effort to get the child to take a turn. For example, adults respond to the child with great consistency. This could be seen as simple reinforcement of the child's behavior in the hope that the adult response will cause the child's behavior to be repeated, or even as a kind of modeling of responsive behavior in the hope that it eventually will be emulated by the child. An infant can return a "vocal volley" by about 2 months of age, and can initiate vocally by 3 to 4 months of age (Bates, O'Connell, & Shore, 1987). Recognizable vocal imitation begins at about 5 months, but is not frequent or systematic until about 10 months of age. During all of this time, the adult consistently initiates and responds to the child's behaviors (including a number of nonvocal behaviors), and thus frames the exchanges so that they seem to be conversational. Adults also make frequent attempts to engage the child in conversation, and adult speech to young children includes a large proportion of speech acts (e.g., expansions, questions, and requests) that are intended to elicit responses from the child (Brinton & Fujuki, 1982; Kaye, 1982; Scherer & Olswang, 1984). In fact, all of the *motherese* alterations adults make in speaking to young children can be viewed as at least partly related to the adult's efforts to keep the child involved in the turn-taking process.

It is probably through such repeated interactive experiences that the child gradually acquires knowledge of when to take a turn, as well as how to signal that the other person can take a turn. Children have mastered *terminal gaze* by 24 months of age. Terminal gaze is the common practice (in speakers in mainstream North American culture) of looking up at the listener at the end of a message to signal that the floor is about to be offered. Once this practice has become part of the child's repertoire (apparently at 24 months of age), the turn-taking proceeds smoothly, with few interruptions of the other partner. However, the adult continues to take a leading (albeit gradually lessening) role in maintaining conversations with young children at least through 3 years of age.

Signaling of Intention

The third preverbal development that seems critical to the acquisition of language is the intention to convey an idea or message to someone else. What follows is a description of the hypothesized major milestones in the child's development of intentionality, where the involvement of both partners is required (Bates et al., 1987; Harding, 1983; Sugarman, 1984).

In the first few months of life, the child's actions are oriented in simple unitary fashion toward either a person or an object. What the child does is grasp, drop, mouth, manipulate, or look at *either* a person or an object. It is widely agreed that these very early infant behaviors are not intentionally communicative. However, in that they quite consistently elicit reactions from the parent, they are viewed as having communicative effect. Soon, by about 4 months of age, some behaviors occur repetitiously or with persistence and the parent begins to infer that the behaviors are communicative.

The simple unitary actions become more complex as they are used in tandem with one another to achieve a goal (e.g., child looks at a toy, reaches for it, grasps it, and finally pulls it into his mouth). Adult interpretation of this goal-directed behavior as communicative is increasingly frequent between 4 and 8 months of age. During this time, also, the parent consistently responds to the child's vocalizations as if they were meaningful conversation. Gradually, the child begins to expect certain behaviors of the adult to follow particular behaviors of his. He might be viewed as beginning to make inferences of his own about which of his behaviors cause particular adult behaviors to follow.

Eventually, by about 8 to 10 months, the child combines an action toward an object with an action toward a person, such as looking at the mother while reaching for a toy. The child is now using people to get objects, as well as using objects to get attention from people, rather than acting on either objects or people separately. That is, rather than simply persisting in reaching toward a hard-to-attain toy, the child now reaches *as well as* looks at the mother, or looks back and forth between the two. This is considered to be a major milestone in the child's communicative development, the beginning of the child's encoding of intent for someone else and the first visible demonstration of the child purposefully conveying a message to another. The reaching and looking are soon combined with simultaneous vocalizing and more conventionalized gesturing such as pointing. In her research, Sugarman (1984) has observed that spontaneous use of words began just after coordinated object and person behaviors were being used with some frequency. From then on, to oversimplify, the developmental process basically consists of an increasing proportion of verbal (rather than nonverbal) communications, and increasing length and complexity of communicative episodes.

This description of the development of the discourse structures of joint reference, turn-taking, and communicative intentionality provides a complementary framework for the notion that separately developing threads of abilities converge at transition points. Add to this the warm, responsive, nurturant affective environment, and the early language learning scene is nearly complete. The missing piece is a description of the nature of parent talk in responding to the child, and/or in initiating interaction with him or her. Because caregiver interactive behaviors may be one of the most important elements of the language learning environment for a child with a hearing loss (as well as one of the most eligible for modification), they will be described in some detail.

It should be noted that this discussion is based on research where the subjects were mainstream American, British, or Australian mothers and children. The degree to which any or all of these features are present in the talk addressed to young children in other cultures is outside the scope of this book. Clearly, children with normal hearing in all cultures learn to talk, and not all cultures use the specific motherese characteristics that are described here. However, the motherese findings are robust for the populations that were represented in the studies, which provides validity to their likely importance when the goal is to create an optimal environment for a child with hearing loss who is learning spoken language in one of the cultures included.

Characteristics of Caregiver Talk

Mothers, fathers, and other caregivers have a special manner or register that they use when talking to infants and young children, at least from birth to age 3. Features of this "baby talk," motherese, or "parentese" register are described below, as they appear in the talk of mainstream North American mothers to their children. To simplify, the term *motherese* will be used here. Not surprisingly, the degree of the mother's incorporation of the various features in her talk changes as the child moves from birth through childhood. Specific changes are mentioned within the discussion of particular features.

1. Content: What Gets Talked About?

The vast majority of topics in the mother's talk from birth to 3 months tend to be about the child's feelings and experiences (e.g., the infant's feeling happy, sad, sleepy, hungry, getting fed, getting diapered, getting picked up) (Snow, 1977). Many of these utterances are in the form of single word "greetings" such as *Hi, OK, Yes, Oh, Aw, Sure, What, Well, Hm* (Kaye, 1980). The topics in the mother's talk begin to shift after about 3 months of age, so that by 7 months of age, topics tend to be more evenly divided between the child's internal experiences and objects/events in the immediately surrounding environment. After 7 months, there is a steady increase in the proportion of the mother's utterances about immediately present objects and people, actions presently occurring or actions just recently completed (Newport et al., 1977; Snow, 1977). With infants between 11 months and 24 months, more than three quarters of the mother's talk was about toys and objects which were actually being manipulated by either mother or child. This means, for example, that when the child is about 1 year of age, measures of motherese lexicon tend to yield sets of words reflecting the 1-year-old's world. This is likely to include names of family members and pets, terms of endearment, words for body parts and functions, words for basic qualities and conditions (e.g., pretty, dirty, good), names of toys and games (Collis, 1977; Collis & Schaefer, 1975).

The contingency between the topics in the mother's talk and the child's likely interests decreases sharply when the child begins using multiple word utterances. It has been hypothesized that at that time, the adult senses that the child's cognitive and linguistic abilities are capable of supporting discussion of less immediate topics and events in the past and future (Bellinger, 1980; Cross, 1977; Lasky & Kopp, 1982; Newport et al., 1977).

The above discussion has been devoted to referential redundancy, or the parallel between the mother's verbal utterance and the child's interests in a particular context (sometimes also referred to as verbal contextual redundancy). A related but somewhat different notion is that of the caregiver's semantic contingency. This refers to the tendency for the mother's utterances to be based on what the child is talking about. Research on parental semantic contingency shows that it correlates positively with children's progress in acquiring a number of language features. In fact, this is one of the most consistent and robust findings regarding motherese and its effects (Barnes, Gutfreund, Satterly, & Wells, 1983; Cross, 1978; Nelson, 1973; Newport et al., 1977; Rocissano & Yatchmink, 1983). The key to a child's very early language acquisition (nonverbal or verbal) may lie in the many situations where the immediately present focus of attention is encoded linguistically in the adult's utterance. The adult utterance thus provides syntactic and semantic information within a conversational frame focused directly on whatever the child is interested in. This concept is closely related to Vygotsky's (1978) notion that higher mental functions, presumably including language, emerge in the child as a result of social mediation.

The Takeaway Message: *Talk about what the child is focused upon or interested in. Or, alternatively, attract the child's attention to something, and then talk about it.*

2. Phonology: What Does Motherese Sound Like?

Relative to adult-adult speech, characteristic delivery in motherese tends to have higher overall pitch, more varied intonational contours, a slower pace, more rhythmic phrasing (it has been described as "singsongy"), longer pauses between utterances, and clearer enunciation. Typical motherese also includes phonological simplification processes such as reduplication (e.g., the mother referring to the child's father as "Dada" in speaking to the child); and lengthened vowels (e.g., a prolonged "Hiiiiii!" or "You want some moooooore?") (Newport, 1977; Phillips, 1973; Sachs, 1979; Snow, 1972, 1977; Stern, Spicker, Barnett, & MacKain, 1983). These phonological changes seem to be more frequent in the mother's speech when the baby is from about 2 to 4 months of age. This is a time of rather intense face-to-face, playful interactions, where the mother is busy trying to keep the infant alert, interested, and happy. To carry out this role, she uses speech features that are most likely to get and hold attention such as a greater range of intonational contours, higher overall pitch, and greater terminal and transitional pitch contrasts. Then, as the child begins to be increasingly interested and able to explore objects and communicate about them, the mother's role shifts to facilitating those interests and abilities. For this new task, the pitch variation and sound repetition no longer need to be quite as exaggerated as they were when the mother was trying to get and keep the child's attention for face-to-face interactions. However, the mother's prosodic features are still (even at 2 years) significantly different from adult-adult speech. This may be related to a continuing fairly frequent need to catch the child's attention, and/or to cue the child that he is being addressed. It may also be part of an attempt to cue the child to take a turn, similar to pausing, as discussed in the next paragraph.

Maternal pausing between sequential utterances is greatest at birth and declines somewhat by 2 years of age. The mother may be using elongated pauses to provide for the infant's slower processing time, as well as to arouse the infant, heighten affect, or to cue the child to take a turn (Arco & McCluskey, 1981; Stern et al., 1983). The need for long "invitational" pauses decreases somewhat after the basic turn-taking rules have been established, but the postmaternal-utterance pauses at 2 years of age are still approximately twice as long as they are in adult-adult conversation.

In contrast to that, however, most maternal responses to infants occur with a one-second interval, and infants also generally respond to their mothers' utterances within a one-second interval (Beebe, Jaffe, Mays, & Alston, 1985; Beebe & Stern, 1977). It may be that when the child is not responding for some reason, the mother simply increases the pause time before producing another utterance herself.

> **The Takeaway Message:** *Motherese has a great range of intonational contours and relatively long invitational pauses after the adult utterance, which probably catches children's attention and cues them that they are being addressed.*

3. Semantics and Syntax: What About Complexity?

Compared with adult-adult talk, motherese is generally shorter in length. The mean length of the mother's utterances to infants between 2 days and 2 years of age varies from about three to four and a half morphemes. This is in contrast to a mean length of utterance in adult-to-adult talk of about eight morphemes (Phillips, 1973; Stern et al, 1983). In addition, motherese exhibits a restricted number of sentence types, as well as simplifications in both semantics (fewer semantic relations expressed in each utterance) and in syntax (fewer subordinate and coordinate clauses; fewer transformations, embeddings, conjoinings, function words).

Changes do occur in the complexity of the mother's semantics and syntax throughout childhood. However, there is marked disagreement among researchers concerning exactly which aspects change, when, in response to what, and in what manner. Some of the conflict may be related to the manner in which individual mothers adjust the complexity of their talk. For example, some mothers seem to match the child's mean length of utterance, and some stay four or five morphemes in advance of the child. It may also be that semantic/syntactic adjustments are made at one or more stages in the child's development, and not at others. Keeping in mind that this topic continues to need clarification, there does seem to be some consistency in two findings. The first is that the mother's syntax demonstrates the most change (increasing mean length of utterance) when the child is moving from 18 to 24 months of age. The second consistent finding is that the complexity of the semantic relations in the mother's talk does not increase during that same time period.

> ***The Takeaway Message:*** *Talk to very young children (birth to 2 years of age) in short, simple phrases, about two or three words in length (not in single words). The adult's utterance length should increase as the child's linguistic complexity increases, staying slightly ahead of the child's abilities.*

4. Repetition: Say It or Play It Again

Two types of repetition have been observed in mother's talk to young children. First, mothers immediately repeat their own utterances (in full) much more frequently in motherese than they do in talk to other adults. This is especially true in the first months of life with an apparent peak in repetition at about 4 months of age. This repetitiveness gradually declines over the next 2 years to become more and more like that found in adult-to-adult conversation (Kaye, 1980; Snow, 1972; Stern et al., 1983).

The other type of repetition has to do with the repeated occurrence of well-practiced sequences of exchanges or routines in interactions between mothers and young children. Research has shown the value of repeated patterned events that help the child discover how language is used appropriately in different contexts (Bruner, 1980; Conti-Ramsden & Friel-Patti, 1987; Peters & Boggs, 1986; Snow et al., 1987). In essence, these are ordinary interactions where the adult and child do things with each other with a great deal of regularity. This includes both the routines of everyday life (such as the routines for getting dressed, for eating, for bedtime) and the routines that occur within play. The responses of each interactant are contingent on the other's behaviors. In the North American context, these routines can be nursery rhymes, songs, tickling games, peek-a-boo games, book-reading, puzzle play, eating, bath, bedtime. The same (or nearly the same) words and phrases are used each time, which makes it easy for the child to predict the next move or utterance in the sequence. After several repetitions, the adult begins to expect child participation at appropriate moments. Less structured routines occur around a wide variety of daily events, where there can be subroutines embedded in longer-term routines. Here also, the patterned nature of the event helps the child discover how language is used appropriately within each event.

> ***The Takeaway Messages:*** *(a) Adults frequently repeat themselves with young children when they are trying to get a message across and they are not sure of the child's attention, focus, or understanding. (b) The routines of everyday life and play provide a multitude of opportunities for varied repetition that promote the child's language development.*

5. Negotiation of Meaning: Huh?

Much of adult talk with young children can be described as attempts to negotiate meaning. In these instances, the adult is most often attempting to resolve the child's unclear, imprecise, incorrect, or incomplete utterance(s). At the same time, it is often the case that the adult's attempt to understand maintains the child's participation in the conversation (Snow, 1984).

Two specific strategies that adults can use in negotiating meaning with young children are expansions (see next section) and seeking clarification. Here are some of the ways adults can seek clarification of meaning in a conversation with a child (Brinton & Fujiki, 1982; Gallagher, 1981; Garvey, 1977; Olsen-Fulero & Conforti, 1983; Peterson, Donner, & Flavelli, 1972):

1. Indicate lack of understanding through a puzzled facial expression and/or through gestures(s) such as lifting the shoulders and hands in a questioning manner. This can be done by itself, or in combination with any of the other clarification questions.
2. Use a neutral request for repetition such as, "What?" "Pardon?" "Huh?" "What did you say?" or "I didn't understand you."
3. Use a yes/no (or "choice") question to solicit confirmation that the adult's interpretation is correct. Several varieties of these requests for confirmation occur:
   a. Adult simply repeats child's utterance with rising intonation.

   Example:

   Child says: "Look! Teapot turn up!"

   Adult says: "The teapot turned upside down?"

   b. Adult repeats part of the child's utterance with rising intonation.

   Example:

   Child says: "Look! Teapot turn up!"

   Adult says: "Up?"

6. Participation-Elicitors: Let's (Keep) Talk(ing)

Snow (1977) said that one of the primary goals in adult-child conversation seems to be to get the child to take a turn. Clearly, the effect of the requests for clarification (described above) is to do just that. But, in fact, any questioning could be expected to include that same participation-eliciting intent (McDonald & Pien, 1982). Naturally, other intents are also likely to be there, such as truly soliciting information. However, any adult utterance that is followed by certain nonverbal cues such as an expectant pause and/or adult facial expression and/or slight lean toward the child could be viewed as participation-eliciting in intention. This may, in fact, describe nearly all of the prosodically highly marked adult utterances in face-to-face interaction with infants during at least the first 6 months of life. Two types of adult utterances to children after they begin talking bear particular mention in this regard, since they have received much research and intervention attention. These are *acknowledgments* and *expansions*.

Acknowledgments are utterances that acknowledge and/or accept the child's previous utterance without adding anything to it. This may take the form of simple confirmatory repetition of the child's utterance or it may be short phrases such as "Right," "Oh," "Um-hmm."

In certain instances, the effect of an acknowledgment may be to give the speaker (child) positive feedback regarding the utterance's truth value or clarity, and/or the child's success in communicating his idea. In any case, acknowledgements tend to serve as an encouragement to the child's continued participation in the conversation (Cross, 1984; Ellis & Wells, 1980; Furrow, Nelson, & Benedict, 1979; Snow et al., 1984).

Expansions (or recasts) and extensions are adult utterances that incorporate part or all of the child's previous utterance in a syntactically and/or semantically better formed sentence. Expansions provide an improved or corrected alternative way of saying whatever the child said. Extensions also provide the improved or corrected alternative, but in addition, amplify the topic in some way. Extensions can request or provide new information about the same topic, or can apply the same information to a new topic.

Examples

Child says: "Zak" (tapping dog's bowl with his foot).

Expansion: "Yes, that's Zak's."

Note: Expansions tend primarily to be syntactic corrections.

Extension: "Yes, it's Zak's bowl, and it's empty." or

"Yes, it's Zak's bowl, and this is Zak's toy."

Note: Extensions provide both syntactic and semantic additions.

In any case, expansions of child utterances may be one of the most frequently suggested and employed strategies in language intervention settings. They are likely to be more effective in eliciting improved responses from children who are at least at the two-word utterance level of syntactic-semantic development (Fey, Krulik, Loeb, & Proctor-Williams, 1999; McNeil & Fowler, 1999). Their use is based on observations that expansions occur frequently in normal caregiver talk, as well as on evidence that expansions and extensions have been associated with increases in grammatical development and in sentence length. Research has also shown that children are most likely to imitate expansions over any other type of adult utterance (Scherer & Olswang, 1984). It may be that an expansion has particular salience and motivating value for a child since it is based directly on the child's utterance, and simply introduces an element of relevant, moderate novelty to it.

7. Responsiveness

In face-to-face interactive play, mothers tend to be very consistently responsive to their children's behaviors (Snow, 1977; Stern, 1974; Trevarthen, 1977). Whatever the infant does will be interpreted as if she has taken a turn in a conversation, including burps and sneezes.

Example:

Context: Mother holding 2-month-old baby on shoulder after child has nursed; mother is patting baby on back gently.

Mother: "OK . . . Time for burpies. Ok now . . . Yeah! Sooooo full . . . Yes, you are. Yeah . . . What a baby! Um-hmmmm . . . "

Baby: [burps]

Mother: "Ooooh! Wow! What a big burp! Good job! Yes . . . Now you feel better."

The parent incorporates the child's behaviors in such a way that a semblance of dialogue is created even in these very early encounters. Kaye and Charney (1980) describe it as follows, " . . . the rule seems to be that if an infant gives his mother any behavior which can be interpreted as if he has taken a turn in conversation, it will be; if he does not, she will pretend he has" (p. 227).

Starting when the child is about 7 months of age, the mother begins to require a bit more from the child in terms of vocalizations and motoric behaviors before she will accept them as conversational turns (Newson, 1977; Snow, 1977; Snow, deBlauw, & van Roosmalen, 1979). She will still often respond to smiles, laughs, burps, and crying as if they were turns, but the vocalizations now tend to be ignored unless they include some consonantal or vocalic babble. The mother is also now more likely to ignore simple kicking or arm flailing. She will respond more selectively to more advanced motoric behaviors such as taking a bite of food, looking toward an object after it has moved or been talked about, or reaching for an object. These requirements for more sophisticated behaviors clearly reflect the mother's recognition of the child's increasing abilities. Through the 7-month to 36-month period, the mother continues to "up the ante" in terms of requiring communicative behaviors from the child. The child's developing abilities and the maternal requirements run parallel to each other, so that the mother continues to be quite consistently responsive to a large proportion of the child's behaviors throughout the birth to 3-year-old age range. Interestingly, starting at about 3 months of age, babies are twice as likely to repeat a vocalization if the parent has responded vocally to the initial vocalization by the child.

The back-and-forth cycles of responsiveness in conversation are similar to a game of catch (Kaye & Charney, 1980, 1981). A competent participant in either event both catches and throws with ease. The type of interactional turn which both (a) responds to the previous turn by the partner, and (b) attempts to elicit a response from the partner has been called a *turnabout* or a *verbal reflective*. Turnabouts seem to be more frequent in adult talk to children than to other adults. Turnabouts are considered to be very powerful language learning devices, since a turnabout by the mother has the properties of relating directly to the child's previous topic, of being responsive to it, and also of positing an expectation of further response from the child. It should be noted that turnabouts may take the form of any of the utterance types described above as being used for negotiation of meaning and/or for eliciting the child's participation. Mothers respond initially to very minimal child behaviors as if they were conversationally meaningful. In catching such minimal behaviors *and* tossing the conversational ball back, the mother is creating a situation where the child appears to be much more of an active participant than she may actually be. Interestingly, of course, the child eventually *does* become an active participant. This process certainly has all the markings of a self-fulfilling prophecy!

Issues About Motherese

How Long Is Motherese Used?

Motherese alterations continue to be used throughout the preschool years, although changes occur as the child's abilities emerge (Girolometto, Weitzman, Wiigs, & Pearce, 1999; McNeil & Fowler, 1999). Caregivers continue to provide a nurturing environment, to engage in topics of mutual interest (and attention) within their mutual experience, to encourage the child to take turns and to talk more through generous use of acknowledgements ("Oh!" "Good."), praise, repetition of own or child utterances with expansions, and use of turnabouts, often with yes/no questions. Prosodic alterations are also often present.

Motherese: Why?

The period from birth to 3 years of age is marked by consistent maternal responsiveness and the framing of interactive events toward the appearance of more and more sophisticated conversations. This creates a situation of some contrast between adult-adult and adult-child conversation. This seems to fit with Snow's (1977) contention that the purpose of adult-adult conversation appears to be to get to take a turn; in adult-child conversation, the purpose is to get the child to take a turn. There is a special significance to this differentiation as it has become one of the primary explanations for why adults "do" motherese. The adult's accepting minimally meaningful behaviors from the child as communicative may be part of an effort to provide a conversational frame to the encounter, and to facilitate the child's participation in the dialogue. The adult's frequent use of imitations of the child's productions, continuates, invitations to vocalize, and turnabouts also seem aimed at guaranteeing the conversational flow (Bruner, 1977; Kaye & Charney, 1980, 1981; Newport et al., 1977; Snow, 1977; Wanska & Bedrosian, 1985).

Another reason why adults use motherese register is that the modifications are fine-tuned to meet the child's developing linguistic and attention levels. The mother's talk is continually adjusted in order to maintain an optimal fit with what the child can understand. The mother is using motherese primarily to ensure the effectiveness of her utterances in terms of the child's understanding and learning. Naturally, this should also enhance the chances of the child's participating in the conversation, which suggests that the feedback and conversation-promoting motivations for motherese are ultimately not so dissimilar (Bellinger, 1980; Cross, 1977, 1978; Snow, 1972).

Other explanations for the motherese register are that it is used to convey a warm, loving, nurturing affect (Sherrer, 1974); to make oneself and one's talk interesting to the child in order to attract and maintain the child's attention (Kaye, 1980; Snow, 1972); and to help the child learn specific linguistic items and vocabulary (Gleitman, Newport, & Gleitman, 1984). All of these explanations have theoretical explanatory merit for at least some features of motherese at some steps in the developmental process; the explanations seem to be complementary, rather than in conflict.

Motherese: Immaterial or Facilitative?

Researchers have demonstrated that the child's receptive and expressive language benefits from having a parent who talks frequently to him or her and who uses a variety of vocabulary (Fey, Krulik, Loeb, & Proctor-Williams, 1999; Hart & Risley, 1999; McNeil & Fowler, 1999; Weizman & Snow, 2001). In addition, children's language is positively affected by parents talking about what the children are attending to, rather than the parents redirecting the child's attention elsewhere and talking about that other topic (Kaiser & Hancock, 2003; Yoder, McCathen, Warren, & Watson, 2001). Although no one disputes the fact that absent or greatly impoverished adult input has a devastating effect on language learning, there is much disagreement about the nature of the adult input that is necessary and/or facilitative of language development in normally developing children. Researchers have not been especially successful at establishing robust relationships between particular semantic, syntactic, or pragmatic features of motherese and subsequent language growth for normal language learners.

One of the sources of confusion is the fact that there is a great deal of individual variability in normal maternal interactional styles (Clarke-Stewart, 1973; Kaye, 1980; Kaye & Charney, 1980, 1981; Newport et al., 1977; Snow et al., 1987). Other sources of variability are related to the variety of contexts being observed in the various studies of interacting, and to changes identified in characteristics of the mother's style at different developmental stages of the child (Conti-Ramsden & Friel-Patti, 1987; Snow et al., 1987). Differences in the *children's* cognitive, learning, and/or interactive style and temperaments could also easily influence the mothers' styles (Bates et al., 1987; Spiker, Boyce, & Boyce, 2003).

As if this were not enough confusion, cross-cultural studies demonstrate that children can become competent language users without experiencing the same adult adjustments typical of middle class motherese in English (Crago, 1988). However, it is difficult to entertain the notion that all of those well-documented motherese adjustments are irrelevant, at least for children similar to the research subjects who are learning language in middle-class English-speaking culture.

It also seems possible that the language learning process for the normally developing child is well cushioned by the child's intact "intake" and "output" systems, and perhaps by the strength of hypothesized drives toward being like her parents or toward communicating in the most efficacious manner possible. The normal child will probably develop language in the face of a number of adverse conditions. For the child with hearing loss (similar to any child with language learning problems), however, the cushioning is not there. In order to assist the child to reach a maximal level of achievement, it makes sense to try to create an optimal set of interactive conditions for facilitating the growth of the child's language.

10

Interacting in Ways That Promote Listening and Talking

Key Points Presented in the Chapter

- The term *aural habilitation* refers to intervention aimed at helping young children with hearing loss learn to listen and talk, where the parents are the primary agents of change in helping the child learn.
- The parents need to absorb a great deal of information about hearing loss and its implications, as well as internalize ways of interacting that will promote the child's use of audition and the child's acquisition of intelligible spoken language.
- For many parents, discovery of the child's hearing loss is a shock, and is accompanied by a whole host of feelings that need to be discussed in order for the parents to be able to cope with all of the demands on their time, energy, thinking, and patience.
- The aural habilitationist may feel pressure to move quickly to minimize any additional loss of hearing or listening time for the child. However, the intervention will be most effective when the professional works with sensitivity and respect for the degree to which the parents' emotional well-being and feelings of efficacy may have been impacted by the discovery of hearing loss in their child, as well as by the ongoing

---

requirements imposed by the reality of addressing the unanticipated needs of the child.

■ The most important intervention tool is properly selected and maintained assistive technology, since it provides the child's brain with access to sound.

■ Putting on hearing aids or cochlear implant(s) is not enough. The child also needs the parent to provide an abundance of developmentally appropriate, auditorily-based verbal interacting.

■ Routine, normal, everyday caregiving and play events provide natural contexts for learning language through listening.

■ The Framework for Maximizing Caregiver Effectiveness in Promoting Auditory/Linguistic Development in Children with Hearing Loss provides guidelines for desirable caregiver behaviors.

■ Normal, everyday interacting needs to be "embellished" to help the child learn spoken language the most effectively, as well as to teach the child specific auditory/linguistic targets. What the parent does is perfectly normal interacting—just more deliberately, and more frequently.

■ Preplanned parent guidance or auditory-verbal sessions are typically structured to provide confirmation of the child's hearing status, diagnostic practice of auditory/linguistic targets, discussion between parent and aural habilitationist, homework for the coming week, and a closing routine.

■ General intervention principles for preplanned parent guidance sessions are similar to those for embellished interacting.

Introduction

In this chapter, intervention aimed at helping young children learn to listen and talk is referred to as *aural habilitation*. The assumption here is that this work will be carried out by a parent, who is being guided and supported by a certified Auditory-Verbal Therapist, a teacher of the hearing impaired, a pediatric audiologist, or a speech-language pathologist. The professional's title matters much less than the professional's expertise and experience.

In its most enlightened and efficacious form, aural habilitation is a collaborative process between parents and professionals. Parents and aural habilitationists should be natural collaborators as they both are striving for the same thing: a better-communicating child. The efficacy of intervention which views the parent as the primary client has long been supported by research, as well as by logical arguments regarding the amount of parent contact with the child, and consequent opportunities for continuity and generalization (Clarke-Stewart, 1973; Dunst, Boyd, Trivette, & Hamby, 2002; Dinnebeil & Hale, 2003; Peterson, Carta, & Greenwood, 2005). What follows is centered around intervention for very young children with hearing loss whose parents or caregivers are considered to be the primary agents of change.

Discovery of a child's hearing loss is likely to evoke a tangle of feelings in the parent that can be long-lasting and recurring as the parent comes to terms with life experiences that are different from those he or she had expected. However, parents will be required to act, even though they are in turmoil, in order to minimize or avoid any additional loss of listening and learning time. The aural habilitationist has a great deal of information and many skills to impart to the parents or caregivers. This must be accomplished with sensitivity and respect for the fact that the learning and skills are not things the parents were always just dying to acquire. They are learning out of love and hope for their child's present and future life. The fortunate thing is that often, the child's progress helps the parents' emotional state begin to lift.

The Emotional Impact of a Child's Hearing Loss on the Family

As parents are expected to take on major roles in the child's learning to listen and talk, the parents' ability to do that needs to be carefully considered. Teaching a child to listen and talk may be easier for parents than teaching the child to sign from one perspective, at least: the hearing/speaking parent does not need to learn a new language in order to teach the child, as they might in order to teach the child to sign. However, the ability to function well in both the parenting and listening-and-language-facilitating roles requires at least a moderate sense of well-being. For many parents, discovery of the child's hearing loss is a shock, and is accompanied by a whole host of feelings that need to be addressed in order for the parent to be able to cope with all of the new demands on their time, energy, thinking, and patience.

In many countries, infants have their hearing screened at birth, so that early identification and early intervention both are a reality for many of today's children who have hearing loss. Although research suggests that parents feel positively about having discovered the hearing loss when the baby was very young, early identification brings with it psychological complexities for parents as they experience waves of grief, reassurance, hope, and distress (Young & Tattersall, 2007).

Approximately 90 to 95% of babies with hearing loss are born to parents who have normal hearing (Mitchell & Karchmer, 2004). Not surprisingly, for the vast majority of those parents the discovery of the child's hearing loss is a crisis, or creates one, for the parents and family. The child is just as he or she was the day before, but much is changed for the parents. For a minority of parents, it is a relatively small crisis, where the parents rapidly and relatively smoothly accept the child's hearing loss, and become implicated in the habilitation process. For the vast majority, however, the child's hearing loss is initially experienced as a catastrophe. Later, the presence and implications of the hearing loss become a simmering crisis that can be coped with, but which periodically returns to an acutely painful stage. Re-eruptions of the emotional crisis often coincide with events such as audiological testing times; or educational transitions into preschool, kindergarten, grade school, or high school; or at graduations; at puberty; at young adulthood; and/or at the parent's retirement. These events sometimes precipitate a reworking of the feelings surrounding the continuing implications of the child's hearing loss (Lukerman, 2006).

The emotional turmoil surrounding the discovery and presence of hearing loss in a child has been likened to grieving, not unlike the process described some time ago by Kubler-Ross (1969). Moses (1985) and Moses and Van Hecke-Wulatin (1981) were some of the first authors to apply grieving process theory to hearing loss. What is being grieved by the parents is the loss of their dreams and fantasies about what the child would be like. Both prior to and after the child's birth, parents have dreams and expectations for the child's future, most of which require an unimpaired child. When those dreams are shattered by the diagnosis of hearing loss, the parent needs to have a chance to grieve about the situation, to separate from the dreams and to let them go. In the process, grieving may stimulate a reevaluation of a number of aspects of one's existence including social, emotional, environmental, and philosophic attitudes and beliefs. This may include unconscious biases such as fear, pity, or revulsion that the parent has toward people who experience disabilities. Alternatively, it may involve a strong desire for things to remain as they were, a very normal fear of change.

According to Luterman (1984), this process may be an existential "boundary experience" that may force the parent into a more intense awareness of reality and of the transitory nature of existence. The consequence may ultimately be a rearrangement of priorities, an abandonment of trivialities and timidity, and the selection of a different set of meanings for one's existence. Again, though, this is not to imply that one embarks on a linear journey through suffering to a final nirvana of acceptance, coping, and purpose. Being able to accept the situation enough to cope with it and move on does not signal a magical end to the recurrence of painful feelings or to the need to work and rework the surrounding issues.

The following emotional states are generally accepted as part of the parental grieving process. These occur in no specific order, nor even necessarily by themselves—even though writing about them requires that they appear to do so.

Denial—The denial may be denial of the accuracy of the diagnosis, of the permanence of the hearing loss, and/or of the impact of the hearing loss on the child's life or on the lives of those around him or her.

Guilt—The parents may feel guilt because they believe they caused the hearing loss. Or, they may believe they are being punished for being "bad" or for something they did or did not do in the past.

Depression—The parents may feel impotent at not being able to cure or take away the hearing loss. They may be enraged at themselves for not having been able to prevent the loss to start with. They may also feel incompetent to deal with what is seen as the impossible demands being imposed by the hearing loss, such as dealing with the technology, and having to do different things with this child than they had expected to do.

Anger—Anger may be felt by the parents at the injustice of it all. They also may be angry at the unasked-for demands on their time, energy, finances, and emotions. The demands all emanate from the child with hearing loss, but the parent's anger is often displaced to other family members and to professionals.

Anxiety—Parents may feel overwhelmed at the added pressures and responsibilities of having a child with a hearing loss. They may also feel anxious about the need to juggle the added responsibilities with their own needs to have an independent life.

These feelings are natural, normal, and perhaps even necessary in order for the parent to deal with the situation and to move on. Each of the emotional states serves a function that eventually allows parents to separate from their shattered dreams for their child to be "perfect," and for themselves to be the parents of that perfect child. Then new dreams can be generated, incorporating the child's hearing loss. The parent begins to feel that coping is, at least occasionally, possible. The reader is strongly urged to seek out Flasher and Fogel's excellent book (2004) for further explanation.

So what is the aural habilitation professional supposed to do with all of this emotional turmoil? On a practical level, the turmoil may occasionally get expressed in a "pure" form with a parent so upset that he or she cannot function at a given moment. Or it may get expressed in a slightly more subtle form such as combinations of alarm, sadness, and frustration about the baby having to receive therapy to learn things other babies learn naturally, about having to learn a lot about something the parent never wanted to learn about in the first place, about having to participate actively in sessions, about having too many or too few sessions, and/or about the difficulty of finding a parking space near the clinic or school. According to Flasher and Fogel (2004), Luterman (1984), Moses (1985), Moses and Van Hecke-Wulatin (1981), and Rogers (1951), the most facilitative thing the professional can do is to convey an attitude of acceptance of whatever the parents' emotional states happen to be.

This is one obvious time when the professional's interpersonal skills will be drawn upon. The idea is not to become a psychotherapist. Indeed, one of the essential aspects of intervention with families of children who are deaf or hard of hearing is to know when the parents' emotional needs exceed the aural habilitationist's skills, and to refer the parents elsewhere for professional counseling. However, it is not practical, possible, or desirable to refer all upset parents for psychiatric care. The aural habilitationist must accept responding empathically as a part of his or her professional responsibilities (Flasher & Fogel, 2004; Figure 10-1).

In the vast majority of instances, what is required is direct, honest, and personal confirmation of the other person's "normalness" and "humanness." This means being genuinely empathic and conveying that intent through active listening. Pickering (1987) calls it "listening as a *receiver* rather than as a critic": accepting rather than evaluating and trying to control (p. 217). Based on Pickering (1987), Tables 10-1 and 10-2 list and illustrate two general types of responses that the aural habilitationist can make in encounters with parents. Responses that reflect empathy are those that acknowledge and attempt to understand the feelings, perceptions, and interpretations of the parent. These responses increase the parent's feelings of autonomy and self-efficacy. They ultimately have a "freeing" effect. The others, the controlling responses, have the opposite

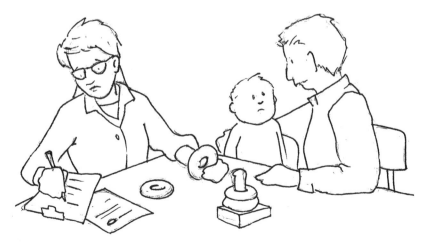

Figure 10-1. The parent has a feeling! Quick—call the psychiatrist! (Phil Youker drawing)

Table 10–1. Empathic Responses (in Encounters of the Interpersonal Kind).

- Reflecting back what was heard, restating, paraphrasing (e.g., If I heard you correctly, you said . . . ?)

- Extending, clarifying what the other said (e.g., Then? And? Tell me more about that. Give me an example. I didn't understand that. What did you mean when you said . . . ?)

- Using supportive, open-ended, exploratory questions—as nonthreatening as possible! (e.g., What happened to make you feel that way? What do you think of when you hear . . . ?)

- Summarizing, synthesizing (e.g., It must be very overwhelming/frustrating/frightening to . . .)

- Perception checking (e.g., You seem to be . . . Does this fit with the way you see things?)

- Acknowledging, without taking the conversation in a different direction (e.g., Um-hmmm. I see what you mean. I can appreciate what you went through.)

- Encouraging expression of an idea or feeling (e.g., How did *you* feel about that?)

- Being quiet

Reprinted with permission from *Listening and Talking: A Guide to Promoting Language in Young Hearing-Impaired Children*, by E. Cole, 1992. Copyright 1992 Alexander Graham Bell Association for the Deaf.

effect of diminishing the parent's feelings of autonomy and self-worth. The outcome of a professional's (even unconscious) attempts to control parents in this way may be either parental resistance (Lowy, 1983) or an overdependence upon the aural habilitationist. The preferred manner of interacting is obvious.

It is through the acceptance and personal confirmation of significant others that the parent may be able to constructively cope with the emotional impact of the child's hearing loss. The professionals involved may have a powerful impact on the parents in this regard, but this support may also come from friends, religious groups, and community and/or parent groups. Parental coping will strengthen the parents' feeling of competence and, in turn, positively affect the child's development.

Table 10–2. Responses That Control (in Encounters of the Interpersonal Kind).

- Changing or diverting the subject without explanation, particularly to avoid discussing the other person's feelings.

- Interpreting, explaining, or diagnosing the other person's behavior (e.g., You do that because . . .).

- Giving advice, insisting, or trying to persuade (e.g., What you should do is . . .).

- Agreeing vigorously. This binds the other person to his present position.

- Expressing own expectations for the other person's behavior. This type of response can bind the other to the past (e.g., You never did *that* before!) or to the future (e.g., I'm sure you will . . .).

- Denying the existence or importance of the other's feelings (e.g., You don't really mean that! You have no reason to feel that way. You shouldn't feel that way.).

- Praising the other for thinking, feeling, or acting in ways you want him or her to; approving on your own personal grounds.

- Judging, disapproving, admonishing on your own personal grounds; blaming, censuring the other for thinking, feeling in ways you do not approve of; imputing unworthy motives.

- Commanding, ordering. (This includes, "Tell me what you want me to do!")

- Labeling, generalizing (e.g., She's always shy. He's aggressive and hyperactive.).

- Controlling through arousing feelings of shame and inferiority (e.g., How can you do this to me when I have done so much for you?).

- Giving false hope or inappropriate reassurance (e.g., It's not as bad as it seems.).

- Focusing inappropriately on yourself (e.g., When my dog died, I felt terrible, too.).

- Probing aggressively, interrogating, asking threatening questions (Tell me how you think a child learns language.).

Reprinted with permission from *Listening and Talking: A Guide to Promoting Language in Young Hearing-Impaired Children*, by E. Cole, 1992. Copyright 1992 Alexander Graham Bell Association for the Deaf.

> *Often, early indications or clues of the child progressing are the most effective and immediate catalysts for giant leaps in the parents' ability to cope with it all. In order for that to happen, intervention tasks, such as hearing aid selection, fitting, and wearing, clearly need to be carried out—and parents need to be guided in what to look for as early indicators of the child listening. These indicators include alerting to sound, turning to sound, quieting to sound, increased vocalizing, decreased vocalizing (while listening), and/or an increased variety in vocalized sounds.*

Intense feelings will unavoidably come up in aural habilitation sessions with individual parents and their children, so the aural habilitationist must be prepared to address them. Parent networks or parent groups also can be extremely valuable and supportive. Parent groups can provide mutual support in a way that the aural habilitationist cannot. The parents may gain hope, relief, and a feeling of cohesiveness with the other parents. The reader is referred to Luterman (2001) and Luterman & Maxon (2002) for an in-depth and eloquent treatment of this topic.

However, intervention for the child cannot be delayed until the parent reaches some mythical level of perfect coping. Hearing aids must be immediately selected, fitted, worn, and maintained. Children must be exposed to spoken language, expected to listen, and vocalize or verbalize—as well as to conform to behavioral expectations. The point is that as the content agenda unfolds, the aural habilitationist must interact with the parent sensitively and empathically, without rejecting, denying, or criticizing how the parents are feeling or behaving.

What Parents Need to Learn

Parents here is used in a generic sense and includes any and all persons associated with the child's well-being or caregiving. This can mean babysitters, grandparents, older siblings, and other relatives and friends. The words *parent* and *caregiver* are used interchangeably here.

There is a lot for the parent to learn. Parents need to absorb information about topics such as the nature and implications of hearing loss; the functioning, benefits, and maintenance of hearing aids and other amplification systems; educational choices and child advocacy; and the development of intelligible spoken language. They also need to internalize ways of interacting that will promote the child's use of audition, and the child's acquisition of intelligible spoken language. The emphasis here is on what can be done to assist parents or other caregivers accomplish what is needed for the child.

Components of Intervention for Babies and Young Children with Hearing Loss

Intervention for a child with a hearing loss has two components of paramount importance. These are:

1. Providing the child's brain with access to auditory information through proper selection and maintenance of technology for the child; and
2. Providing the child with an abundance of developmentally appropriate, auditorily-based, verbal interacting.

The first five chapters of this book have focused on what needs to be understood and done in order to address the first component. The child's hearing technology is *the most important intervention tool*! Assuming that the child's hearing technology has been properly selected, and is being carefully monitored and maintained, most of the professional and parent effort can then be directed toward delivering the other component: providing abundant, developmentally appropriate, and auditorily-based communicative experience.

Providing abundant, auditorily-based communicative experience is not an especially easy task. There are no universal cookbooks or surefire formulas or even particular language, auditory, or speech-training exercises or activities to be uniformly applied in order to guarantee an outcome of a perfectly intelligible, independent, socialized, and happy child. In fact, in intervention with very young children with hearing loss, there is no clear separation among language, auditory, and speech work. Any interactive event necessarily taps and exercises both areas to some degree—which is a wonderful thing! The adult's job is to be aware of the existence and importance of the synergism of language, auditory, and speech elements to which the child is being exposed in any routine event, and to emphasize them, provide another example, push it all just one more step, make certain the event occurs again, and most of all reinforce and encourage the child by keeping it all meaningful and fun.

The first part of this chapter begins with a discussion of the types of routine, normal, everyday events that provide natural contexts for language learning. The chapter then turns to possible effects of the hearing loss on adult-child interactions, and sets out clear procedures for examining those normal, everyday interactive events in order to determine areas in the parent's usual interactive behavior that may be facilitating or hindering the child's language growth. This is followed by discussion of ways of emphasizing particular language, auditory, or speech elements in the course of normal, but slightly "embellished," interacting and pre-planned play.

When to Talk with Your Child and What to Talk About

Babies and very young children with hearing loss typically can learn language in the course of normal, everyday events, as do normally hearing children. The essential difference is that for children who have hearing loss, it is important to maintain an *optimally* rich environment or an embellished environment. That is, verbal interaction must occur frequently and consistently and be framed within the use of auditory strategies in order to establish a desirable level of support. However, sometimes there may be omissions or gaps in the child's linguistic knowledge that will need to be learned from preplanned adult instruction. Preplanned instruction with very young children is most effective when it is focused on something of interest to the child, and when it is playful, brief, and highly rewarded.

In this regard, then, much of the job of the aural habilitationist is to heighten the parents' awareness of how much they are already naturally doing, and to encourage them to do more of it. Simple, everyday routines and play can form the basis for the provision of abundant, auditorily based communicative experience. Particularly in the birth to 2-year-old period, the necessities of household functioning (including especially baby care) work to support the establishment of regular routines. Since these are frequently repeated, the child is provided with nearly the same meaningful experiences with nearly the same language over and over. Examples of some of those ordinary, everyday routines and playful activities can be found in Table 10–3.

As mentioned in Chapter 9, some children without identified disabilities of any kind will learn language under all kinds of conditions. However, at least in mainstream middle class North American, British, and Australian culture, children develop spoken language in the course of interactions with fluent-speaking adults. Because the child with hearing loss is operating with reduced quality, quantity, and intensity of auditory/linguistic input, it makes sense to provide an environment that has enriched levels of facilitative stimuli.

Actually, any time the caregiver is with the child is a possible time for normal, everyday interacting and language "input." The basic idea is to respond to the child's communicative attempts, and to talk about whatever interests the child about the events or materials at hand. The idea is not to intrude into the child's self-absorbed exploratory play in order to engage him or her in talk every waking minute, but to select (or create) opportune moments for verbal interaction. This may be through observing the child carefully, and joining in when the child looks up and appears interested in having the parent's involvement. Or, it may be at a moment when the parent has something genuinely exciting, interesting, or important to tell the child. For some parents, these embellishments are already natural behaviors. For others, the notions are easily internalized and expanded upon. For still others, who may be less experienced or less talkative with young children, more guidance and conscious behavior change may be required.

Table 10–3. Examples of Ordinary, Everyday Routines that Can Be the Scene for Providing Abundant, Auditorily-Based Communicative Experience for Children

---

Birth to 6 Months:

Feeding, getting diapers changed, having baths, getting dressed; getting put to sleep; manipulating simple toys and objects; watching parents, siblings, pets; being fastened into strollers, car seats, infant seats; being engaged in visual/vocal games with adults and siblings (including peek-a-boo games).

---

6 to 12 Months:

Feeding, getting diapers changed, having baths, getting dressed; being put to sleep; being engaged in simple nursery rhymes involving manipulation of the child and, often, anticipation of tickling, such as "This Little Piggy," "Round and Round the Garden," "Pattycake"; being watched and helped as gross motor skills improve and the child crawls (both on the floor and up the stairs), stands, takes a few steps; being fastened into strollers, car seats, infant seats; taking walks and observing the world; increasingly active play with objects and toys (banging, dropping, throwing, turning, pulling, squeezing); verbal greeting routines, animal sound imitation.

---

12 to 18 Months:

Feeding, getting diapers changed, having baths, getting dressed; being put to bed; playing with balls, active motoric play (climbing, bouncing, walking, running); container play (filling and pouring, especially), block play, picture books and stories; drawing with crayons.

---

18 to 36 Months:

Feeding, getting diapers changed, using the potty (some), having baths, getting dressed, going to bed; active motoric play; play with balls, water, sand, blocks, play dough, crayons; picture books and stories; "helping" with bed-making, dusting, setting the table, sweeping, filling and emptying the dishwasher, cooking, shopping; going to the park; playing on playground toys; nursery rhymes and songs.

---

3 to 5 Years:

Eating snacks and meals; taking trips in the car; doing errands; putting dishes in the dishwasher, folding laundry, setting the table, cooking, making beds, sweeping; shopping; going to the park; picking up brothers and sisters, watching siblings' sports practices; cleaning up; getting dressed, toileting, bathing; going to bed; active play outside; play with balls, water, sand, blocks, play dough; drawing, painting; reading picture books and stories, nursery rhymes and songs; being polite, making friends with peers.

Once the child has appropriate audiologic technology and noise in the environment has been managed, what can caregivers do to provide an enriched auditory/linguistic environment? The Framework for Maximizing Caregiver Effectiveness in Promoting Auditory/Linguistic Development in Children with Hearing Loss (in the next section) was developed to provide concrete information about exactly that. The Framework clearly lays out interactive behaviors that are language facilitating for caregivers (including teachers and therapists) to use from birth to age 6. The intention is that the Framework will be used to reinforce or affirm language promoting behaviors that caregivers are already using, as well as to encourage the addition of ones of which they may not been aware. The Framework is not intended to be used to correct "mistakes" that parents are making, but to help them provide an interactive environment with enriched levels of auditory/linguistic facilitation in an attempt to compensate for the impact of the disadvantages imposed by the hearing loss.

A Framework for Maximizing Caregiver Effectiveness in Promoting Auditory/Linguistic Development in Children with Hearing Loss

Background and Rationale

Sometimes a child's hearing loss seems to have little or no effect on the interactive relationship with his or her parents. But the intactness of those interactions *can* be threatened in several ways. First of all, when a child has an undetected hearing loss, he is not receiving auditory/linguistic stimulation in the same manner as his normally hearing peers. And even after a sensorineural loss is detected and appropriate hearing aids worn consistently, the input is reduced in quality, quantity, and intensity. That is, the hearing aid and the cochlear implant both provide access to speech, but are unlike corrective lenses for eyes: they do not restore listening abilities to normal threshold levels and make speech clear. Speech still lacks the clarity and intensity of the speech received by a normally hearing

> *There are frustrations and problems inherent to trying to understand and be understood by any young child who is only just beginning to learn that adult signals (e.g., words) have consistency and significance. If the child is the physical size of a 2-year-old with normal learning abilities, but is understanding and producing language at a much younger age level, a developmental dysschrony is created which sets up the interactive scene for frustration and problems.*

infant. Further, the young child with a severe to profound hearing loss needs to *learn* that he can benefit from "overhearing" conversations directed toward others in his environment; the child with hearing loss may not automatically overhear the speech of others. These are the physiologic and psychoacoustic reasons that the process of learning spoken language can be so long and arduous for children who are deaf or hard of hearing. These are also reasons that the child with a hearing loss may not respond in expected ways to parent messages or cues, and may not send out expected cues. This mismatch of expectations can disrupt interactional events from the very beginning. In addition, as mentioned earlier in this chapter, the caregiver's ability to interact "normally" may also be influenced by emotional turmoil that can surround the discovery, as well as the continuing presence, of the hearing loss. In the course of this process, a number of powerful emotions are experienced by the parent that may interfere with the parent's normal ability to be sensitive to the child's communicative cues, to respond to them, and to send appropriate cues to the child.

To summarize, the lack of expected audition-based responses from the child, the slowness of the process due to the reductions in quality and quality of the auditory-linguistic input, and the parent's emotional turmoil all may contribute toward limiting the child's access to precisely the kind of auditory, linguistic, and social interaction that he or she needs. Furthermore, these factors may explain some of the research findings regarding caregiver talk to children who are deaf or hard of hearing which suggest that parent speech to children with hearing loss varies considerably from parent speech to normally hearing children as shown in Table 10–4.

Table 10–4. Summary of Research Findings Regarding Adult Talk to Young Children with Hearing Loss.

- Reduced amount of talk directed toward child
- More exact self-repetitions
- Fewer expansions
- Shorter sentences
- Simpler grammatical constructions
- More frequent rejecting, critical, or ignoring responses
- More direct imperatives (attempts to control child's behavior)
- More adult topic changes away from child's focus of attention, activity, or previous utterance
- Speech which is faster, less fluent, less intelligible, less audible

(Note: See review in Cole, E. (1992). *Listening and Talking: A Guide to Promoting Spoken Language in Young Hearing-Impaired Children* (pp. 42–46). Washington, DC: Alexander Graham Bell Association for the Deaf.)

All of those findings may be normal responses to the child's not understanding or responding in expected ways, to the parent not being able to understand the child's utterances, and to the parent's feelings of frustration, sadness, or hopelessness. But however normal these responses may be, they are of concern since many of them are not interactive behaviors that promote listening and language at all stages of development. Although physiologically intact children may learn fluent language in less-than-optimal conditions, children with sensory impairments such as hearing loss require more supportive conditions to achieve in accordance with their potential.

The child with hearing loss is likely to progress best with more frequent and direct access to social and verbal interactions, more consistent adult responsiveness, more repetition in varied ways, and sometimes more consciously planned input. As a consequence, it becomes imperative that the parent and aural habilitationist understand the features of optimal, growth-promoting interactions between caregivers and their young babies and children in order to foster them. The Framework that follows is offered as an attempt to augment that understanding (Table 10-5).

Table 10–5. A Framework for Maximizing Caregiver Effectiveness in Promoting Auditory/Linguistic Development in Children Who Have Hearing Loss

Behavior	Comments

I. Sensitivity to Child

   1. Handles child in a positive manner.

   2. Paces play and talk in accordance with child's tempo.

   3. Follows child's interests much of the time.

   4. Provides appropriate stimulation, activities, and play for the child's age and stage.

   5. Encourages and facilitates child's play with objects and materials.

II. Conversational Behaviors

  A. In responding to the child

   6. Recognizes the child's communicative attempts.

   7. Responds to child's communicative attempts.

   8. Responds with a response which includes a question or comment requiring a further response from the child.

   9. Imitates child's productions.

  10. Provides child with the words appropriate to what he or she apparently wants to express.

  11. Expands child's productions semantically and/or grammatically.

  B. In establishing shared attention

  12. Attempts to engage child.

  13. Talks about what the child is experiencing, looking at, doing.

  14. Uses voice (first) to attract child's attention to objects, events, self.

Table 10–5. *continued*

Behavior	Comments
15. Uses body movement, gestures, touch appropriately in attracting child's attention to objects, events, self.	
16. Uses phrases and sentences of appropriate length and complexity.	
C. In general	
17. Pauses expectantly after speaking to encourage child to respond.	
18. Speaks to child with appropriate rate, intensity, and pitch.	
19. Uses interesting, animated voice.	
20. Uses normal, unexaggerated mouth movements.	
21. Uses audition-maximizing techniques.	
22. Uses appropriate gesture.	

Source: Adapted from Cole, E. B. (1992). *Listening and Talking: A Guide to Promoting Spoken Language in Young Hearing-Impaired Children.* Washington, DC: Alexander Graham Bell Association for the Deaf. (Reprinted with permission)

Structure of the Framework

Items on the Framework are intended to provide a guide to the major components of optimal caregiver communication-promoting behaviors, with several additions specific to interacting with a child who is deaf or hard of hearing. All of the items in Section I are related to being sensitive to the child in some way. This section is intended to highlight specific adult behaviors that can promote a positive affective environment. Section II of the Framework outlines the interactive mechanics of the situation: the "how" of establishing a shared focus, of responding, and of talking to the child. This section includes items from the language intervention literature that are believed to be facilitative of language development in children with language learning problems. Detailed explanations for all components can be found in Appendix 4.

Getting a Representative Sample of Interacting

This Framework is intended to be used in the study of videotaped samples of the parent and child interacting in a normal, everyday fashion. Videotaping is the method of choice for collecting the sample as it provides a retrievable record of both the auditory and visual components of the events. Because much early communicating occurs through nonvocal, nonauditory means such as changes in gaze direction, body orientation, and gesture, it is especially important to have the visual record available. Videotaping also allows for multiple reviewings of the interactional sample. This is necessary in order to account for social, physical, and linguistic dimensions of the context that contribute to the interactants' co-construction of meaning in a given instance.

The usefulness of the sample depends very heavily on the degree to which it is representative of normal interacting between this particular parent and child. Often the presence of the equipment and the observational aspects of the videotaping event mitigate against "naturalness." It is not unusual for the parent to feel a bit shy and embarrassed at the first taping session, or for either the parent or the child to "perform," sometimes unconsciously. Some of the measures listed in Table 10-6 may be helpful in counteracting these possibilities and attempting to set everyone at ease so that the sample will be as representative as possible.

Discussing the Framework with Parents

The interpersonal skills of the aural habilitationist are enormously important in the process of discussing something as personal and sensitive as the way a parent interacts with his or her child. The aural habilitationist will need to guard carefully against any possibility of conveying unspoken censure of the parent, since collaboration will be impossible if the parent feels judged or blamed. Some practical suggestions for addressing the items with sensitivity include the following:

Table 10–6. Steps to Consider in Trying to Get a Representative Sample of Interactive Behaviors When Videotaping

- Videotaping should take place in the child's home or in some other setting which is very familiar to the child.

- The interventionist should discuss the purpose and planned use of the tape with the caregiver. The purpose is to get a good sample of how the caregiver and child play and talk together, which will then be studied by both the interventionist and the parent to be certain that the interactions are as language-promoting as they can be. If taping is done on a routine basis and copies made for the parents, then the parents will have a record of their child's progress.

- The caregiver's help should be enlisted in order to decide which toys or activities to have available for the taping so that the caregiver and baby or toddler will be likely to interact a great deal (e.g., feeding or lunchtime; diaper-changing, bathing; playing in a swing; playing with play dough, tea set, dolls and clothes, building blocks, doctor kit, etc.).

- The interventionist should mention to the parent that he or she will be trying not to interact with either participant during the taping. The usefulness of the tape will be greatly compromised if much of the parent's talk is directed to the interventionist rather than to the child. It will also be compromised if the child is constantly looking off-camera at the interventionist, or walking over to him or her.

- The interventionist can set up the equipment, and then wait 5 or 10 minutes before actually beginning the taping in order to let some of the novelty wear off. It will depend upon the particular child whether or not it is most useful to allow some (limited) exploration of the equipment, or simply not to allow the child to touch it.

- The videotaping should be at least 10 or 15 minutes in duration. Usually adults' camera consciousness abates after about 5 minutes; children often forget about the camera immediately if the activity holds enough interest for them. After that occurs, the sample of normal, natural, everyday interacting needs to be at least 5 to 10 minutes in duration.

1. The caregiver can take home the tape and the Framework, and simply view the tape with the Framework items in mind. Or, the aural habilitationist could suggest that the caregiver look for specific target items, such as what the baby does every time the mother leans in and smiles.

2. In viewing the tape with the caregiver, the aural habilitationist can purposely point out examples of instances on the videotape where the parent demonstrates desired behaviors. Together, the aural habilitationist and the parent note the effect that the parent's behavior has on the child.

3. The aural habilitationist can check his or her perceptions with those of the parent. "I don't see a great deal of X in this little segment we videotaped. Is that what happens other times too?" or, "It looks to me as if you are working very hard to get Johnny's attention. Does it seem that way to you, too?"

4. As part of discussing a particular event or item, the aural habilitationist can ask open-ended, exploratory questions concerning that item. Examples might be, "How do you think you (or the child) were feeling at that point?" or, "What occurred to make that happen right there?" or, "How well does Johnny seem to imitate you when you sit beside him and speak close to his microphone?" These questions must be carefully phrased, so that they are not perceived as threatening or critical.

The Framework provides a *guideline* for desirable caregiver behaviors. It can be used to help parents become aware of how much they are already doing. It can also be used to identify behaviors they wish to change. In this regard, Luterman's words are relevant when he says, "People will learn just what they are ready to learn and absorb. The best indication of readiness is a parent-asked question: gratuitous information usually serves to increase confusion and is rarely helpful" (1984, p. 65). Behaviors the parents themselves identify as problematic are most likely to be the ones about which they will be ready to absorb suggestions. This does not mean that the aural habilitationist has to wait until the parent discovers every problem before bringing it up, but it does mean that the targets will not meet with much success if they are summarily selected and imposed by the aural habilitationist. A way needs to be found to help the parent discover the problematic areas in such a manner that they can "hear" the suggestions for change.

Ways of Addressing Parent-Chosen Targets

Once interactive targets for change have been identified, the next step is to determine how the targets will be worked on. Clearly, this is another instance of something that is most likely to be effective if it comes from the parent, rather than being imposed by the aural habilitationist. However, the aural habilitationist needs to be ready with suggestions to offer for the parent's consideration, if there is a need. Methods of achieving adult behavior change vary widely depending on the behaviors and the individuals involved. Simply becoming aware of the importance of a particular behavior (perhaps as a result of using the Framework) may be enough to cause a change in some behaviors. For example, a parent may notice that her voice was very high when she spoke to the child. To change it, the parent may just decide to try to keep her voice pitched lower, and be able to make that change simply from having decided to do it. Or, the parent may have a means for helping him- or herself to make the change. For example, the parent may decide to leave an audiotape recorder running as she is playing with the child at home in order to remind herself to keep her pitch down, and to provide a check of how well she is doing in that regard. Another idea is for the parent to ask someone at home to provide reminders or feedback regarding the behavior—including particularly instances where the change has occurred.

Other behaviors initially may be changed more easily if there is a period of focused feedback from the aural habilitationist. One way to do this is to examine in detail one or more instances where the behavior was problematic on the videotape. This examination might include consideration of what was happening just before the parent behavior occurred, exactly what the parent did, what the parent intended to accomplish by the action, and what effect the parent's behavior had on the child. Then a number of possible alternate behaviors for that instance could be generated. This focused feedback can be extended into an on-the-spot coaching event, also. This occurs when the parent and child play at some normal activity, and the aural habilitationist quietly interjects a suggestion at the exact moment the behavior either is or is not occurring. Using an FM system for this activity to connect parent and aural habilitationist may be a good idea with some parents, assuming there is a one-way mirror arrangement so that the aural habilitationist can be coaching from outside of the room. This kind of intense feedback may be useful for many of the behaviors on the Framework, but to be effective it must be done with the parent's full agreement.

The possible ways of helping a parent change behaviors are limited only by the particular behaviors involved and by the

> *Probably one of the most common strategies used in intervention is that of "expert" demonstration. The parent is expected to learn how to behave in a certain way from observing the expert do it. In this case, the aural habilitationist would interact with the child while being videotaped, and the parent and aural habilitationist would use the Framework to analyze what just occurred on the taped segment. Demonstration can be quite effective (and, in this context, it certainly makes you put your money where your mouth is), but it does have several inherent dangers. For example, the demonstration may leave the parent feeling overwhelmed and inadequate. It may also have looked so smooth and easy, and occurred so quickly that the parent may have missed the essential point of the demonstration. In order to counteract these possibilities, it may be useful to have the parent take over in interacting with the child immediately after the demonstration, and attempt to replicate it or to perform the desired behavior at the next opportunity, with the aural habilitationist right there to adjust or confirm.*

creativity of the parent and aural habilitationist. The key element in all of this, however, is that the effectiveness of any behavior change plan is directly dependent upon the parent's commitment to it. Adults respond most favorably when they are actively involved in designing and implementing their own learning. This is the reason that it is optimal for the parent to be the one who recognizes the problematic nature of a particular behavior, and who generates and enacts the plans for change. It is also the reason that the aural habilitationist needs to interact with the parent in ways that contribute to the *parent's* feeling of autonomy, confidence, and competence (DesJardin& Eisenberg, 2007).

Teaching Through Incidental and Embellished Interacting

This section of the chapter describes ways that parents and teachers can use everyday interactions to help babies, toddlers, and young children learn spoken language through listening. Two ways of teaching spoken language through normal, everyday interacting are incidental teaching and embellished teaching through playful interacting. Both incidental teaching and embellished teaching have a very high ecological validity in that what is being learned is totally related to normal natural learning by the child in the situational context in which the teaching is occurring (Barnett, VanDerHeyden, & Witt, 2007). Both situations involve individual teaching and learning (which generally is considered to be the most intense), although the instructional intensity might be seen to be less for situations where incidental teaching is occurring. On the other hand, that does not necessarily mean that learning is less. Each is explained in turn.

Teaching Through Incidental Interacting

Babies and young children are sponges for incidental learning, and adults who are interested in children are teaching them every time they interact with them, whether or not they are aware of it. Take a look at the following normal, everyday event that occurred between a parent and a 2½-year-old child who has a hearing loss.

The parent and child take a walk after an early summer rain shower, and they come upon a live worm on the sidewalk. The child points it out, "Look! Worm!" The parent leans down to see and replies, "Yes—I see it. Look! The worm is wiggling!"

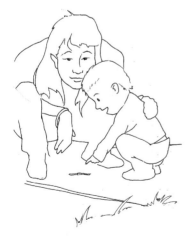

The child is fascinated by a wiggly worm on the sidewalk.

Without even trying, the parent is incidentally teaching the child an enormous variety of things. For example, she is teaching the child that what he says is meaningful and of communicative value to the parent; that people respond to each other in conversations; that the responding is generally related to the semantic content of the previous speaker's utterance. She is teaching him through repeated natural exposure that the "mover" (the worm) can perform an (intransitive) "action"; that the "mover/subject" is mentioned first, and then the "action/verb"; that the presently occurring action is coded by the use of a present progressive form of *be* + verb-*ing*; and that the subject is preceded by a definite article *the* that signals that the noun *worm* that follows it is known to both conversational partners. The event is, furthermore, an auditory one, since the parent leaned down to within about 18 inches of the child's hearing aids, and since the child was looking at the worm as they were talking, not at the parent's face. With regard to incidental speech-teaching in this event, the parent's intonation was animated and naturally varied, and thus provided auditory exposure to a normal speech pattern. There were no phonemes being particularly emphasized in the parent's utterance, unless one counts the /w/ since it was used in two words. However, any time the parent uses spoken language with the child, the child is being incidentally taught phonemes simply through exposure. All of these teaching aspects of the event can be considered to be by-products of the unrelated worm finding event, and thus fit the definition of incidental teaching and learning.

Teaching Through Embellished Interacting

Now, let's make this an embellished interaction. After having spoken, the parent realizes that the child probably does not know the word "wiggling." On the spot, the parent decides it is probably a useful word for this particular child to learn because "wiggling" is an action likely to continue to catch the child's fancy in a number of everyday contexts (worms, strings, spaghetti, the child—all wiggle). So, in the next breath, the parent says:

"Wiggle, wiggle, wiggle. The worm is *still* wiggling!" (Pause for the child to respond.) "Oh look! There's another worm that's wiggling." (Pause—the child finds a third worm.) "Oh—you found another one! Is that worm wiggling?" (Pause.) "Yes, it is! Oh, that's funny. Can you wiggle like a worm?" (And so on.)

In the parent's mind, "wiggle" has become a vocabulary goal. The parent is intentionally providing varied, repetitive exposure to that goal, and attempting to elicit it. The goal is specific and deliberately sought after, and the adult's actions are intended to reduce the time period required for the child to learn the word through depending entirely on the vagaries of totally natural exposure.

However, the teaching is incidental in that it is occurring with the child and parent focused on a normal, everyday activity, and the adult is employing ordinary language appropriate to that event (taking a walk and finding a worm). *This kind of incidental seizing-of-the-teachable-moment is embellished interacting, or embellished teaching by the adult.*

Teaching Spoken Language Through Embellished Interacting

The Framework for Maximizing Caregiver Effectiveness in Promoting Auditory/Linguistic Development in Children with Hearing Loss (see Table 10-5) lays out the components of embellished incidental teaching of spoken language. The idea is for the caregiver to make every effort to create a positive, accepting, and interesting communicative environment, and to interact with the child in ways that will promote the child's motivation to communicate verbally with increasing effectiveness. All of the items of the Framework relate to those objectives. Ways of better understanding the components, as well as improving them when needed, can be found in Appendix 4. Some additional important concepts for guiding the choices of items to embellish will be discussed below.

Underlying informal teaching embellishments that can be used to facilitate the child's learning of specific aspects of language is a time-honored language learning principle: the *Informativeness Principle* of Greenfield and Smith (1976). The idea stems from an observation that, at the one-word stage of linguistic development, when the child is going to talk, he or she is most likely to verbally encode the most informative (interesting, novel, uncertain, dynamic) element of the situation. So, for example, if the child's cookie falls off the table, the most likely utterance will concern the "fell down" business, not the "cookie" part. And if the child says nothing, the preferred adult utterance might be, "It fell down," rather than, "Oh! The cookie!" Of course, the aspect which is the most informative to the child may not always be obvious and predictable. For example, if the cookie falls off the table and the dog rapidly gobbles it up, one is faced with the quandary of whether "fell down," "all gone," or "doggie!" is the most interesting aspect of the situation to the child.

This means that, in providing the child with the words appropriate to what he or she wants to express, the parent needs to be observing keenly in order to encode (talk about) the most informative aspect of the situation which is presumably what the child would be trying to express (Paul, 2007). (See Framework items 2, 3, 6, 7, 10, 13.) The Informative Principle also has implications for the use of expansions. Extended expansions (which provide related and new ideas to the child's original utterance) fit well with the concept of informativeness. Minimal syntactic expansions fit less well since the addition of a plural *s* or an *-ing* probably has low informativeness value to the child. (See Framework item 11.)

Responding with a response that includes a question or comment for the child (Framework item 8) will also be most effective if the question or comment is purposefully centered on some salient, novel, or uncertain aspect. If one stretches the principle to include being informative, dynamic, and interesting, it could also include speaking in phrases and sentences of appropriate length and complexity, as well as speaking in an interesting and animated voice. (See Framework items 16 and 19.)

Several other language intervention techniques that are not on the Framework merit particular mention. They are excellent examples of ways of carrying out embellished incidental teaching, and they also adhere to the Informativeness Principle. They can be used to emphasize any language feature(s) that fit with the expectations for that child's age and stage. One of the techniques is the use of multiple examples. When an event occurs where the child has produced a target item or an approximation to it, the parent recreates and repeats the event paralleling what the child has done. For example, if the child is pretending to make a stuffed elephant jump off a chair and says, "Jump!" the adult [immediately thinking either of extended expansions or of mover-action, intransitive sentence frames (!)] could then say:

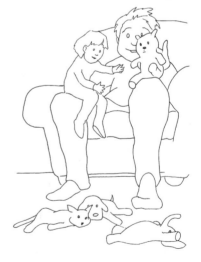

"Yes, the elephant jumped right off the chair!" (picking up a stuffed dog) "And then the doggie jumped." (making dog jump) "And the kitty cat jumped." (making cat toy jump off)

Father and child are having a great time making all the animals jump off the chair.

"And then the bear said, 'I want a turn!' (getting the bear ready to jump, and then pausing) "So then . . . " (And, one hopes, the child would say at least some part of, "The bear jumped.")

It should be noted that this is an auditory activity, in that the child is sitting on the parent's lap and is focused on the animals that are jumping, not watching the parent's face all of the time. This "jumping" scenario could also be used with a child who is not yet using words. The adult would similarly observe the child's play, provide the words, and vary one aspect of the play in an interesting and fun manner. The scenario could be simplified to be "Uh-oh—the (animal) fell down!" each time, with the expectation that the child might imitate the "Uh-oh" or the "fell down."

Another variation on this multiple example theme would be to provide several instances of exactly the same event, followed by one different one. Here, the adult would participate in the toy bear jumping off of the chair several times (while talking about it), and then have the bear *climb up* the chair to create a related, but new and remark-worthy event.

Other intervention techniques which conform to the Informativeness Principle require an already established routine or "script" (Weismer, 2000) between the adult and the child. Consequently, this technique would not be appropriate with a very small infant until the child has enough experience with the event to have built up an expectation regarding the way things *should* go. These strategies are based on Fey, Long, and Finestack (2003), Owens (2004), and Warren and Yoder's (1998) idea of the adult being a "saboteur" of routine events in order to stimulate communication or entice the child into communicating. One way to do this is to violate the order of the steps of a task or to omit one. For example, in making orange juice with the child, the parent could have the child pour the frozen juice into a container, and add the cans of water. Then the adult would act as if he or she was going to pour it into glasses (skipping the step of stirring). Or, object function can be violated through getting ready to pour the juice into a shoe or a hat. As mentioned above, the success of these techniques hinges on the child's knowledge that there is a "right" way for these events to occur. Otherwise, nothing will be said as the child will innocently accept what the adult is doing as normal behavior. But when sabotage works, it can be great fun since any harmless violation of expectations of this sort is likely to evoke laughter.

> *To reiterate, then, the parents' job is to provide an abundance of appropriate verbal interacting in the course of normal, everyday events. Within the course of this normal-but-embellished interacting, there are some strategies that the parent can use to emphasize particular language elements which are appropriate for the child's age and stage. These include providing the child with the words to describe what the child is likely to think is the most interesting aspect of the situation; providing expansions and extensions; using various kinds of multiple example techniques; violating the order of events or the function of objects; and purposefully setting up the environment so that a target is likely to be used (e.g., hiding objects). The notion underlying all of these strategies is that language is used for communicating—and all of these strategies create a meaningful reason to communicate. The possibilities are limited only by one's ingenuity.*

Other strategies are perhaps more obvious such as hiding objects in order to stimulate "Where?" questions, or to stimulate guesses as to the object's location. (It is not necessary to fake this situation in most households.) Another strategy, long recommended by teachers of the deaf, is to require that the child vocalize or speak in order to get something. This operant strategy is probably acceptable for phrases and situations well known to the child, similar to the common practice of saying, "You have to say 'please' before I'll give it to you." But the inherent danger is that it can turn into a power struggle, which the parent never wins no matter what the outcome.

Teaching Listening (Audition) Through Embellished Interacting

The explicated examples in Chapter 7 clearly illustrate the ways in which normal, everyday activities can be embellished in order to provide the child with opportunities to auditorily attend selectively; localize; discriminate; identify, categorize, associate; integrate, interpret, and comprehend. The suggestion was made that parents need to be aware that these "listening events" are occurring and are important. Then they will be able and motivated to create similar listening opportunities whenever possible in order to enhance the child's automatic and full use of residual hearing. Caregiver and interventionist auditory strategies need to be internalized and used in all interactions with the child. These strategies are listed in Table 10–7.

The reader is referred to Cole, Carroll, Coyne, Gill, and Paterson (2005), Estabrooks (2006), and Rossi (2003) for further additional examples of auditory strategies being used in the course of everyday activities. One caveat: there will be occasions when it is appropriate to smile and interact when your baby or young child *is* watching your face, and it is important to have fun and enjoy these moments without feeling guilty! The idea is to become more and more conscious of times when you can employ auditory strategies, and to do so as often as possible. Each time the child relies on hearing alone to listen and understand, he builds confidence in his auditory abilities.

Table 10–7. Auditory Strategies for Everyday Use

- Reduce or eliminate all extraneous noise. (Turn off the TV!)
- Get down on the child's level.
- Place yourself behind or beside the child near the microphone of the child's equipment.
- Talk, and expect the child to understand even when he or she is not watching your face.
- Keep the child's visual attention on the toys or objects in front of you both.
- If you do allow the child to watch your face, look for an opportunity to say it again right afterwards without allowing the child to watch.
- Present your message auditory-only the first time, and every time that you possibly can.
- Remember that by employing these strategies you are helping the child to gain confidence in his or her ability to understand based on listening alone.
- Be a parent who says "Listen!" (– not "Look at me!")

Teaching Speech Through Embellished Interacting

Phonating/Vocalizing

With some exceptions, very young children who are deaf or hard of hearing are usually vocalizing to some extent at the time that the hearing loss is detected. The task of the parents is to encourage an abundance of vocalizing by the child through consistently and positively responding to it (Brady, Marquis, Fleming, & McLean, 2004; Gazdag & Warren, 2000; Ling, 1989, 2002; Paul, 2007; Poehlman & Fiese, 2001; Yoder & Warren, 1998, 2002). The encouragement often takes the form of the parent smiling, looking interested, moving closer to the child, and imitating the child's vocalization. The child may also be encouraged to vocalize as a result of hearing and experiencing others talking around him or her. This would include the interactive nonsense babbling that parents sometimes initiate with babies, as well as humming and singing near the child. In fact, simply hearing language spoken to and around him or her may be a motivation for the child to vocalize.

Not all children are natural imitators, but having a child who imitates speech sounds can be very useful for a variety of reasons. One use is for planning which phonemes (speech sounds) or prosodic features (the features that make up the melody of speech: intonation, pitch, loudness, rhythmic patterns) should become the next targets for deliberate stimulation. Another reason imitation by the child is useful is that the child is extremely likely to imitate only sounds that he can hear. If the child cannot imitate a particular sound at all, or does it incorrectly, then it may be time to make adjustments to the child's hearing aids, earmold system, or cochlear implant programming in order to improve the child's access to that sound (usually it is a set of sounds similar to the missed one).

On the other hand, an incorrectly imitated speech sound could occur because the child has not learned to listen for its essential features. For example, the child might be confusing the *b* and the *m* sounds. These are two sounds that he can hear, but they sound the same to him or her because he has not learned to listen for their distinguishing features. The child's family or aural habilitationist can use auditory-based techniques to help him perceive the salient differences and to produce the sounds differently.

Another reason that the child being able and willing to imitate is useful is for checking whether or not the child's cochlear implant or digital hearing aids have been appropriately programmed. If the child could hear and imitate a particular sound, and then suddenly is unable to, then it is likely that the child no longer has adequate auditory access to the acoustic information necessary for perceiving it. In this case, improvements to the program are likely to result in immediate restoration of the child's ability to hear and imitate the target sound(s). If the child has never been able to hear or produce the sound, when auditory access is provided he is unlikely to suddenly produce it correctly (although that sometimes does happen). However, with a few days of focused attention on the sound in playful speech activities, he is likely to show major improvement.

How to Encourage a Child to Imitate

If the child is 2 to 5 months old and is wearing hearing instruments that provide him or her with appropriate access to speech, then engaging in playful speech is usually easy. Infants at this age will often babble back and forth with an adult, if the adult has playfully imitated a sound that the infant just produced. Mealtimes and diaper-changing times are great times to get a vocal volley of this nature going.

If the child is no longer an infant, then playful speech activities can become one of the ways in which caregivers and toddlers interact with each other. The child vocalizes; the adult smiles, leans toward the child, imitates the vocalization, and waits expectantly for the child to vocalize again; the child vocalizes; and the adult imitates whatever the child said; and so on. If the child does not seem to have the idea of this kind of back-and-forth babbling game, then try nonverbal imitative games. These imitative games can be "speechy," such as imitating mouth movements (raspberries, sticking out the tongue in different goofy directions, pursing the lips, kissing), or imitating hand motions and facial expressions for "Mmmmm" or "Yuck!" or imitative singing games such as "Eensy Weensy Spider." Taking turns kissing small plastic animals one at a time and tossing them in a fishbowl (no fish in it!) or a glass carafe filled with water is another playful imitative game. After the plastic toys are in the water, it can be stirred to make a whirlpool bath. The idea is to catch the child's fancy, keep it playful, and have him imitate without thinking about it.

Another way to elicit imitation is using a toy that can be operated with a switch or a squeeze ball that is out of sight, such as a hopping frog or Oscar coming out of his garbage can. The adult models the motion or words ("Hop hop hop" or knocking on Oscar's garbage can, and saying, "Oscar, come out!"). Then the toy is moved toward the child, and the child is encouraged to imitate the adult's model. Nothing happens until the child does what's needed, or unless the adult repeats the model. Then the toy needs to be put away so that the child does not discover what was actually making the frog hop or Oscar come out.

Once the child will play imitative turn-taking games, start to build specific speech sounds into the play. It is important to vary the length of the speech sound strings, as well as to vary the intonation and loudness. Listening for and imitating increasingly longer strings of reduplicated and alternated syllables has the added bonuses of helping build the child's auditory memory (listening and remembering) and practicing the automaticity needed for articulation in running speech.

Sound-Toy Associations

One frequently suggested early intervention strategy is to associate a deliberately selected sound with a particular toy or with a frequently occurring event (Cole et al, 2005; Estabrooks, 2006; Ling, 2002). Sound-toy association has several benefits, including enhancing the child's perception and production of speech sounds. (It also teaches a consistent sound/word for each of the toys or activities.) Examples follow of sound-toy and sound-event associations that can be used in many daily situations, but the caregiver can make up others that will recur frequently in their particular home routines.

To Highlight Intonational Variation

Use dramatic expressions such as "Uh-oh" (for things falling down), "All gone" (for food being finished or toys rolling under furniture), "Oh no!" (for toys colliding or breaking or accidents of all kinds), "Wow!" (for delightful events), "Mmmm" (for anything smelling or tasting good), "Aaaaaaa" or Aaaaaaaeeeeeee" or "Aaaeeeaaaeee" of long duration (to signify flying of airplanes or birds). Produce the phrases with very marked high/low contrasts of the intonational contours.

To Highlight Variations in Intensity

Use "Shhhh!" and a whisper for any quiet events such as a baby or doll sleeping. Play the "wake up" game where one person closes his eyes and pretends to sleep ("Shhhh! X is sleeping."). The other one shouts ("Boo!" or the person's name) to wake him up.

To Highlight Variations in Rhythmic Patterns (Duration)

Use expressions that have interesting contrasts of rhythmic patterns such as "So . . . big!"; or "Drip drip drip" for a faucet or for rain falling off of a flower versus "Shhhhhhhh" (sound of water coming out of faucet quickly) or "Pitter-patter" for ongoing rain; or "Mmmm" for something smelling or tasting good, versus "Yuck!" for the reverse; or "Up up up up—down . . . " for a small doll climbing up a slide and then coming down; "Choo-choooo . . . " for the train's whistle, and "Ch-ch-ch-ch" for the train moving (pretend they still sound like that).

To Highlight Specific Vowel Sounds

For /a/   "Hop hop hop" (a rabbit or a frog) or "Hot!"

For /i/   "Peek-a-boo!" or "Peek!" or "Go to sleep!" "Whee!"

For /u/   "Boo!" or "Mooooooooo" or "Ooooooo" (train whistle)

For /au/   "Meow" or "Bowwow" or "Ow!" or "Round and round"

For /ai/   "Bye-bye" or "eye" or "Hi!"

For /ɛ/   "bed" or "wet"

For /ʊ/   "push" or "woof woof"

For /ae/   "quack quack" or "Daddy"

For /ʌ/   · "up" or "cut"

For /o/   "nose" or "No no!" or "It broke." "It's broken."

To Highlight Specific Consonant Sounds

For /b/   "Bye-bye" or "Boo!"

For /p/   "Ppppppp" (boat sound) or "Pop!" (bubbles)

For /w/   "Walk, walk, walk" (any toy or person walking)

For /m/   "Mmmmmmm!" (for something smelling or tasting good)

For /h/   "Hi!" or "Ho ho ho!" (Santa Claus)

For ʃ   "Shhhhh!"

For /f/   "Off!" or "foot"

For tʃ   "Ch-ch-ch" (train sound)

---

*To be effective, the sound should be used consistently whenever the child plays with the toy or the event occurs. The child can thus learn in a very natural manner to associate the toy or event with both listening for and producing the chosen sound. Once the child can, using audition alone, select or indicate the toy or activity for a set 6 to 8 items, he has demonstrated that he can associate a sound with a toy, and understands how to do auditory selection using sounds, words, or phrases. It is important always to surround the targeted sound with talk about the toy or activity ("I hear a boat that's going ppppp very quietly."), so that the child doesn't begin to think that a "ppppppp" is a boat. When the child has demonstrated that he or she can say "ppppp," it is time to drop that sound as a label for the boat, and time to use the real word for **boat**, pairing it with the "ppppp" but soon insisting on usage of the word, not just the sound.*

Parent Guidance Sessions or Auditory-Verbal Therapy Sessions

When the goal is for the child with hearing loss to learn to talk, the child's parents need information and guidance from professionals who specialize in developing spoken language through listening. Often, that support occurs through Auditory Verbal Therapy or through parent guidance sessions. Parent guidance sessions or Auditory-Verbal Therapy sessions should be part of the intervention plan for any family with a young child who has hearing loss. For children in the birth to three age range, federal law currently requires that sessions occur in naturalistic environments. This generally is interpreted to be the child's home or day care center. The principle of providing intervention in comfortable, normal settings is a valid one for children with many types of disabilities. However, for children with hearing loss who are learning spoken language through listening, the home or daycare can sometimes present so much noise that the child cannot hear anything but the noise. If the noise cannot be reduced or eliminated, a different, quiet setting must be found to be able to provide an appropriate listening and learning environment that takes into account the unique listening needs of a child with a hearing loss. This is the only way that the parent will be able to know that the child really *can* learn through listening.

The same concern about noise exists for children in the 3- to 6-year-old age range who are in preschool group settings, as described in Chapter 6. Individual sessions for children in the 3- to 6-year-old range also need to take place in a quiet setting. For children in group preschool settings, individual sessions with the aural habilitationist may take place on a daily basis. However, parents of preschoolers need to be involved in the sessions at least once a week so that all of the child's team is working on the same goals and objectives in a similar manner, and so that the parent can engage in ongoing discussion about the child's equipment, instructional program, and progress. This is very important for most parents of preschoolers with hearing loss, and crucial for parents whose child's hearing loss was discovered late.

The sessions are carefully preplanned by the professional to include time to talk with the parent about how the child is doing, as well as time for diagnostic therapy with the child for checking progress, for determining what's next in stretching the child's abilities, and for demonstrating techniques and activities to teach targets. Parents are present and participating for all of each session, since the parent is expected to implement suggestions and activities at home. Here is a list of the kinds of things that need to be accomplished in a session.

Components to Be Accomplished in a Typical Preplanned Session

- Confirmation that the child has access to sound.
- Checking with parent about child's progress and the parent's homework.
- Diagnostic practice through play on specific auditory-linguistic targets with aural habilitationist and parent changing roles throughout as the person interacting with the child; aural habilitationist coaches, as appropriate. Activities are playful, geared to child's needs, paced to child's interest/stamina level, and interspersed with songs, books, gross motor movement, and play, as appropriate. Depending on the child's age and attention span, there could be as many as 10 or 12 toys played with in a preplanned fashion, or as few as 4 or 5 toys or preplanned activities.
- Parent and aural habilitationist discuss any of the following:
  — Issues of concern to parent
  — Information that needs to be taught
  — What will be done at home during the next week by parent and child (homework)
- Closing routine with child; could include turning off lights, picking up toys, saying good-bye, walking to door.

The aural habilitationist's job is to create activities that will both teach and test the child's ability to meet the target(s) that are on his agenda. Experienced therapists say that they approach that task from two different directions. One is to start from the direction of the target or goal. In considering the target, what playful and enticing activity could be done that would cause the child to "fall over" the target multiple times? The other way of approaching the planning of the session is to consider first the kinds of activities and toys that the child will enjoy, and then to see how those toys can be used to provide playful practice on the child's targets. The challenge of solving this puzzle for assisting each child to achieve multiple auditory, language, and speech targets playfully is at the heart of preplanned intervention for children who have hearing loss.

Not surprisingly, general principles for intervention include many of the same strategies discussed above for embellished interacting. A list follows:

- Using motherese (except not using a higher vocal pitch)
- Providing reasons to talk
- Keeping the communication meaningful and informative
- Using multiple exemplars
- Enticing the child to communicate
- Using routines or "scripts" for certain activities (includes songs and rhymes)
- Providing choices for the child to make so that communication is meaningful
- Expanding the child's utterances
- Extending the child's utterances
- Encouraging imitation
- Encouraging initiations and self-generated language from the child
- Always pushing on to the next step (If the child can say *big*, teach him *huge*, *gigantic*, *mammoth*, and even *gi-normous*.)
- Using literature
- Keeping it playful

Sample Preplanned Scenario

An example of a preplanned core activity with a 20-month-old and his mother follows. The event took approximately 15 minutes from beginning to end. This is an example of diagnostic practice on specific auditory and linguistic targets. The child's equipment has already been checked, and the parent's homework from the previous week discussed.

The Context

The aural habilitationist, the mother, and the child are sitting at a small table. This particular child has a severe hearing loss that was identified 4 months before this session. He is just beginning to produce vowels with some variety and on demand. The aural habilitationist has three small toys hidden in a box: a rabbit (for /a/ in *hop hop hop*); a cow (for /u/ in *mooo*); and a dog (for /au/ in *bow wow*). The specific speech goals in the aural habilitationist's mind are for the child to imitate /a/, /u/, and /au/ in the course of the activity; the auditory goals are to participate in the routines for listening, and to select correctly each toy when its sound is produced. The language goals include learning *hop*, *moo*, and *bow wow* as lexical items of a sort, as well as more informal goals of being optimally exposed to language and communication.

The choice of *hop hop hop* and *moooo* and *bow wow* as three words using the three target phonemes was not random. The three words provide salient contrasts in duration which may be the acoustic parameter that the child first utilizes in discriminating among them. Further, they are all mid- to low-frequency, intense sounds, which enhances the likelihood of the child easily detecting them and attending to them. And finally, /au/ is a diphthong requiring rapid tongue movement (always a desirable target) from the /a/ part to the /u/ part of the diphthong.

The Action

The aural habilitationist shakes the box, looking intrigued, and says, "I hear something. I think there's something in the box . . . Listen, Mommy!" The aural habilitationist hands the box to the child's mother.

The mother also shakes the box, looks interested and curious, and says, "I hear something too! Here, Alan—you want to listen too?" She hands the box to the child.

Alan shakes the box with vigor, vocalizing with a central vowel sound he frequently uses.

The mother smiles and says, "You hear that too, don't you!"

Explanation

The box-shaking routine is done to encourage the child to listen and to be curious about sounds he hears. By having the mother listen, and then react to hearing the sound, the aural habilitationist has provided the child with a model of listening and of being interested and excited about listening. Also, by having the parent immediately take over and perform the same activity, the aural habilitationist demonstrated an embellished informal strategy for the parent that could be used in other everyday instances. If there was some problem in the parent's ability to carry out the activity, the aural habilitationist could gently coach the parent right at that moment.

The Action

Alan starts to try to open the box. The box is purposely fastened in such a way that a child cannot open it. Alan hands the box to the aural habilitationist, looks her in the eye, and vocalizes.

Explanation

The box is "child-proofed" so that the child will be required to ask for help in order to get it open. This creates a need for the child to express a request for an action, and allows exposure to an "Open the _____" routine.

The Action

The aural habilitationist accepts the box and says, "Oh, okay. You want me to open the box. Here, I'll open it for you." The aural habilitationist quickly removes the rabbit from the box and conceals it in her hand. She says, "I found a little bunny rabbit! This rabbit goes hop hop hop." As she says "hop hop hop," she brings up her hand holding the rabbit to partially conceal her mouth. She says "hop hop hop" again in this way, and then reaches her hand out (still holding the rabbit) toward the mother's face.

The mother recognizes this as a cue to repeat what the aural habilitationist said and did. The mother immediately says, "The rabbit goes hop hop hop," and makes the rabbit hop. The child's eyes are on the rabbit, not on the mother's lips, so the mother does not try to conceal her mouth.

The aural habilitationist then says, "Yes! It goes hop hop hop," holding the hand-concealed rabbit in front of her mouth again, smiling, and looking pleased. She then reaches it toward the child's mouth, as she had just done with the mother, as a cue for the child to produce (imitate) the sounds. The child says "A a a," and the aural habilitationist smiles and says, "Yes, that's right. The rabbit goes hop hop hop right over to you!" She gives the rabbit to the child to play with for a few minutes.

(The action to this point has taken about 60 seconds, at most; the child plays with the rabbit for another minute or two.)

Explanation

The aural habilitationist's actions are intended to encourage the child to listen to and imitate the *hop hop hop*. She conceals the rabbit to add an element of mystery. She speaks in phrases and sentences of normal length, and uses the *hop hop hop* target in a sentence, not just in isolation. The aural habilitationist covers her mouth in order to require that the child listen to the target. The hand cue is consciously used in order to signal the moment when the other person is supposed to imitate. The mother is again used as a model for the child's behavior. If the child had not imitated, the mother could have demonstrated *hop hop hop* again; then the child could be given one more opportunity to produce the target prior to being given the toy. The child needs to be given the toy as a reward for staying involved in the activity, even if he does not produce the sound!

The Action

Then the aural habilitationist brings out a toy barn and places it on the table in front of the child. The aural habilitationist says, "Alan, the rabbit is *so* sleepy. He wants to go to sleep. He wants to go to sleep in the barn." She opens the barn door and puts the rabbit inside. The aural habilitationist says, "Night night, rabbit. Go to sleep. Shhhh!" She shuts the barn door, pushes the barn to the far side of the table out of the child's reach, while saying, "Night night, rabbit. Shhhh!" again.

(The going-to-sleep episode takes 10 to 20 seconds. It could be more if the child participated a great deal, or if he objected to giving up the toy.)

Explanation

This same routine is repeated for the other two toys (the cow and the dog), with the parent being the one who controls the toys, exposes the child to the targets, and attempts to elicit them.

The Action

After all three animals are safely sleeping in the barn, the aural habilitationist glides right into an auditory selection activity. While Alan is looking at the barn where the last animal just disappeared, the aural habilitationist can say, "Uh-oh. Time to wake up, cow! Can you wake up the cow, Alan? I want the one that goes 'Moooo!' Can you wake up the one that goes 'Moooo'?" Alan looks blankly at the aural habilitationist. The aural habilitationist says, "Let's see if Mommy can help. Mommy, can you get me the one that goes 'Moooo'?"

The mother does, saying "Come on, cow. Wake up. Time to go! Moooo!" The mother puts the cow back in the box the aural habilitationist is holding and says, "Bye-bye, cow! Moooo!" The exit of the other animals is similarly handled, with the child being given every opportunity to select the correct toy based on the auditory message alone, as well as to produce the sound. The activity is over when the last animal is inside the box.

The aural habilitationist and the mother then discuss all the ways in which "hop hop hop" and "shhhhh" might come up during the next week, and how the parent will try to emphasize these two words through daily play and interacting.

Explanation

This part of the activity allows the toys to be left on the table but out of sight, and out of immediate consideration. It also allows for exposure to the routines for "Go to sleep" (for the /i/ sound) and to "Shhhh!"

Most of the basic principles for effective language facilitation are there. The context is play; the language is normal; the targets are generally incorporated into complete sentences; much repetitive but varied exposure to the targets is provided; at the aural habilitationist's request, the mother demonstrates auditory and speech behaviors for the child; the aural habilitationist demonstrates strategies for the parent to use to encourage the child to listen and to imitate; the parent attempts the activities immediately after the aural habilitationist; and the parent, rather than the aural habilitationist, does the majority of the interacting with the child.

Substructure

Preplanned teaching events generally have three parts: (a) getting the toys or materials out in front of the participants, (b) playing with the toys or materials, and (c) getting the toys or materials put away again. Each part of the event has auditory, speech, language, and management routines associated with it which, once learned by all the participants, make the event flow smoothly.

In this example, the speech and language routines are centered on consistent use of the sound-toy and sound-event associations. Examples from the session include the box-opening episode ("Open the X") and the episode where the animals were put to sleep in the barn ("Go to sleep. Shhhh!"). One auditory routine in the illustration occurs at the outset where the box is shaken, making a noise, and the aural habilitationist and the mother model listening behavior while talking about it. When the aural habilitationist and the mother conceal their mouths, it is a routine intended to require the child to listen carefully. But it also could be considered a management routine, whereby the child is being cued to listen as a preface to being asked to imitate or respond. Using the mother to model correct responding behavior probably also provides the same sort of management cue ("Be alert—you are next!") as does the practice of holding a closed hand near the mouth of the person whose turn it is to speak.

It should be noted that these are *not* routines until the child and parent have participated in them a number of times!

About the Benefits and Limitations of Preplanned Teaching

For the child who cooperates easily, there is likely to be one major benefit: The time required for the child to acquire the targets through natural exposure may be reduced. This may happen because of the greater amount of repetition provided, and because of the increased demands for imitative practice that occur in a teaching event of this kind, which is surely instructionally intense. For the aural habilitationist who employs this kind of activity, there may accrue a feeling that tangible progress is being carefully crafted, and that "real" teaching is going on. The parent may also feel comfortable with preplanned activities for those reasons.

However, one concern about direct teaching of specific targets is that the child's learning may not generalize to other situations, or in the worst case, the targets learned may not even be appropriate for use in situations other than in therapy. This is clearly something to guard against in planning.

In addition, the adult is very much in charge of this kind of activity, and the child's primary role is to cooperate by listening, imitating, and doing what he or she is told. For some children, even at 5 years of age, these are very exacting demands! However, although the period from 18 months to 3 years (and older) is notorious as a time for children to be asserting their independence through the full variety of noncooperative tactics, a number of young children really enjoy short periods of adult-directed play. The success of this type of activity seems to hinge on the child's desire to comply, and on teacher or parent ability to keep the child's interest and enthusiasm high.

Strategies for maintaining the child's interest and enthusiasm are ones that promote the activity's naturalness and informality. These include playing with vigor and enthusiasm; smiling, patting, and hugging the child; joking; using age-appropriate toys; creating mystery and curiosity (hiding the toys); letting the child be as active as possible (letting the child shake the box and eventually play with the toys); giving the child choices to make; judging the pace of the steps appropriately (moving quickly from one step to the next, but at the same time pausing to allow the child sufficient time to participate); and recognizing and responding in a positive manner to all of the child's attempts to communicate. These strategies mask the adult-directiveness and make the preplanned teaching event communicative and fun.

The most important thing to remember in implementing intervention intended to help the parent help the child learn to talk is to *listen to the parent and to the child.* Plans are meant to be carefully prepared, and then tossed rapidly out the window if competencies or interests were improperly estimated, or if other needs arise that are more pressing, such as a grandma coming to visit, or the child not responding auditorily as well as several days ago, or the child having learned how to pump on the swing, or the parent having a meltdown from trying to keep hearing aids on very tiny pliable ears, or a family of turkeys walking by the window. Don't ever let lessons get in the way of life!

How to Grow Your Baby's/Child's Brain

This is a handout that can be given to all families who have infants or children with any type and degree of hearing problem.

Above all, love, play, and have fun with your child!

1. The *quieter* the room and the *closer* you are to your child, the better you will be heard. The child may have difficulty over-hearing conversations and hearing you from a distance. You need to be close to your child when you speak. Keep the TV and CD player off when not actively listening to them.

2. Your child must *wear his or her hearing aid or cochlear implant during all waking hours* (except bathing or swim-ming, of course), every day of the week. The brain needs con-stant, detailed auditory input in order to develop. Knowingly depriving your child of this access is a form of neglect. The technology is your access to the brain and your child's access to full knowledge of the world around him. If your child pulls off the devices, promptly, persistently, and calmly replace them.

3. Check your child's technology regularly. Equipment malfunc-tions, often. Become proficient at *troubleshooting*.

4. *Use an FM system at home* to facilitate distance hearing and incidental learning. An FM system can be used during reading, too, to improve the signal-to-noise ratio and to facilitate the development of auditory self-monitoring. Place the FM micro-phone on the child so that she can clearly hear her own speech, thereby facilitating the development of the "auditory feedback loop."

5. *Focus on listening*, not just seeing. Call attention to sounds and to conversations in the room. Point to your ear and smile, and talk about the sounds you just heard and what they mean. Use listening words such as "You heard that," "You were listening," and "I heard you."

6. *Maintain a joint focus of attention* when reading and when engaged in activities. That is, the child looks at the book or at the activity while listening to you.

7. Speak in sentences, not single words, with *clear speech* using lots of melody. Speak a bit slower to allow the child time to process the words. Many adults speak faster than most children can listen.

8. *Read aloud* to your child, daily. Even infants can be read to, as can older children. Try to read at least 10 books to your baby or child each day. We should be reading chapter books by preschool.

9. *Sing and read nursery rhymes* to your baby or young child every day. Fill her days with all kinds of music and songs to promote interhemispheric transfer.

10. Name *objects* in the environment as you encounter them during daily routines. Constantly be mindful of expanding vocabulary.

11. Talk about and *describe* how things sound, look, and feel.

12. Talk about where objects are *located*. You will use many prepositions such as *in, on, under, behind, beside, next to, and between*. Prepositions are the bridge between concrete and abstract thinking.

13. Compare how objects or actions are *similar and different* in size, shape, quantity, smell, color, and texture.

14. *Describe sequences*. Talk about the steps involved in activities as you are doing the activity. Sequencing is necessary for organization and for the successful completion of any task.

15. Tell *familiar stories* or stories about events from your day or from your past. Keep *narratives* simpler for younger children, and increase complexity as your child grows.

APPENDIX

2

Application and Instructions for the Ling 6-7 Sound Test

The Ling 6-7 sounds are /oo/, /ah/, /ee/, /s/, /sh/, and /m/. The seventh is a silent interval.

For a child 18 months of age and older, start out sitting next to the child about three inches away, and encourage the child to drop a toy or block into a container when he or she detects each sound. You may need to have parents and/or older siblings model this behavior or provide a "hand-over-hand" facilitation for the child before he or she begins to listen and drop independently. Continue saying the sounds and gradually, one step at a time, move away from the child. Note the distance cutoffs. Once you know the child's distance hearing, administer the test only at that distance. There is no need to start close because the issue is the monitoring of distance hearing. Distance hearing depends on the hearing loss, hearing for that day, ambient room noise, and hearing aid or cochlear implant efficiency. All consonants and vowels should be detected out to 40 feet in quiet with cochlear implants. For children who wear hearing aids, the /sh/ and /s/, due to their weak acoustic energy and high frequencies, may need much closer distances for detection than vowels.

For children between the ages of 6 months and 18 months, have the child sit in a high chair. A test assistant will need to have "quiet toys" for the child to play with or look at to keep the child occupied. With the presenter standing behind the child and out of the child's visual range, present each of the Ling-6 sounds individually.

Note when the child turns to look for the sound presented. The assistant should then regain the child's attention with the quiet toys, so the next Ling sound can be presented.

For children less than 6 months of age, hold the child close to you with the child's best ear or hearing aid nearest you. Sing the Ling 6 Song to the tune of "Wheels on the Bus," while rocking the child back and forth. Include siblings and other family members by using "hand cuing" or "toy cuing" to encourage them to repeat the Ling 6 sounds as presented in the song. This will act as a model for the child and will help to acoustically highlight the Ling 6 sounds for the infant.

> *Take care to produce all sounds at a normal conversational loudness. Do not increase your intensity or sound duration as you increase your distance from the child.*

APPENDIX

3

Targets for Auditory/Verbal Learning

Prerequisite for Auditory Brain Development:

*Child/Student wears hearing aid/implant all waking hours.

*For all distance listening activities, the teacher needs to be sure to know the range of hearing that the child's technology allows (e.g., can the child detect /s/ at 8 inches, 30 feet, or some other distance).

<u>Directions:</u> These are targets for auditory/linguistic learning that, over time, should be demonstrated by a child with hearing loss who is learning spoken language through listening. See Chapter 7 for a more complete explanation of the usage of this chart.

A suggested way of tracking development of the behaviors is to write the observation dates in the corresponding column. "Rarely observed" refers to behaviors that are observed less than 50% of the time, "Emerging" behaviors are those which occur approximately 50 to 75% of the time when they could have occurred, and behaviors which are "Appropriate Demonstrated" are those that occur approximately 80% or more of the time when they could have occurred.

Phase I: Being Aware of Sound

Stage/Skill	Indicators/Examples	Rarely Observed	Emerging	Appropriately Demonstrated
1. Responds reflexively to sound (auditory attention).	*Young child:* May blink or widen eyes; startle; cry; change rhythm of sucking or breathing.			
2. Searches for sound/attempts to lateralize or localize (auditory attention).	*Young child:* May move eyes and/or head in seeking the sound source; look toward a nearby adult or speaker; perform head turning responses for visual reinforcement audiometry. Older child: Looks for sources of sounds.			
3. Sustained attention to sound (auditory attention).	*Young child:* Moves body rhythmically, smiles and coos to talking or music *Older child:* May clap, sing, dance in response to music, nursery rhymes, poems, or clapping patterns; attends to nearby conversations			
4. Demonstrates learned responses to having heard something without seeing the sound source (auditory association).	*Young child:* Points to ear, smiles, looks to adult, claps when sound is heard, participates in Visual Reinforcement Audiometry reliably. *Older child:* Reliably performs the Conditioned Play Task by raising hand, pushing button, or saying "I heard that" for audiologic testing. Takes off equipment and gives/shows to adult.			
5. Indicates that hearing aid/cochlear implant is not working (auditory attention).	*Young child:* Takes off equipment, takes off equipment and gives/shows to adult. *Older child:* Tells adult when equipment is not working.			

312

Phase II: Connecting Sound with Meaning

Stage/Skill	Indicators/Examples	Not Present	Emerging	Appropriately Demonstrated
1. Responds to speech (auditory association).	*Young child:* Smiles or coos responsively *Older child:* Turns toward speaker(s)			
2. Responds to novel sounds (auditory association).	*Young child:* Quiets or excites *Older child:* Searches for sound sources, or may ask what made a novel sound.			
3. Responds to loud, unexpected noises (auditory association).	*Young child:* May cry or indicate displeasure, or simply widen eyes or startle. If sound is repeated without meaning, child may no longer respond.			
4. Responds to hearing aid/cochlear implant being turned on (auditory association).	*Young child:* May quiet, change vocalizations *Older child:* May smile, or point to ear, or say "It's working."			
5. Speechlike vocalizations (early auditory feedback)	*Young child:* Uses some clear vowels/consonants, intonational and rhythmic patterns—child's vocalizing sounds "speechy."			

continues

Stage/Skill	Indicators/Examples	Not Present	Emerging	Appropriately Demonstrated
6. Responds to calling voice (without seeing the speaker).	Searches, turns, stops activity.			
a. in quiet (close by)				
b. in noise (close by) (auditory figure-ground)	N.B. This can be a difficult—if not impossible—task for some children. Practice in controlled conditions may improve the child's ability, but FM should be used in all instances at home and at school where it is important that the speaker's message be heard in order to reduce the detrimental effects of even "small" amounts of noise and of distance on the child's ability to hear and understand.			
c. from another room (distance listening)	This is a very important milestone as it suggests some level of auditory scanning of the environment, and attentiveness to messages that are not directed toward the child within his or her visual field (rudimentary *overhearing*). The child's technology may or may not limit ability to do this; surrounding noise may also make it difficult.			

Stage/Skill	Indicators/Examples	Not Present	Emerging	Appropriately Demonstrated
7. Anticipates what comes next in simple nursery rhymes, finger plays, songs, stories (auditory closure).	*Young child:* Expresses what comes next using body movements vocalizations, words. *Older child:* Expresses what comes next using words.			
a. live voice				
b. recorded voice (somewhat degraded signal)				
8. Engages in vocal turn-taking.	*Young child:* Raspberries, vowel sounds, repeats consonants, intonational patterns			
a. one or two exchanges				
b. three or more exchanges				

Phase III: Understanding Simple Language Through Listening

Stage/Skill	Indicators/Examples	Not Present	Emerging	Appropriately Demonstrated
1. Performs appropriate actions when common, everyday words are used without watching the speaker's face.	*Young child:* Stops activity (words such as "no"), waves (words such as "bye-bye"), looks toward the person (words such "mama"), points (words such as "uh-oh," "all gone"). *Older child:* Responds appropriately to common, everyday phrases or requests (e.g., "Get your shoes," "Time to go!," "Daddy's/Mommy's home!").			
2. Responds to Learning to Listen sounds (up to seven) without watching the speaker's face.	*Young child:* Reaches for toy associated with sound.			
3. Imitates an increasing number and variety of speech sounds with prosodic features varied (auditory feedback).	*Young child:* Imitates a variety of sounds in playful elicited speech activities. *Older child:* Imitates an increasing number of speech sounds with accuracy and ease of production in an increasing number of co-articulated syllable contexts.			

Stage/Skill	Indicators/Examples	Not Present	Emerging	Appropriately Demonstrated
4. Responds to Ling 6 Sounds				
a. detection	*Young child:* Puts rings on a post, claps, throws soft toys in container, raises hand			
b. discrimination/ identification	Imitates sounds.			
5. Responds appropriately to simple questions or requests without seeing the speaker's face.				
a. in a closed set of up to 7 items (identification)	Chooses the correct object or picture from a set of known objects or pictures.			
b. in normal, everyday situations (comprehension)	Follows a few one-step requests or responds to simple questions without watching the speaker.			
6. Engages in brief, spontaneous, pragmatically correct conversations on simple, everyday topics with 1 or 2 exchanges without watching the speaker's face.	Participates in conversation with an adult or peer without watching the other person's face.			

Phase IV: Understanding Increasingly Complex Language Through Listening

Stage/Skill	Indicators/Examples	Not Present	Emerging	Appropriately Demonstrated
1. Responds appropriately to a variety of familiar, everyday phrases and expressions and questions without watching the speaker's face.	Time for lunch, What do you want for lunch, ___ or ___? Where's your ___? Get the ___ ___. (Adjective + Noun)			
a. in quiet				
b. in noise (auditory figure-ground)				
c. at a distance when engaged in play	This is an important milestone, suggesting some level of auditory scanning, and *overhearing*.			
2. Spontaneously imitates familiar, everyday phrases or other peoples' speech, with or without fully understanding what they are saying (auditory memory).	N.B. Can be immediate or delayed imitation (sometimes occurs to the amusement or chagrin of the adults). This is an important auditory/ linguistic/cognitive milestone, since the child is imitating from *overhearing* conversation rather than direct instruction!			
3. Recognizes recordings of familiar songs and rhymes	Sings or fills in familiar parts			

Stage/Skill	Indicators/Examples	Not Present	Emerging	Appropriately Demonstrated
4. Imitates an increasing number of random digits: 4, 5, 6, 7, 8, 9 digits. (auditory memory)	Repeats an increasing number of random digits; try both frontward and backward.			
5. Imitates increasingly longer utterances in accordance with language abilities (auditory tracking and auditory memory).	Imitates words, phrases, sentences			
a. 2–3 words in length				
b. 4–5 words in length				
c. 7–10 words in length				
6. Begins using words or expressions that have not been directly taught.	Uses novel words/expressions, which have not been directly taught— a very important auditory/linguistic/cognitive milestone as it is clear evidence that the child is learning from *overhearing*.			

continues

Phase IV *continued*

Stage/Skill	Indicators/Examples	Not Present	Emerging	Appropriately Demonstrated
7. Without watching the speaker's face, responds appropriately to utterances that increase in grammatical complexity and length from 2-word utterances right through to complex language (8- to 12-word utterances).	Points to pictures or objects; chooses picture or object; manipulates toys or objects in accordance with the spoken message; or responds verbally to statements or questions.			
a. live voice at normal conversational distance				
b. recorded voice				
c. live voice at a distance				
d. over the telephone				
e. at a distance, spontaneously (distance listening; overhearing)	Responds to familiar speech that is or is not directed toward him or her. This is a very important auditory/linguistic/cognitive milestone, since it requires distance listening, auditory scanning and *overhearing*.			

Stage/Skill	Indicators/Examples	Not Present	Emerging	Appropriately Demonstrated
8. Without watching the speaker's face, responds appropriately to requests that have an increasing number of steps indicated by verb changes.	Follows commands, complies with requests.			
a. two-step requests	e.g., Please get the cups and put them on the table.			
b. three-step requests	e.g., Wash your hands, brush your teeth, and pick out a book.			
9. Identifies an object or activity based on clues (riddles) without watching the speaker's face.	Names the object or activity.			
a. simple sentences				
b. complex language				
10. Answers personal questions with the topic given without watching the speaker's face.	Appropriately answers questions.			
a. simple language				
b. complex language				

continues

Stage/Skill	Indicators/Examples	Not Present	Emerging	Appropriately Demonstrated
11. Answers questions with no topic given without watching the speaker's face.	Appropriately answers questions.			
a. simple language				
b. complex language				
12. Re-tells stories or events with 2, 3, or 4 events/ideas/concepts in the appropriate order (auditory-only presentation).				
13. Understands and supplies whole word or message when part is missing (auditory closure).				
14. Listens to a familiar paragraph or story of increasing length and answers questions regarding the main idea and supporting details.	Appropriately answers questions.			
a. live voice				
b. recorded voce (degraded signal)				

Stage/Skill	Indicators/Examples	Not Present	Emerging	Appropriately Demonstrated
15. Carries out a telephone task for a specific purpose.	Examples: Calls the bookstore to ask about a specific book; calls a friend to ask about an assignment; calls parent to find out what time they will be picked up.			
16. Engages in increasingly longer spontaneous, pragmatically correct conversations without having to watch the speaker's face.				
a. with the topic stated ahead of time				
b. without the topic stated ahead of time				
c. while engaged in another task or activity				

continues

Phase IV continued

Stage/Skill	Indicators/Examples	Not Present	Emerging	Appropriately Demonstrated
17. While engaged in an activity of their own choosing, the child demonstrates that they have an awareness of other conversations that have been occurring around them or can spontaneously tune in to conversations that have occurring around them (distance listening, overhearing, listening set, auditory multitasking). **Requirements:** Technology which permits listening at a distance; and curiosity!	It is this ability to tune in and out of conversations that are occurring around them that will give the child the ability to learn from the world around them, without having to be directly taught. This ability underlies the child's ability to use the surrounding world continuously to acquire vocabulary, grammar, pragmatics and sociolinguistic appropriateness, *and* information—thus building the foundation for maturing social-emotional development, theory of mind, and executive function.			

Sources: Caleffe-Schenck, N. S., and Stredler-Brown, A. (1992). Early Steps. Auditory Skills Checklist. Cole, E. (2004). Early Spoken Language through Audition Checklist, *SKI*HI Manual* (Vol. I, pp.137–141). Stredler-Brown, A., and Johnson, D. C. (2003). Functional Auditory Performance Indicators (FAPI).

APPENDIX

4

Explanation for Items on the Framework

I. Sensitivity to Child

Items in this section all require that the caregiver demonstrate a level of awareness of the child's way of being, and a desire to adjust to it in a supportive manner which promotes the child's social/emotional, cognitive, *and* linguistic development. The items can be grouped as follows.

Item 1: Affect

Handles child in positive manner. The parent-child affective relationship is considered to have fundamental importance for a child's language development, as well as for his or her social and cognitive development (Bromwich, 1981, 1997; Clarke-Stewart, 1973; Dore, 1986; Owens, 2005; Paul, 2007). "Handling the child in a positive manner" could include behaviors such as caressing, hugging, and smiling and behaving in a warm, loving, accepting, and joyous fashion with the child. It could also include simply being near the child, watching him or her thoughtfully, and being openly available for interaction. The key question here is, "Does the parent behave in ways which tell the child that the parent loves him and enjoys being with him?"

Sometimes, even if many other areas on the Framework are problematic, this is one area that is not, and the importance of it can be emphasized by the interventionist. Sometimes it is a question of caregivers not knowing how to behave in ways that send the warm, positive message they want to send. Sometimes the caregiver is unaware of the difference that this can make in the child's behavior. And sometimes the caregiver actually is feeling primarily frustrated, angry, or hopeless towards the child, rather than warm and loving. Obviously, this can be a temporary or long-term phenomenon. The interventionist must be aware of the limits of his or her expertise in addressing this particular area, and must know when to draw on the assistance of a social worker or clinical psychologist.

Items 2 and 3: Pacing and Focus

Paces play and talk in accordance with child's tempo. Follows child's interests much of the time. These items relate to the caregiver's ability to read the child's cues quickly regarding such dimensions as the amount of information and stimulation the child can absorb, the kinds of things the child is interested in, and how he or she indicates that interest. What needs to happen is for the caregiver to observe the child frequently and carefully, to follow his or her interests and tempo, and to fit in with both (Bromwich, 1997). With a young child, the cues may lie in such things as rate of body movement, orientation and/or tension of the body, facial expressions, gaze direction, gaze shifts, gestures, and vocalizations (Paul, 2007).

The interventionist and the caregiver may find it useful to study the videotapes of the child interacting to determine what the child's more salient as well as subtle cues are, and to spot moments where the adult responded or interjected comments in synchrony with the child's tempo and focus.

Items 4 and 5: Appropriate Stimulation

Provides appropriate stimulation, activities, and play for the child's age and stage. Encourages and facilitates child's play with objects and materials. According to Clarke-Stewart's seminal work (1973), the environment most growth-facilitating not only will be warm and loving, but also will be stimulating in terms of visual, verbal, and material input. Naturally, what is appropriate will vary throughout the early childhood period. The point is that the caregiver needs to be aware of the child's changing needs and abilities with regard to toys, books, and activities, and needs to be providing for them (Gazdag & Warren, 2000; Thal & Clancy, 2001).

II. Conversational Behaviors

Items in this section relate to what the caregiver does in the course of communicative interactions with the child. This section begins with behaviors associated with responding to the child's communicative attempts, because parental responsiveness is highly associated with the child's language development (Brady, Marquis, Fleming, & McLean, 2004; Gazdag & Warren, 2000; Poehlmann & Fiese, 2001). But clearly, the caregiver cannot (and would not want to) *always* follow the child and respond to him. Consequently, features of efficaciously establishing a shared focus, or initiating interactions, are next in the Framework. The final group of items is those which apply in an overall sense to all caregiver talk in the course of communicative interactions with their hearing-impaired child.

A. In Responding to the Child

Items 6, 7, and 8: Recognizing Cues and Responding

Recognizes the child's communicative attempts. Responds to child's communicative attempts. Responds with a response which includes a question or comment requiring a further response from the child. Adult responsiveness to the child's attempts to communicate is considered to be one of the most important facilitative elements for optimal development of language in young children (Cook, Tessier, Klein, & Armbruster, 2000). In order to respond to the child (item 6), the caregiver must be able to recognize the child's communicative behaviors as such. For the older child, these may be words, with or without gestures. For the younger child, as mentioned above, communicative behaviors may be cued by rate of body movement, orientation and/or tension of the body, facial expressions, gaze direction, gaze shifts, gestures, and vocalizations (Bromwich, 1997; MacDonald, 1989; Rossetti, 2001).

The caregiver can respond to the child's communicative attempts in words and/or by smiling, nodding, gesturing, moving closer (item 7). One of the most effective ways of continuing the conversational exchange is to respond and include a question or comment that encourages the child to respond also (item 8). For example, an infant might reach toward an object and look back and forth between the object and the adult. The adult's response could be to smile, move the object close to the infant, and say, "Oh you want the dolly, don't you?" The expected child response would be to take the dolly and relax body tension, and perhaps put it in his or her mouth or manipulate it. For an older child, the response to the child's "Uh-oh!" might be the adult's visual attention, moving closer, and "What happened?" The child's expected response might be to point at an object and say, "Broke" or "Fell down." These conversational *turnabouts* or *verbal reflectives* are considered to be very powerful learning devices (Kaye & Charney, 1980, 1981; Proctor-Williams, Fey, & Loeb, 2001).

Caregivers of young children with hearing impairments may need some guidance in recognizing and effectively responding to child behaviors which are potentially communicative. Particularly with intervention which begins with children who are over the age of 12 months, caregivers tend to focus on the child's production of *words* as evidence of progress. Long before words appear, there are a multitude of potentially (and actually) communicative behaviors which the caregiver can advantageously promote.

Item 9: Imitation

Imitates child's productions. Obviously, conversation consists of more than the two people imitating each other's contributions. But imitation is a normal and important part of caregiver-child interaction, particularly during the first 12 months. In order to imitate the child, the parent is automatically required to recognize and respond to the child's cues, to follow the child's interests rather than imposing the parent's own agenda, and to sense the child's tempo. By imitating the child, the parent has an excellent chance of successfully establishing a mutual focus of attention, and of engaging in turn-taking. Furthermore, it can be playful and fun!

Item 10: Providing the Words

Provides child with the words appropriate to what he or she apparently wants to express. Providing the child with the words appropriate to what he or she apparently wants to express has some of the same benefits as imitating the child's utterance (Capone & McGregor, 2004). It requires recognizing and interpreting the child's cues, as well as following the child's lead. Snow, Midkiff-Borunda, Small, and Proctor (1984) and Vygotski (1978) have all viewed it as vitally important for cognitive development and language learning that there should be a correspondence between what the adult says and the objects and events in the immediately surrounding environment. If the topic and message expressed by the adult are the child's own, the adult utterance seems likely to have even more significance and impact.

There are two dangers inherent to this activity, however. The first is that the caregiver must be a keen observer of the child's cues, and as accurate an interpreter of the child's intentions as possible. If not, and there is a mismatch between the caregiver's words and the child's real message, it could be at best meaningless, and at worst detrimental (Duchan, 1986). The other danger to guard against is also related to the caregiver's ability to determine which of the child's behaviors are potentially communicative. Providing words to describe every gesture or sound the child makes could clearly become a mindless narration of ongoing events. The idea is to focus on the times when the child is actually trying to express something, and to give him the words he would use in that situation.

Examples

Context: The child peers over the side of the high chair, points downwards, looks sad, and vocalizes.

Adult: "Uh-oh! The cookie fell down."

or

Context: The child points out of the car window and vocalizes excitedly.

Adult: "Oh look! A great big fire truck!"

Item 11: Expansions

Expands child's productions semantically and/or grammatically. Expansions are parental responses that repeat part or all of the child's preceding utterance and add to it either semantically or syntactically or both. They can be minimal replies which basically correct grammar in the child's utterance, or they can be more extended expansions which provide related new ideas or information (Proctor-Williams, Fey, & Loeb, 2001). In both of the following instances, the mother's utterances are extended expansions of the child's preceding utterances that provide the child with both a syntactic alternative and a semantic extension.

Examples

Child: "Broke truck."

Mother: "Tommy broke the truck. Too bad."

or

Child: "Doggie pee-pee!"

Mother: "Oh no! The doggie went pee-pee on the floor!"

Expansions are considered to be of great importance in intervention settings since they occur with great regularity in normal caregiver talk, since they model correctly for the child how to add syntactic or semantic elements to an utterance, and as they are positively correlated with measures of language development. Interestingly, it has been shown that children are more likely to imitate expansions spontaneously than any other type of adult utterance (Folger & Chapman, 1978; Gazdag & Warren, 2000; Scherer & Olswang, 1984; Seitz & Stewart, 1975). This may be because an expansion is directly based on the child's utterance, and thus holds some automatic interest to him. Also, the adult expansion often only adds a moderately novel element to the original utterance, and in fact, often supplies words the child probably understands, but did not use in his original utterance. When the expanded adult's utterance also contains a "hook" intended to clarify the child's message and/or which expects a response from the child, it may be even more powerful as a conversation-promoting strategy. In the examples above, the caregiver could respond with the following expansions which also contain hooks.

Examples

"Tommy broke the truck?"

(an expansion; also a yes/no clarification question)

or

"The doggie went pee-pee *where*?"

(an expansion; also a request for specific additional information)

The examples then become not just expanded responses, but turnabouts as discussed in Kaye and Charney, 1980, 1981, and Proctor-Williams, Fey, and Loeb, 2001. The benefits of these responses are that the caregiver is responding to the child, is on the child's topic, is modeling a semantically/syntactically expanded and correct utterance, is engaged in negotiating communicative meaning, and has made an attempt to elicit continued participation from the child. And, in most cases, none of this requires conscious effort beyond wanting to understand and communicate with the child!

B. In Establishing Shared Attention

Items 12 and 13: Engaging the Child

Attempts to engage child. Talks about what the child is experiencing, looking at, doing. Item 12 is listed separately in order to refocus attention on two important elements of interaction already mentioned above as part of other items. One element relates to the items concerning affect, similar to item 1. Whether the caregiver does or does not occasionally attempt to engage the child in playful interaction or conversation can be a clue to the parent's level of coping and/or commitment to the process (see Chapter 6). If the caregiver does not attempt to engage the child, that could be a bit of behavioral evidence that there are problems in their affective relationship or that the parent is simply feeling too hopeless or frustrated to bother. Or, a lack of attempting to engage the child may be related to the other element upon which item 12 is intended to refocus attention. That element is that with all the emphasis on responding to the child (items 3, 6–11), the caregiver may begin to get the impression that one is *never* supposed to initiate interaction, only to respond to the child's apparent communicative attempts. This simply is not the case. To begin with, it is impractical in terms of the daily events occurring in the child's life: Try dressing or feeding a child in a purely responsive manner! Taken to the extreme, if the adults rarely initiate communication with the child, it could deprive the child of normal opportunities to learn to respond to others' communicative attempts (including others' interests and agendas).

That said, item 13 reiterates that any child-directed utterance is likely to be most successful at capturing and maintaining the child's attention, as well as at eliciting a response, if the adult utterance has some connection with what the child is experiencing, looking at, or doing. That is, the caregiver certainly can initiate at will and on any topic, but can expect the most rewarding child response if the parent's utterance fits in with the child's state and interests at that moment. This requires observation, sensitivity, and insight into the child's behavioral cues to his or her state and interest. (See items 2, 3, and 4, also.)

Items 14 and 15: Sense Modalities

Uses voice (first) to attract child's attention to objects, events, self. Uses body movement, gesture, touch appropriately in attracting child's attention to objects, events, self. Items 14 and 15 concern the caregiver's use of sense modalities in attracting the child's attention. The items here refer to adult strategies used in the course of normal interactive events. Because spoken language is primarily an acoustic event, it can most efficaciously be learned by means of acoustic input (i.e., through listening). Thus, as part of helping the child learn to listen, the caregiver should always attempt to attract the child's attention using voice alone (e.g., through calling the child's name). When the child responds based on listening alone, do make sure that the child knows that that was a great thing to do! If the child does not respond, get closer to the child's microphone and call again. If the child still does not respond after three tries or so, then catch the child's visual attention and let him know that you were calling him, and that he was supposed to listen and respond.

One of the important aspects to consider is: "To *what* does one attract the child's attention?" There should be a meaningful reason for the child to turn, such as to look at an interesting toy or event. Otherwise, why would anyone continue turning when called?

Item 16: Sentence Complexity

Uses phrases and sentences of appropriate length and complexity. This item needs to be interpreted with caution and some latitude. Research fairly consistently reports that adults use sentences of approximately eight morphemes when speaking with each other, and of about three to five morphemes when speaking with children from birth through toddlerhood (Fey, Long, & Finestack, 2003; Owens, 2005; Phillips, 1973; Sheng, McGregor, & Xu, 2005; Stern, Spieker, Barnett, & MacKain, 1983).

However, research results are markedly inconsistent (see Snow, Perlman, & Nathan, 1987, for a review) regarding the exact nature of the semantic/syntactic changes which occur, and when and why they occur during the birth to 3-year-old age period. For example, with very young infants (i.e., birth to 2 months), some mothers use utterances of adult length as they croon and talk to them. Then, perhaps as the child shows an increasing capability of participating in face-to-face play interactions, some mothers reduce the length and complexity of their utterances to fit more closely with the child's early smiling and babbling exchanges. Other mothers use short utterances from the beginning. And after the child begins using words, some mothers match the child's utterance length, whereas some stay several morphemes in advance.

Lacking whatever certainty research could provide for this item, the interventionist can rely on what seems sensible from a communication and learning point of view. An argument could be made that if an adult is using very long and complex sentences with a young child, it is possible that the adult has no expectation that the child will understand what is being said. With the neonate, the mother's long crooning sentences are likely to be more a part of the mother's efforts to provide a safe and comforting environment for the child, than a part of attempting to communicate specific messages to the child. When an adult uses very long sentences with an older child, it can sometimes actually sound as if the adult is talking to himself or herself, rather than to the child. In intervention settings, the intent generally is to communicate with the child. One is striving for the child's understanding. Consequently, the three- to five-morpheme length is probably a reasonable guideline for most caregiver utterances in most situations.

As for whether the caregiver's utterances should match or stay slightly in advance of the child's utterance length as the child's language grows, it seems sensible for the caregiver's utterance length and complexity to be generally a bit in advance of the child. Certainly, this will automatically be the case if the caregiver is speaking primarily in phrases and sentences (rather than in single words) in order to provide more complete "acoustic envelopes," and if the caregiver is responding to the child's utterances using expansions and/or turnabouts (see Chapter 8)

In General

Items 17, 18, 19, and 20: Manner of Speaking

Pauses expectantly after speaking to encourage child to respond. Speaks to child with appropriate rate, intensity, and pitch. Uses interesting, animated voice. Uses normal, unexaggerated mouth movements. All of these items (17, 18, 19, 20) relate to the manner in which the caregiver delivers the message to the child. They are interrelated, but it is possible for one item to be problematic and not the others.

Pausing after speaking to encourage the child to respond (item 17) is a fundamental part of turn-taking. In practice, it can mean giving the child the space (time) to "get a word in edgewise," or it can mean waiting long enough for the child to process the adult message and to respond to it. According to Stern et al. (1983), maternal pausing between utterances is greatest at birth and declines somewhat after basic turn-taking rules are established. However, between-utterance pauses even at 2 years of age are still approximately twice as long as they are in adult-adult utterances.

The caregiver's rate of speaking (item 18) also tends to be a bit slower in adult-child speech than in adult-adult speech, with enunciation somewhat clearer. Clarifying the message in these ways could be important in many instances as an aid to the child's understanding (Sheng, McGregor, & Xu, 2005). But it would be most reasonable to maintain a normal rate of about three to five syllables per second (Ling, 2002) in order to avoid distorting the message. At slower rates, there can be a tendency to overenunciate: to mouth the articulatory movements to an excessive extent. And this can create a situation where the child can only understand people who make exaggerated mouth movements. (Not surprisingly, these are also often the *children* who overenunciate.) If the rate is careful but normal, the mouth movements are also likely to be normal and unexaggerated (item 20).

Intensity (item 18) should be normal (not shouting and not murmuring) in order to avoid inadvertently distorting the acoustic signal, and must take into account the child's hearing range (Ling, 1981). The closer the speaker's mouth is to the child's hearing aid microphone, the louder it will be for the child. The generally accepted optimal distance is four to six inches from the microphone. However, in normal conversational situations the optimum speaking distance is entirely dependent on the degree of the child's hearing loss, the level of background noise, the social context, and the presence or absence of FM devices.

In normal motherese, the overall pitch is generally higher and the intonational contours more varied than in adult-adult talk. If the overall pitch is too high (item 18), it may give a less-than-optimal signal to a child with a high frequency hearing loss. However, varied intonational contours and an interesting, animated voice (item 19) are likely to be well within the hearing capabilities of nearly all children with hearing loss. As these voice features are used to get and maintain the child's attention (Stern et al., 1983), as well as to cue constituent boundaries, sentence types, and speech acts, it is especially important that caregivers incorporate them when talking to children with hearing loss.

Items 21 and 22: Sense Modalities Again

Uses audition-maximizing techniques. Uses appropriate gesture. Items 21 and 22 concern the caregiver's use of sense modalities in situations other than attracting the child's attention (see items 14 and 15). The principles are the same, in that auditory input is the preferred choice for receiving an acoustically based communication modality (i.e., spoken language).

Strategies for maximizing the child's listening abilities include speaking well within the child's hearing range; using a normal overall pitch and rate of speaking; using an animated, interesting voice with varied intonational contours; speaking while sitting behind or beside the child; obscuring the child's view of the lips using the hand or a piece of paper; and attracting the child's visual focus away from the face and to the toys or activities at hand while speaking.

The amount of gesture that is appropriate (item 22) will need to be interpreted with some flexibility according to the individual case and contexts observed. Research suggests that most child communications include gestures throughout the birth to 3-year-old time period (Carpenter, Mastergeorge, & Coggins, 1983; Lasky & Klopp, 1982). When the goal is for the child to learn spoken language through listening, natural gestures on the adult's part are fine, as long as they are not excessive and it is still acoustics (spoken language) that is conveying the message, not gestures. The item has been included on the Framework to encourage discussion in case the caregiver's gestures seem to be the major mode of conveying messages.

APPENDIX
5

Checklist for Evaluating Preschool Group Settings for Children With Hearing Loss Who Are Learning Spoken Language

Federal law (IDEA, 2007) says that the educational program for any child with an identified disability must be individually determined by the child's placement team, which includes the parents and representatives from the child's school district. For some children, a preschool setting may not be the most appropriate educational setting, if, for example, the parents will be continuing to provide auditory-verbal therapy, guided by an Auditory-Verbal Therapist. For other children, the child's placement team may decide that a preschool will be the most appropriate educational setting for that child. The Checklist which follows is offered as a way of assisting with the process of evaluating the appropriateness of preschool settings under consideration, and of assuring that the necessary elements are present in order that the child will have appropriate auditory access to the curriculum, and will have instruction which will address his or her unique auditory and language-learning needs.

Children with hearing loss have listening and language learning needs that are unique, and that make placement in preschool group settings a different process than it is for a child with a different disability (Alexander, 1992; Joint Committee on Infant Hearing, 2007). When considering placement in a preschool group setting for any child with hearing loss who is learning to listen and talk, the child's team (parents and school personnel) needs to take into account the elements of that setting that will appropriately address those unique listening and language learning needs. Without these elements, the placement is likely to provide restrictions on the child's access to the curriculum and to the instruction from which he or she is intended to benefit.

If the goal is for the child to (continue to) develop spoken language through audition, the following elements need to be present in any preschool group learning setting, in order to address the unique listening and language-learning needs of a child with hearing loss.

Listening Needs

1. **Child needs appropriate auditory access to spoken communication.**
   - Through appropriate educational activities and classroom management techniques, teacher generally keeps classroom quiet enough that children can hear whomever is speaking.
   - All preschool staff members are vigilant about maintaining as quiet a learning environment as is possible.
   - Classroom has acoustic treatments, such as the following:
     - Acoustic tiles in the ceiling
     - Carpeting or chair slippers
     - Sound absorbent surfaces on at least some walls (e.g. bulletin boards) so that reverberation is reduced.
     - Sound absorbent window coverings
     - Very quiet HVAC system (unnoticeable)
   - Classroom is located in a quiet spot away from city traffic, hallway noise, gym
   - Child has properly selected and fit personal FM equipment for use in all group activities where it is important for the child to hear the person who is speaking.
   - Teacher is committed to wearing the FM transmitter with appropriate microphone placement, and uses it in all appropriate settings, being vigilant to turn it off in inappropriate settings.
   - Training for all school staff is given prior to the child's arrival at school by an educational audiologist, teacher of the hearing-

impaired or other knowledgeable professional regarding the child's FM equipment and regarding the child's needs related to the hearing loss.

■ One adult in the child's school takes responsibility for daily checks of the child's personal audiologic technology and FM equipment, as well as for troubleshooting, and requesting additional technical help when needed.

■ In case the child's school FM malfunctions, school system has provisions for loaner FM equipment to be available within 48 hours.

2. **Child needs to have his/her hearing status closely monitored, with systematic changes in child's technology made in response to changes in thresholds and/or changes in child's auditory perceptual abilities as reported by parents or professionals who work with the child.**

■ Educational audiologist is an integral part of the child's team. The audiologist is the only professional with the expertise and licensure to select, fit, and monitor the child's audiological technology (including personal FM technology). Typically, preschoolers need to have their hearing evaluated at least 2 to 4 times during the school year, and more frequently when parents or teachers are concerned about changes in the child's responses

Spoken Language Learning Needs

1. **Child needs to continue to develop spoken language through listening.**

■ Intervention services are available from professionals with expertise in working with children who have hearing loss and who are learning spoken language through listening. This expertise includes knowledge of current audiological technology, as well as knowledge and skills in aural habilitation/auditory verbal therapy.

■ If child receives services at school, a quiet space is available for intervention focused on the child's individual auditory-linguistic targets.

■ School staff expect to work as a team with parents to continue to develop child's spoken language through listening by means of (for example) weekly parent guidance sessions, regular team meetings, regular communication with parents so that parents can assist with pre- and post-teaching, as well as with vocabulary expansion and practice on new linguistic structures.

2. **Child needs a linguistically enriched environment.**
   - ■ Teacher frequently encourages all children to interact verbally in class.
   - ■ Teacher bases most of her activities and conversation around developmentally appropriate activities that capture the children's interest and curiosity.
   - ■ Play centers, tables, chairs are arranged in a way that encourages verbal interaction in small groups.
   - ■ Teacher repeats, summarizes other children's comments and questions.
   - ■ Teacher checks for comprehension, without asking, "Do you understand?"
   - ■ Teacher's pace reflects student understanding.

3. **Child needs excellent models of spoken language.**
   - ■ Teacher's usual rate, pitch, vocal intensity, and articulation make teachers' speech easy to hear and understand.
   - ■ Teacher uses facial expression and natural gestures to aid comprehension in talking to preschoolers.
   - ■ Most of the children in the class are typically developing children whose behavior and spoken language are within normal limits for their ages.

4. **Child needs to learn appropriate ways of interacting with typically developing peers (e.g., how to start/carry on/close a conversation or play; how to negotiate ownership of toys or materials; how to take turns; how to initiate play with a peer)**
   - ■ Preschool offers frequent opportunities for play and verbal interacting with typically developing peers.
   - ■ Adults are available to expedite verbal interactions among the children, but to step back, when appropriate.

APPENDIX
6

Selected Resources

Normal Development of Spoken Language: Textbooks

Gleason, J. B., & Ratner, N. B. (2009). *The development of language* (7th ed.). Boston, MA: Allyn & Bacon.

Hoff, E. (2008). *Language development* (4th ed.). Belmont, CA: Thomson Wadsworth.

Hulit, L. M., Howard, M. R., & Fahey, K. P. (2011). *Born to talk: An introduction to speech and language development* (5th ed.). Toronto, Canada: Pearson Education.

Otto, B. W. (2009). *Language development in early childhood education* (3rd ed.). Boston, MA: Merrill.

Owens, R. E. (2008). *Language development: An introduction* (7th ed.). Boston, MA: Allyn & Bacon.

Paul, R. (2006). *Language disorders from infancy through adolescence* (3rd ed.). St. Louis, MO: Mosby Elsevier.

Assessment of Auditory Abilities

Targets for Auditory/Verbal Learning (See Appendix 3)
Infant-Toddler Meaningful Auditory Integration Scale (IT-MAIS)

Language Assessment Tools

Boehm 3–Preschool
Boehm, A. E. (2001). Austin, TX: Pro-Ed.
- Assesses knowledge of concepts, receptive only; provides percentiles, T-scores, age equivalents.

Brigance Early Childhood Development Inventory
Brigance, A. H. (2010). North Billerica, MA: Curriculum Associates, Inc.
- Curriculum-based assessment from birth to 7 years in six developmental areas.

Carolina Curriculum for Infants and Toddlers (3rd ed.)
Johnson-Martin, N., Hacker, B., & Attermeier, S. (2004). Baltimore, MD: Paul H. Brookes.
- Provides assessment and intervention for children birth to 24 months; includes prelinguistic and verbal communication, as well as cognition, social skills, and fine and gross motor abilities.

Clinical Evaluation of Language Fundamentals—Preschool (2nd ed.) (CELF-Preschool)
Wiig, E. H., Secord, W., & Semel, E. (2004). San Antonio, TX: Harcourt.
- Assesses receptive and expressive language, provides standard scores, percentile scores.

Cottage Acquisition Scales for Listening, Language, and Speech (CASLLS)
Wilkes, E. (2003). San Antonio, TX: Sunshine Cottage.
- Criterion-referenced assessment of listening, language, speech, and cognition; based on normal development of children, birth to 8 years.

Peabody Picture Vocabulary Test (4th ed.) (PPVT-4)
Dunn, L., & Dunn, L. (2006). Circle Pines, MN: American Guidance Service.
- Assesses receptive vocabulary, ages 2½ years to adult; provides standard scores, percentiles, age equivalents, stanine; widely recognized.

Preschool Language Scale (4th ed.)
Zimmerman, I., Steiner, V., & Pond, R. (2002). San Antonio, TX: Psychological Corporation.
- Assesses receptive and expressive language abilities, provides standard scores, percentile ranks, and age equivalents.

MacArthur-Bates Communicative Development Inventories
Marchman, V. A., Fenson, L., Thal, D., Dale, P., Reznick, S., Bates, E., et al. (2006). Baltimore, MD: Paul H. Brookes.
- Assesses receptive and expressive vocabulary and early language from nonverbal gestures through use of word combinations; parent report.

Receptive-Expressive Emergent Language Scale (REEL) (3rd ed.)
Bzoch, K., League, R., & Brown, V. (2003). Austin, TX: Pro-Ed.
- Assesses receptive and expressive language; provides standard scores.

Reynell Developmental Language Scales
Reynell, J. K., & Gruber, C. P. (1999). Los Angeles, CA: Western Psychological Services.
- Assesses receptive and expressive language abilities; provides standard scores.

Test for Auditory Comprehension of Language (TACL-3)
Carrow-Woolfolk, E. (1999). Austin, TX: Pro-Ed.
- Comprehension of word classes and relations, grammatical morphemes, complex sentences; provides percentiles, standard scores, age equivalents, ages 3 to 10 years.

Mainstream Assessment of Readiness for Children Over Five (MARCOF)

Developed by Cynthia Robinson for MED-El
(http://Medel.at/US/Rehabilitation).
- Provides a numerical scoring sheet for important factors in determining a child's readiness for mainstreaming, identifies strengths and challenges, needs for supports in the mainstream.

Books and Materials of Interest to Parents and Interventionists

Beyond Baby Talk
Apel, K., & Masterson, J. (2001). New York, NY: Prima Publishing.
■ Book for parents about speech and language development.

The SKI-HI Curriculum
■ See the section entitled Early Spoken Language through Audition by Cole, E. B., Carroll, E., Coyne, J., Gill, E., & Paterson, M. (2005). (Vol. I, pp. 137–141; Vol. II, pp. 1279–1394), Logan, UT: Hope, Inc.

Estabrooks, W. (Ed.). (2001). *50 FAQs about AVT.* Toronto, Canada: Learning to Listen Foundation.

Estabrooks, W., & Samson, A. B. (2003). *Songs for listening! Songs for life!* Washington, DC: Alexander Graham Bell Association for the Deaf and Hard of Hearing.

Hollinger, P., & Doner, K. (2003). *What babies say before they can talk.* New York, NY: Simon & Schuster.

Human Development: The First Two-and-One-Half Years: Program 7—Language and Program 4—Infant Communication
Concept Media, P.O. Box 19542, Irvine, CA 92713.
■ Videos showing stages of language development.

It Takes Two to Talk: A Practical Guide for Parents of Children with Language Delays (3rd ed.)
Pepper, J., & Weitzman, E. (2004). Toronto, Canada: The Hanen Centre.
■ Book with specific suggestions for parents about how to promote their child's language development through ordinary, everyday routines and play.

Let's Learn around the Clock: A Professional's Early Intervention Toolbox
Rossi, K. (2005). Washington, DC: Alexander Graham Bell Association for the Deaf and Hard of Hearing.
■ Comprehensive intervention program for use through everyday activities, birth to 3 years of age.

Ling, D. (2002). *Speech and the hearing-impaired child: Theory and practice* (2nd ed.). Washington, DC: Alexander Graham Bell Association for the Deaf and Hard of Hearing.

Listen, Learn, and Talk (Videos and Printed Materials) Cochlear Limited (2003)

Poland, C., & Chouinard, A. (2008). *Let's talk together: Home activities for early speech and language development.* Maple Grove, MN: Talking Child, LLC.

Pollack, D., Goldberg, D., & Caleffe-Schenck, N. (1997). *Educational audiology for the limited-hearing infant and preschooler: An auditory-verbal program.* Springfield, IL: Charles C. Thomas.

A Few Favorite Web Sites for Parents and Interventionists

http://agbell.org

http://agbellacademy.org

http://babyhearing.org

http://listen-up.org

http://cochlearamericas.com/Support

http://dltk-teach.com

http://hearingjourney.com/Listening_Room

http://release-on-reading.com

http://johntracyclinic.org

http://magickeys.com

http://medel.at/US/Rehabilitation

http://naturallearning.com/fingerplays.shtml

http://oraldeafed.org

http://preschoolexpress.com/toddlerstation.shtml

APPENDIX

7

Description and Practice of Listening and Spoken Language Specialists: LSLS Cert. AVT and LSLS Cert. AVEd.

Listening and Spoken Language Specialists

Listening and Spoken Language Specialists (LSLS) help children who are deaf or hard of hearing develop spoken language and literacy primarily through listening.

LSLS professionals focus on education, guidance, advocacy, family support, and the rigorous application of techniques, strategies, and procedures that promote optimal acquisition of spoken language through listening by newborns, infants, toddlers, and children who are deaf or hard of hearing.

LSLS professionals guide parents in helping their children develop intelligible spoken language through listening and coach them in advocating their children's inclusion in the mainstream school. Ultimately, parents gain confidence that their children will have access to the full range of educational, social, and vocational choices in life.

Listening and Spoken Language Approaches

The two main Listening and Spoken Language approaches, historically, have been the Auditory-Verbal Approach (AV) and the Auditory-Oral Approach (A-O). Today, as a result of advances in newborn hearing screening, hearing technologies, early intervention programs, and the knowledge and skills of professionals, these two approaches have more similarities than differences and they can lead to similar outcomes.

The AG Bell Academy for Listening and Spoken Language certifies Listening and Spoken Language Specialists (LSLS).

Currently, the designations of the LSLS certification program are: LSLS Cert. AVT (Certified Auditory-Verbal Therapist) and LSLS Cert. AVEd (Certified Auditory-Verbal Educator). The LSLS must provide services in adherence to the A G Bell Academy Code of Ethics and the Principles of Auditory-Verbal Therapy or the Principles of Auditory-Verbal Education (available in the LSLS Candidate Handbooks and online at http://www.agbellacademy.org).

Listening and Spoken Language Practice

Listening and Spoken Language Specialists have similar knowledge and skills and work on behalf of the child and family.

The LSLS Cert. AVT works one-on-one with the child and family in all intervention sessions.

The LSLS Cert. AVEd involves the family and also works directly with the child in individual or group/classroom settings.

The LSLS Cert. AVT and the LSLS Cert. AVEd both follow developmental models of audition, speech, language, cognition and communication.

The LSLS Cert. AVT and the LSLS Cert. AVEd both use evidence-based practices.

The LSLS Cert. AVT and the LSLS Cert. AVEd both strive for excellent outcomes in listening, spoken language, literacy and independence for children who are deaf or hard of hearing.

APPENDIX

Principles of LSLS Practice*

Principles of LSLS Auditory-Verbal Therapy

1. Promote early diagnosis of hearing loss in newborns, infants, toddlers, and young children, followed by immediate audiologic management and Auditory-Verbal therapy.
2. Recommend immediate assessment and use of appropriate, state-of-the-art hearing technology to obtain maximum benefits of auditory stimulation.
3. Guide and coach parents to help their child use hearing as the primary sensory modality in developing listening and spoken language.
4. Guide and coach parents[1] to become the primary facilitators of their child's listening and spoken language development through active consistent participation in individualized Auditory-Verbal therapy.
5. Guide and coach parents[1] to create environments that support listening for the acquisition of spoken language throughout the child's daily activities.

---

*An Auditory-Verbal Practice requires all 10 principles.
[1]The term "parents" also includes grandparents, relatives, guardians, and any caregivers who interact with the child.
Adapted from the Principles originally developed by Doreen Pollack (1970).
Adopted by the AG Bell Academy for Listening and Spoken Language®, July 26, 2007.

6. Guide and coach parents[1] to help their child integrate listening and spoken language into all aspects of the child's life.
7. Guide and coach parents[1] to use natural developmental patterns of audition, speech, language, cognition, and communication.
8. Guide and coach parents[1] to help their child self-monitor spoken language through listening.
9. Administer ongoing formal and informal diagnostic assessments to develop individualized Auditory-Verbal treatment plans, to monitor progress and to evaluate the effectiveness of the plans for the child and family.
10. Promote education in regular schools with peers who have typical hearing and with appropriate services from early childhood onward.

Principles of LSLS Auditory-Verbal Education (LSLS Cert. AVEd)[1]

A Listening and Spoken Language Educator (LSLS Cert. AVEd) teaches children with hearing loss to listen and talk exclusively though listening and spoken language instruction.

1. Promote early diagnosis of hearing loss in infants, toddlers, and young children, followed by immediate audiologic assessment and use of appropriate state of the art hearing technology to ensure maximum benefits of auditory stimulation.

2. Promote immediate audiologic management and development of listening and spoken language for children as their primary mode of communication.

3. Create and maintain acoustically controlled environments that support listening and talking for the acquisition of spoken language throughout the child's daily activities.

4. Guide and coach parents to become effective facilitators of their child's listening and spoken language development in all aspects of the child's life.

5. Provide effective teaching with families and children in settings such as homes, classrooms, therapy rooms, hospitals, or clinics.

6. Provide focused and individualized instruction to the child through lesson plans and classroom activities while maximizing listening and spoken language.

7. Collaborate with parents and professionals to develop goals, objectives, and strategies for achieving the natural developmental patterns of audition, speech, language, cognition, and communication.

8. Promote each child's ability to self-monitor spoken language through listening.

9. Use diagnostic assessments to develop individualized objectives, to monitor progress, and to evaluate the effectiveness of the teaching activities.

10. Promote education in regular classrooms with peers who have typical hearing, as early as possible, when the child has the skills to do so successfully.

---

[1]Reprinted with Permission from: AG Bell Academy for Listening and Spoken Language®.

APPENDIX

Knowledge and Competencies Needed by Listening and Spoken Language Specialists (LSLS)

AG BELL ACADEMY
INTERNATIONAL CERTIFICATION PROGRAM FOR
LISTENING AND SPOKEN LANGUAGE SPECIALISTS (LSLS)

Certified Auditory-Verbal Educator® – LSLS Cert. AVEd®
Certified Auditory-Verbal Therapist® – LSLS Cert. AVT®

Core Competencies/Content Areas/Test Domains for the LSLS[1]

This is a list of the core competencies/content areas/test domains and their body of knowledge that a professional must have to qualify for and pass a test to earn the Listening and Spoken Language Specialist (LSLS) Certification. The nine content areas/domains covered in the LSLS test include:

Domain 1. Hearing and Hearing Technology

Domain 2. Auditory Functioning

Domain 3. Spoken Language Communication

Domain 4. Child Development

Domain 5. Parent Guidance, Education, and Support

Domain 6. Strategies for Listening and Spoken Language Development

Domain 7. History, Philosophy, and Professional Issues

Domain 8. Education (The focus of this domain is on the development and expansion of the auditory and language skills that underlie and support the child's progress in the general education curriculum.)

Domain 9. Emergent Literacy (The focus of this domain is on the development of the auditory and language skills that underlie and support the acquisition and advancement of literacy.)

Following is a list of the nine content areas/test domains with the addition of their competencies to classify the LSLS body of knowledge. Questions on the LSLS test will address these competencies.

Domain 1. Hearing and Hearing Technology

A. Hearing Science/Audiology

1. Anatomy of the ear and neural pathways
2. Physiology of hearing
3. Physics of sound (e.g., decibel; frequency; sound waves)
4. Psychoacoustics (e.g., HL; SPL; SL)
5. Auditory perception (e.g., masking; localization; binaural hearing)
6. Speech acoustics

7. Environmental acoustics
   a. Signal-to-noise ratio
   b. Distance
   c. Noise
   d. Reverberation
8. Causes of hearing impairment
9. Types of hearing impairment and disorders (e.g., site of lesion; age of onset)
10. Early identification and high risk factors
11. Audiogram, audiogram interpretation and implications to speech perception
12. Audiologic assessments
    a. Behavioral
    b. Speech perception testing
    c. Electrophysiologic (e.g., OAE, ABR ASSR, acoustic immittance)
    d. Hearing aid evaluation (e.g., real ear/probe microphone; electroacoustic analysis)
    e. Cochlear implant candidacy, surgery, activation, functional application of programs

B. Hearing Technology

1. Sensory devices (e.g., hearing aids; cochlear implants; vibro-tactile aids; transposition aids)
2. Assistive listening devices (e.g., personal FM/auditory trainers; soundfield FM and infrared (IR) systems)
3. Earmold acoustics (e.g., impact of the earmold characteristics on the transmission of sound)
4. Hearing technology troubleshooting strategies

Domain 2. Auditory Functioning

1. Auditory skill development
2. Infant auditory development (e.g., neural development; plasticity)
3. Functional listening skill assessments and evaluations, both formal and informal
4. Acoustic phonetics as related to speech perception and production
5. Functional use of audition

Domain 3. Spoken Language Communication

A. Speech

1. Anatomy of speech/voice mechanism
2. Physiology of speech/voice mechanism
3. Suprasegmental, segmental, coarticulation aspects of speech production
4. Sequences of typical speech development (e.g., pre-verbal; articulation; phonology; intelligibility)
5. Sequence of speech development in clients with various sensory devices (e.g.,hearing aids; cochlear implants; vibrotactile aids; transposition aids)
6. Speech production assessment measures (both formal and informal)
7. Teaching techniques in speech production
   a. Prerequisite skills for phoneme production
   b. Developmental (habilitative) and remedial (rehabilitative) speech development
   c. Suprasegmental and segmental aspects of speech facilitation
   d. Auditory strategies for speech facilitation
   e. Visual and tactile strategies for speech facilitation
   f. Integration of speech targets into spoken language
8. Speech characteristics of children without auditory access to the full speech spectrum
9. International Phonetic Alphabet (IPA)
10. Impact of auditory access on speech production

B. Language

1. Impact of auditory access on language development
2. Aspects of language (e.g., phonology; pragmatics; morphology; syntax; semantics)
3. Sequence of typical language development (e.g., prelinguistic; communicative intent; linguistic)
4. Language assessment measures (both formal and informal)
5. Teaching techniques in receptive and expressive language
6. Impact of speech acoustics on choice of language targets (e.g., inside/beside; he/she)
7. Development of complex conversational competence

8. Development of divergent/convergent thinking
9. Figurative language and higher level semantic usage

Domain 4. Child Development

1. Sequence of typical child development
   a. Cognitive
   b. Gross and fine motor
   c. Self-help
   d. Play
2. Influence of associated factors on child development (e.g., cultural; community; family)
3. Conditions that are present in addition to hearing impairment (e.g., sensory integration deficits; visual challenges; Autism Spectrum Disorders; neurological disorders; learning disabilities)

Domain 5. Parent Guidance, Education, and Support

1. Family systems (e.g., boundaries; roles; extended family; siblings)
2. Impact of hearing impairment on family (e.g., coping mechanisms, family functioning; stages of grief)
3. Family counseling techniques (e.g., active listening; reflective listening; questioning; open ended statements)
4. Family coaching and guidance techniques (e.g., demonstration; modeling; turning over the task; providing feedback; co-teaching)
5. Impact of associated factors on parent guidance (e.g., cultural; language in the home; economic; lifestyle; community)
6. Behavior management techniques
7. Adult learning styles

Domain 6. Strategies for Listening and Spoken Language Development

1. Learning to listen strategies (e.g., creating optimal listening environment; positioning to maximize auditory input)
2. Pausing (wait time) appropriately

3. Language facilitation techniques (e.g., expansion and modeling)
4. Prompting techniques (e.g., linguistic; phonological; acoustic; physical; printed written prompts)
5. Responsive teaching (e.g., listening to the client and modifying according to the client's language and speech production)
6. Creating a need for the child to talk
7. Acoustic highlighting techniques
8. Auditory presentation prior to visual presentation (e.g., say before seeing)
9. Spoken language modeling
10. Meaningful, interactive conversation
11. Experience-based, naturalistic language activities
12. Experience and personalized books

Domain 7. History, Philosophy, and Professional Issues

A. History and Philosophy

1. History of education of individuals who are deaf or hard of hearing
2. Historical perspective of communication approaches
3. Current communication approaches and principles for individuals who are deaf or hard of hearing

B. Professional Issues

1. Ethical requirements and issues
2. Professional development requirements and opportunities
3. Evidence-based practice and research findings

Domain 8. Education

(**The focus of this domain is on the development and expansion of the auditory and language skills that underlie and support the child's progress in the general education curriculum.**)

1. Continuum of educational and community (e.g., child care; respite care) placements

2. Curricular objectives that meet local standards in areas of instruction
3. Strategies for pre-teaching and re-teaching (post-teaching) the academic curriculum
4. Strategies for pre-teaching and re-teaching (post-teaching) language needed for academics
5. Strategies to integrate auditory speech language goals with curriculum
6. Cognitive and academic assessments
7. Process for developing individualized educational plans
8. Collaborative strategies with school professionals

Domain 9. Emergent Literacy

(The focus of this domain is on the development of the auditory and language skills that underlie and support the acquisition and advancement of literacy.)

1. The learning sequence and pedagogy related to teaching the following skills in accordance with the child's level of language development:
   a. Reciting finger plays and nursery rhymes
   b. Telling and/or retelling stories
   c. Activity and story sequencing
   d. Singing songs and engaging in musical activities
   e. Creating experience stories/experience books
   f. Organization of books (e.g., cover; back; title; author page)
   g. Directionality and orientation of print
   h. Distinguishing letters, words, sentences, spaces and punctuation that mark text
   i. Phonics (e.g., sound-symbol correspondences and letter-sound correspondences)
   j. Phonemic awareness (e.g., sound matching; isolating; substituting; adding; blending; segmenting; deleting)
   k. Sight of word recognition
   l. Strategies for the development of listening, speaking, reading and writing vocabulary
   m. Contextual clues to decode meaning
   n. Oral reading fluency development

o. Text comprehension strategies (e.g., direct explanation; modeling; guided practice; and application)

p. Abstract and figurative language (e.g., similes; metaphors)

q. Divergent question comprehension (e.g., inferential questions; predictions)

Reprinted with Permission from: AG Bell Academy for Listening and Spoken Language®.

10

Listening and Spoken Language Domains Addressed in This Book

Domain	Chapter	Competencies
1	1	A. 1, 2, 7, 10
		B. 1
	2	A. 1, 2, 3, 4, 6, 7
	3	A. 1, 2, 3, 4, 5, 8, 9, 10
	4	A. 1, 2, 3, 4, 5, 6, 7, 10, 11, 12
	5	A. 3, 4, 5, 6, 7, 10, 11, 12
		B. 1, 2, 3, 4
	7	A. 6, 7
	Appendix 1	A. 7
		B. 2
	Appendix 2	A. 6
	Appendix 5	A. 7
2	1	1, 2, 5
	2	4
	5	3
	7	1, 3, 4, 5
	10	5
	Appendix 1	1, 5
	Appendix 2	3, 4, 5
	Appendix 3	1, 3, 4, 5

continues

Domain	Chapter	Competencies
3	7	A. 3, 4, 10
		B. 1
	8	B. 2, 3, 7
	9	A. 3
		B. 5, 7
	10	A. 3
		B. 5, 7
	Appendix 1	B. 5
	Appendix 3	A. 3, 10
		B. 5, 7
	Appendix 4	B. 3, 5, 7
	Appendix 5	B. 1
	Appendix 6	B. 3, 4, 5
4	3	3
	6	2, 3
	10	1
	Appendix 4	1
5	10	2, 3, 4, 5
	Appendix 4	4
6	7	1, 2, 7, 8
	9	2, 3, 5, 6, 9, 10, 11
	10	1, 2, 3, 4, 5, 6, 7, 8, 9, 10, 11, 12
	Appendix 1	3, 10, 11
	Appendix 4	1, 2, 3, 4, 5, 6, 7, 8, 9, 10, 11
	Appendix 6	1, 2, 3, 4, 5, 6, 7, 8, 9, 10, 11, 12
7	1	B. 3
	5	B. 3
	6	A. 3
	Appendix 7	A. 3
		B. 2
	Appendix 8	A. 3
		B. 2
	Appendix 9	A. 3
		B. 2
	Appendix 10	B. 2
8	6	1
	Appendix 5	1
9	10	1. a, b, d, e, l
	Appendix 1	1. b, c, d
	Appendix 5	1. a, b, d, e, f, g, h, i, j, k
	Appendix 6	1. l

References

Ackerhalt, A. H., & Wright, E. R. (2003). Do you know your child's special education rights? *Volta Voices, 10*(3), 4-6.

Adrian, M. (2009). Acoustical retrofitting for learning spaces. *Volta Voices, 16*(5), 16-21.

Akhtar, N., Jipson, J., & Callanan, M. A. (2001). Learning words through overhearing. *Child Development, 72*(2), 416-430.

Alexander, L. (1992). Notice of Policy Guidance, Deaf Students Education Services. *Federal Register, 57*, 49274-01.

Alexiades, G., & Hoffman, R. A. (2008). Medical evaluation and management of hearing loss in children. In J. R. Madell & C. Flexer, (Eds.), *Pediatric audiology: Diagnosis, technology, and management* (pp. 25-30*)*. New York, NY: Thieme.

Allegretti, C. M. (2002). The effects of a cochlear implant on the family of a hearing-impaired child. *Pediatric Nursing, 28*, 614-620.

American Academy of Audiology. (2004). *Pediatric Amplification Guideline.* [Position statement of the American Academy of Audiology]. *Audiology Today, 16*(2), 46-53.

American National Standards Institute. (2002). *Acoustical performance criteria, design requirements, and guidelines for schools* (S12.60-2002). New York: American National Standards Institute (ANSI S12.60).

American Speech-Language-Hearing Association. (2000). *Guidelines for fitting and monitoring FM systems.* Available from http://www.asha.org/members/deskref-journals/deskref/default

American Speech-Language-Hearing Association. (2004). *Cochlear implants.* Available from http://www.asha.org/members/deskref-journals/deskref/default

American Speech-Language-Hearing Association. (2004). *Guidelines for the audiologic assessment of children from birth to 5 years of age.* Available from http://www.asha.org/members/deskref-journals/deskref/default

American Speech-Language-Hearing Association. (2005). *Guidelines for addressing acoustics in educational settings.* Available from http://www.asha.org/members/deskref-journals/deskref/default

American Speech-Language-Hearing Association. (2006*). Roles, knowledge, and skills: Audiologists providing clinical services to infants and young children birth to 5 years of age.* Available from http://www.asha.org/members/deskref-journals/deskref/default

Anderson, K. (1989). *Screening instrument for targeting educational risk* (SIFTER). Tampa, FL: Educational Audiology Association.

Anderson, K. (2000). *Early listening function (ELF).* Retrieved October 16, 2006, from http://www.hear2learn.com

Anderson, K. (2004). The problem of classroom acoustics: The typical classroom soundscape is a barrier to learning. *Seminars in Hearing, 25*(2), 117-129.

Anderson, K., & Matkin, N. (1996). *Screening instrument for targeting educational risk in preschool children (Age 3-kindergarten)* (Preschool SIFTER). Retrieved October 16, 2006, from http://www.hear2learn.com

Anderson, K., & Smaldino, J. (1998). *The listening inventory for education: An efficacy tool.* (LIFE). Retrieved October 16, 2006, from http://www.hear2learn.com

Anderson, K., & Smaldino, J. (2000). *Children's home inventory for listening difficulties.* (CHILD). Retrieved October 16, 2006, from http://www.hear2learn.com

Anderson, K. L. (2001, April). Voicing concern about noisy classrooms. *Educational Leadership,* 77-79.

Anderson, K. L., Goldstein, H., Colodzin, L., & Inglehart, F. (2005). Benefit of S/N enhancing devices to speech perception of children listening in a typical classroom with hearing aids or a cochlear implant. *Journal of Educational Audiology, 12,* 14-28.

Arco, C. M. B., & McCluskey, K. A. (1981). "A change of pace:" An investigation of the salience of maternal temporal style in mother-infant play. *Child Development, 52,* 941-949.

Arjmand, E. M., & Webber, A. (2004). Audiometric findings in children with a large vestibular aqueduct. *Archives of Otolaryngology-Head and Neck Surgery, 130,* 1169-1174.

Baguley, D. M., & McFerran, D. J. (2002). Current perspectives on tinnitus. *Archives of Disease in Childhood, 86,* 141-143.

Baldwin, S. M., Gajewski, B. J., & Widen, J. E. (2010). An evaluation of the cross-check principle using visual reinforcement audiometry, otoacoustic emissions, and tympanometry. *Journal of the American Academy of Audiology, 21*(3), 187-196.

Barnes, S., Gutfreund, M., Satterly, D., & Wells, C. (1983). Characteristics of adult speech which predict children's language development. *Journal of Child Language, 10,* 65-84.

Barnett, D. W., VanDerHeyden, A. M., & Witt, J. C. (2007). Achieving science-based practice through response to intervention: What it might look like in preschools. *Journal of Educational and Psychological Consultation, 17*(1), 31-54.

Bates, E., Benigni, L., Bretherton, I., Camaioni, L., & Volterra, V. (1979). *The emergence of symbols: Cognition and communication in infancy.* New York, NY: Academic Press.

Bates, E., & Goodman, J. (1999). On the emergence of grammar from the lexicon. In B. MacWhinney (Ed.), *The emergence of language* (pp. 29-80). Mahwah, NJ: Lawrence Erlbaum.

Bates, E., O'Connell, B., & Shore, C. (1987). Language and communication in infancy. In J. D. Osofsky (Ed.), *Handbook of infant development* (pp. 149-203). New York, NY: John Wiley & Sons.

Bateson, M. C. (1979). The epigenesist of conversational interaction: A personal account of research development. In M. Bullowa (Ed.), *Before speech: The beginning of interpersonal communication* (pp. 63-77). Cambridge, UK: Cambridge University Press.

Beck, D. L. (2010). Shifting paradigms: Bone-anchored hearing systems. *Hearing Review, 17*(1), 22-26.

Beebe, B., Jaffe, J., Feldstein, S., Mays, K., & Alson, D. (1985). Matching of timing: The application of an adult dialogue model to mother-infant vocal and kinesthetic interactions. In T. Field (Ed.), *Infant social perceptions* (pp. 217-241). Norwood, NJ: Ablex.

Beebe, B., & Stern, D. (1977). Engagement-disengagement and early object experience. In N. Freedman & S. Grant (Eds.), *Communicative structures and psychic structures* (pp. 35-55). New York, NY: Plenum Press.

Bellinger, D. (1980). Changes in the explicitness of mother's directives as children age. *Journal of Child Language, 6*, 443-455.

Bellis, T. J. (2003). *Assessment and management of central auditory processing disorders in the educational setting: From science to practice* (2nd ed.). Clifton Park, NY: Thomson Delmar Learning.

Bench, J., Hoffman, E., & Wilson, I. (1974). A comparison of live and video-record viewing of infant behavior under sound stimulation. I. Neonates. *Developmental Psychology, 7*, 455-464.

Bentler, R. (2010). Frequency-lowering hearing aids: Verification tools and research needs. *ASHA Leader, 15*(4), 14-16.

Berg, F. S. (1993). *Acoustics and sound systems in schools.* San Diego, CA: Singular Publishing Group.

Berlin, C. I., Hood, L. J., Morlet, T., Wilensky, D., Li, L., Mattingly, K. R., et al. (2010). Multi-site diagnosis and management of 260 patients with auditory neuropathy/dys-synchrony (auditory neuropathy spectrum disorder). *International Journal of Audiology, 49*(1), 30-43.

Berlin, C. I., Hood, L. J., Morlet, T., Wilensky, D., St. John, P., Montgomery, E., et al. (2005). Absent or elevated middle ear muscle reflexes in the presence of normal otoacoustic emissions: A universal finding in 136 cases of auditory neuropathy/dys-synchrony. *Journal of the American Academy of Audiology, 16*, 546-553.

Berlin, C. I., & Weyand, T. G. (2003). *The brain and sensory plasticity: Language acquisition and hearing.* Clifton Park, NY: Thomson Delmar Learning.

Bertolini, P., Lassalle, M., Mercier, G., Raquin, M. A., Izzi, G., Corradini, N., et al. (2004). Platinum compound-related ototoxicity in children: Long-term follow-up reveals continuous worsening of hearing loss. *Journal of Pediatric Hematology and Oncology, 26*(10), 649-655.

Bess, F. H., Dodd-Murphy, J., & Parker, R. A. (1998). Children with minimal sensorineural hearing loss: Prevalence, educational performance, and functional status. *Ear and Hearing, 19*, 339-354.

Bess, F. H., & Humes, L. E. (2003). *Audiology: The fundamentals* (3rd ed.). Philadelphia, PA: Lippincott Williams & Wilkins.

Blair, J. C. (2006). Teachers' impressions of classroom amplification. *Educational Audiology Review, 23*(1), 12-13.

Bloom, L. (1973). *One word at a time: The use of single word utterances before syntax.* The Hague, The Netherlands: Mouton.

Bloom, L. (1983). Of continuity, discontinuity, and the magic of language development. In R. M. Golinkoff (Ed.), *The transition from prelinguistic to linguistic communication* (pp. 79-92). Hillsdale, NJ: Lawrence Erlbaum.

Bloom, L., & Lahey, M. (1978). *Language development and language disorders.* New York, NY: John Wiley & Sons.

Bloom, L., & Lo, E., (1990). Adult perception of vocalizing infants. *Infant Behavior and Development, 13*, 209-213.

Boothroyd, A. (1997). Auditory development of the hearing child. *Scandinavian Audiology, 26*(Suppl. 46), 9-16.

Boothroyd, A. (2002, April). *Optimizing FM and sound-field amplification in the classroom.* Paper presented at the American Academy of Audiology National Convention, Philadelphia, PA.

Boothroyd, A. (2004). Room acoustics and speech perception. *Seminars in Hearing, 25*(2), 155-166.

Brady, N., Marquis, J., Fleming, K., & McLean, L. (2004). Prelinguistic predictor of language growth in children with developmental disabilities. *Journal of Speech, Language, and Hearing Research, 47*, 663-677.

Braine, M. D. S. (1988). Modeling the acquisition of linguistic structure. In Y. Levy, I. M. Schlesinger, & M. D. S. Braine (Eds.), *Categories and processes in language acquisition* (pp. 217-259). Hillsdale, NJ: Erlbaum.

Braine, M. D. S. (1994). Is nativism sufficient? *Journal of Child Language, 21*, 9-32.

Brinton, B., & Fujiki, M. (1982). A comparison of request-response sequences in the discourse of normal and language disordered children. *Journal of Speech and Hearing Disorders, 47*, 57-63.

Bromwich, R. (1981). *Working with parents and infants: An interactional approach*. Baltimore, MD: University Park Press.

Bromwich, R. (1997). *Working with families and their infants at risk*. Austin, TX: Pro-Ed.

Bruner, J. (1975). The ontogenesis of speech acts. *Journal of Child Language, 2*, 1-19.

Bruner, J. (1977). Early social interaction and language acquisition. In H. R. Schaffer (Ed.), *Studies in mother-infant interaction* (pp. 271-289). London, UK: Academic Press.

Bruner, J. (1983). The acquisition of pragmatic commitments. In R.M. Golinkoff (Ed.), *The transition from prelinguistic to linguistic communication* (pp. 27-42). Hillsdale, NJ: Lawrence Erlbaum.

Caleffe-Schenck, N. S., & Stredler-Brown, A. (1992). *Auditory Skills Checklist*. (Available from the Colorado School for the Deaf and Blind, 33 N. Institute St., Colorado Springs, CO 80903).

Camarata, S., & Nelson, K. (2006). Conversational recast intervention with preschool and older children. In R. McCauley & M. Fey (Eds.), *Treatment of language disorders in children*. Baltimore, MD: Paul H. Brookes.

Campbell, K. C. M. (2009). Emerging pharmacologic treatments for hearing loss and tinnitus. *ASHA Leader, 14*(6), 14-17.

Capone, N., & McGregor, K. (2004). Gesture development: A review for clinical and research practices. *Journal of Speech, Language, and Hearing Research, 47*, 173-187.

Carpenter, M., Tomasello, M., & Striano, T. (2005). Role reversal, imitation and language in typically developing infants and children with autism. *Infancy, 8*, 253-278.

Carpenter, R. L., Mastergeorge, A. M., & Coggins, T. E. (1983). The acquisition of communicative intentions in infants eight to fifteen months of age. *Language and Speech, 26*, 101-116.

Chermak, G. D., Bellis, J. B., & Musiek, F. E. (2007). Neurobiology, cognitive science, and intervention. In G. D. Chermak & F. E. Musiek (Eds.), *Handbook of central auditory processing disorder: Comprehensive intervention* (Vol. II, pp. 3-28). San Diego, CA: Plural.

Chermak, G. D., & Musiek, F. E. (Eds.). (2007). *Differential diagnosis, related neuroscience, and multidisciplinary perspectives on central auditory processing disorder*. San Diego, CA: Plural.

Chermak, G. D., & Musiek, F. E. (Eds.). (2007). *Handbook of central auditory processing disorder: Comprehensive intervention* (Vol. II). San Diego, CA: Plural.

Ching, T. C., Hill, M., & Psarros, C. (2000, August). *Strategies for evaluation of hearing aid fitting for children (PEACH and TEACH)*. Paper presented at the International Hearing Aid Research Conference, Lake Tahoe, CA.

Chomsky, N. (1993). On the nature, use and acquisition of language. In A. J. Goldman (Ed.), *Reading in philosophy and cognitive science* (Vol. C, pp. 511–534). Cambridge, MA: MIT Press.

Christensen, L. (2009). New bone-anchored amplification options for children. *ASHA Leader, 14*(9), 5–7.

Christensen, L., Smith-Olinde, L., Kimberlain, J., Richter, G. T., & Dornhoffer, J. L. (2010). Comparison of traditional bone-conduction hearing aids with the Baha system. *Journal of the American Academy of Audiology, 21*(4), 267–273.

Clark, G. (2003). *Cochlear implants: Fundamentals and applications*. New York, NY: AIP Press.

Clark, J. L., & Roeser, R. J. (2005). Large vestibular aqueduct syndrome: A case study. *Journal of the American Academy of Audiology, 16*, 822–828.

Clark, M. (2006). *A practical guide to quality interaction with children who have a hearing loss*. San Diego, CA: Plural.

Clarke-Stewart, K. A. (1973). Interactions between mothers and their young children: Characteristics and consequences. *Monographs of the Society for Research in Child Development, 38*(6, 7, Serial No. 149).

Clinard, C., & Tremblay, K. (2008). Auditory training: What improves perception and how? *Audiology Today, 20*, 68–69.

Cohen, N., Roland, J. T., & Marrinan, M. (2004). Meningitis in cochlear implant recipients: The North American experience. *Otology and Neurotology, 25*, 275–281.

Cole, E. B. (1994). Encouraging intelligible spoken language development in infants and toddlers with hearing loss. *Infant-Toddler Intervention, 4*(4), 263–284.

Cole, E. B., Carroll, E., Coyne, J., Gill, E., & Paterson, M. (2005). Early spoken language through audition. In *The SKI-HI Curriculum* (Vol. I, pp. 137–141; Vol. II, pp. 1279–1394). Logan, UT: Hope.

Collis, G. (1977). Visual co-orientation and maternal speech. In H. R. Schaffer (Ed.), *Studies in mother-infant interaction* (pp. 355–375). London, UK: Academic Press.

Collis, G., & Schaffer, H. (1975). Synchronization of visual attention in mother-infant pairs. *Journal of Child Psychological Psychiatry, 16*, 315–320.

Cone, B., & Garinis, A. (2009). Auditory steady-state responses and speech feature discrimination in infants. *Journal of the American Academy of Audiology, 20*(10), 629–643.

Conti-Ramsden, G., & Friel-Patti, S. (1987). Situational variability in mother-child conversations. In K. E. Nelson & A. Van Kleeck (Eds.), *Children's language* (Vol. 6, pp. 43–63). Hillsdale, NJ: Lawrence Erlbaum.

Cook, K. A., & Walsh, M. (2005, May). *Otitis media*. Retrieved August 8, 2006, from Web MD, http://www.eMedicine.com

Cook, R. E., Tessier, A., Klein, M., & Armbruster, V. (2000). Nurturing communication skills. In R. E. Cook, A Tessier, & M. D. Klein (Eds.), *Adapting early childhood curricula for children in inclusive settings* (5th ed., pp. 290–399). Englewood Cliffs, NY: Merrill.

Cox, R. M. (2009). Verification and what to do until your probe-mic system arrives. *Hearing Journal, 62*(10), 10–14.

Crago, M. (1988). *Cultural context in communicative interaction of young Inuit children.* Unpublished doctoral dissertation, McGill University, Montreal, Quebec.

Crandell, C., & Smaldino, J. (2002). *Classroom acoustics.* Paper presented at the American Academy of Audiology National Convention, Philadelphia, PA.

Crandell, C. C., Kreisman, B. M., Smaldino, J. J., & Kreisman, N. V. (2004). Room acoustics intervention efficacy measures. *Seminars in Hearing, 25*(2), 201–206.

Crandell, C. C., Smaldino, J. J., & Flexer, C. (Eds.). (2005). *Sound-field amplification: Applications to speech perception and classroom acoustics* (2nd ed.). Clifton Park, NY: Thomson Delmar Learning.

Cross, T. G. (1977). Mother's speech adjustments: The contribution of selected child listener variables. In C. E. Snow & C. A. Ferguson (Eds.), *Talking to children: Language input and acquisition* (pp. 151–188). Cambridge, UK: Cambridge University Press.

Cross, T. G. (1978). Mother's speech and its association with rate of linguistic development in young children. In N. Waterson & C. E. Snow (Eds.), *Talking to children: Language input and acquisition* (pp. 199–216). Cambridge, UK: Cambridge University Press.

Cross, T. G. (1984). Habilitating the language-impaired child: Ideas from studies of parent-infant interaction. *Topics in Language Disorders, 4*, 1–14.

Cullington, H. E., & Zeng, F. G. (2010). Bimodal hearing benefit for speech recognition with competing voice in cochlear implant subject with normal hearing in the contralateral ear. *Ear and Hearing, 31*(1), 70–73.

Dabrowski, T., Myers, B., & Danilova R. (2009). Identifying enlarged vestibular aqueduct syndrome. *Advance for Audiologists, 11*(6), 46–49.

Davis, J. (Ed.). (1990). *Our forgotten children: Hard-of-hearing pupils in the schools.* Bethesda, MD: Self-Help for Hard of Hearing People.

Davis, W. E. (2001). Proportional frequency compression in hearing instruments. *Hearing Review, 8*(2), 34–39.

Dehaene, S. (2009). *Reading in the brain: The science and evolution of a human invention.* New York, NY: Penguin Group.

Delage, H., & Tuller, L. (2007). Language development and mild-to-moderate hearing loss: Does language normalize with age? *Journal of Speech, Language, and Hearing Research, 50*, 1300–1313.

DesJardin, J. L., & Eisenberg, L .S. (2007). Maternal contributions: Supporting language development in young children with cochlear implants. *Ear and Hearing, 28,* 456–469.

Dillon, H. (2001). *Hearing aids.* New York, NY: Thieme.

Dillon, H. (2006). What's new from NAL in hearing aid prescriptions? *Hearing Journal, 59*(10), 10–16.

Dillon, H., Ching, T., & Golding, M. (2008). Hearing aids for infants and children. In J. R. Madell & C. Flexer, (Eds.), *Pediatric audiology: Diagnosis, technology, and management* (pp. 168–182). New York, NY: Thieme.

Dinnebeil, L., & Hale, L. (2003). Incorporating principles of family-centered practice in early intervention program evaluation. *Zero to Three, 23,* 24–27.

Dobie, R. A., & Berlin, C. I. (1979). Influence of otitis media on hearing and development. *Annals of Otology, Rhinology and Laryngology, 88,* 46–53.

Doidge, N. (2007). *The BRAIN that changes itself.* London, UK: Penguin Books.

Dore, J. (1986). The development of conversational competence. In R. L. Schiefelbusch (Ed.), *Language competence: Assessment and intervention* (pp. 3–60). San Diego, CA: College-Hill Press.

Dore, J., Gearhart, M., & Newman, D. (1978). The structure of nursery school conversation. In K. E. Nelson (Ed.), *Children's language* (Vol. 1, pp. 337–395). New York, NY: Gardner Press.

Duchan, J. F. (1986). Language intervention through sense making and fine tuning. In R. L. Schiefelbusch (Ed.), *Language competence: Assessment and intervention* (pp. 187–212). San Diego, CA: College-Hill Press.

Dunst, C., Boyd, K., Trivette, C., & Hamby, D. (2002). Family-oriented program models and professional help-giving practices. *Family Relations: Interdisciplinary Journal of Applied Family Studies, 51,* 221–229.

Edwards, D., & Feun, L. (2005). A formative evaluation of sound-field amplification systems across several grade levels in four schools. *Journal of Educational Audiology, 12,* 57–64.

Ellis, R., & Well, G (1980). Enabling factors in adult-child discourse. *First Language, 1,* 46–82.

English, K., & Church, G. (1999). Unilateral hearing loss in children: An update for the 1990s. *Language, Speech, and Hearing Services in Schools, 30,* 26–31.

Erber, N. P. (1982). *Auditory training.* Washington, DC: Alexander Graham Bell Association for the Deaf and Hard of Hearing.

Ertmer, E., Strong, L., & Sadogopan, N. (2003). Beginning to communicate after cochlear implantation: Oral language development in a young child. *Journal of Speech, Language, and Hearing Research, 46,* 328–340.

Estabrooks, W. (Ed.). (2006). *Auditory-verbal therapy and practice.* Washington, DC: Alexander Graham Bell Association for the Deaf and Hard of Hearing.

Fabry, D. (2008). Cochlear implants and hearing aids: Converging/colliding technologies. *Hearing Journal, 61*(7), 10-17.

Fey, M., Krulik, T., Loeb, D., & Proctor-Williams, K. (1999). Sentence recast use by parents of children with typical language and children with specific language impairment. *American Journal of Speech-Language Pathology, 8,* 273-286.

Fey, M., & Loeb, D. (2002). An evaluation of the facilitative effects of inverted yes-no questions on the acquisition of auxiliary verbs. *Journal of Speech, Language, and Hearing Research, 45,* 160-174.

Fey, M., Long, S., & Finestack, L. (2003). Ten principles of grammar facilitation for children with specific language impairments. *American Journal of Speech-Language Pathology, 12,* 3-15.

Finkelstein, J. A., Stille, C. J., Rifas-Shiman, S. L., & Goldmann, D. (2005, June). Watchful waiting for acute otitis media: Are parents and physicians ready? *Pediatrics, 115*(6), 1466-1473.

Fitzgerald, D. C. (2001). Perilymphatic fistula and Ménière's disease: Clinical series and literature review. *Annals of Otology, Rhinology, and Laryngology, 110,* 430-436.

Fitzpatrick, E., Angus, D., Durieux-Smith, A., Graham, I.D., & Coyle, D. (2008). Parents' needs following identification of childhood hearing loss. *American Journal of Audiology, 17,* 38-49.

Fitzpatrick, E., Olds, J., Durieux-Smith, A., McCrae, R., Schramm, D., & Gaboury, I. (2009). Pediatric cochlear implantation: How much hearing is too much? *International Journal of Audiology, 48,* 91-97.

Flasher, L. V., & Fogel, P. T. (2004). *Counseling skills for speech-language pathologists and audiologists.* Clifton Park, NY: Thomson Delmar Learning.

Flexer, C. (2004). *Classroom amplification and the brain* [Videotape]. Layton, Utah: Info-Link Video Bulletin.

Flexer, C. (2004). The impact of classroom acoustics: Listening, learning, and literacy. *Seminars in Hearing, 25*(2), 131-140.

Flexer, C., & Long, S. (2003). Sound-field amplification: Preliminary information regarding special education referrals. *Communication Disorders Quarterly, 25*(1), 29-34.

Flexer, C., & Madell, J. (2009). The concept of listening age for audiologic management of pediatric hearing loss. *Audiology Today, 21,* 31-35.

Flexer, C., & Rollow, J. (2009). Classroom acoustic accessibility: A brain-based perspective. *Volta Voices, 16*(5), 16-18.

Flynn, T. S., Flynn, M. C., & Gregory, M. (2005). The FM advantage in the real classroom. *Journal of Educational Audiology, 12,* 35-42.

Foder, J. (1997, May 16). Do we have it in us? [Review of the book *Rethinking innateness*], *Times Literary Supplement*, 3-4.

Folger, J. P., & Chapman, R. S. (1978). A pragmatic analysis of spontaneous imitations. *Journal of Child Language, 5*, 25-38.

Fowler, K. (2008). Congenital CMV infection and hearing loss. *Volta Voices, 15*(6), 16-18.

French, N., & Steinberg, J. (1947). Factors governing the intelligibility of speech sounds. *Journal of the Acoustical Society of America, 19*, 90-119.

Fry, D. B. (1966). The development of the phonological system in the normal and the deaf child. In F. Smith & G. A. Miller (Eds.), *The genesis of language* (pp. 187-206). Cambridge, MA: MIT Press.

Fry, D. B. (1978). The role and primacy of the auditory channel in speech and language development. In M. Ross & T. G. Giolas (Eds.), *Auditory management of hearing-impaired children* (pp. 15-43). Baltimore, MD: University Park Press.

Furrow, D., Nelson, K. E., & Benedict, H. (1979). Mothers' speech to children and syntactic development: Some simple relationships. *Journal of Child Language, 6*, 423-442.

Furth, H. (1966). *Thinking without language.* New York, NY: Free Press.

Gabbard, S. A. (2003, November). *The use of FM technology for infants and young children.* Paper presented at ACCESS Conference, Chicago, IL.

Gallagher, T. (1977). Revision behaviors in the speech of normal children developing language. *Journal of Speech and Hearing Research, 70*, 303-318.

Gallagher, T. (1981). Contingent query sentences within adult-child discourse. *Journal of Child Language, 8*, 51-62.

Garvey, C. (1977). The contingent query: A dependent act in conversation. In M. L. Lewis & L. A. Rosenblum (Eds.), *Interaction, conversation, and the development of language* (pp. 63-93). New York, NY: John Wiley and Sons.

Garvey, C., Garvey, K., & Hendi, A. (2008). A review of common dermatologic disorders of the external ear. *Journal of the American Academy of Audiology, 19*, 226-232.

Gazdag, G., & Warren, S. F. (2000). Effects of adult contingent imitation on development of young children's vocal imitation. *Journal of Early Intervention, 23*(1), 24-35.

Geers, A. (2004). Speech, language and reading skills after early cochlear implantation. *Archives of Otolaryngology-Head and Neck Surgery, 130*, 634-638.

Geers, A., & Moog, J. (1989). Factors predictive of the development of literacy in profoundly hearing-impaired adolescents. *Volta Review, 91*, 69-86.

Geers, A. E., Moog, J. S., Biedenstein, J., Brenner, C., & Hayes, H. (2009). Spoken language scores of children using cochlear implants compared to hearing age-mates at school entry. *Journal of Deaf Studies and Deaf Education, 14,* 371-385.

Geers, A., Nicholas, J., & Sedley, A. (2003). Language skills of children with early cochlear implantation. *Ear and Hearing, 24,* 46-58.

Geers, A. E. (2002). Factors affecting the development of speech, language and literacy in children with early cochlear implantation. *Language, Speech and Hearing Services in Schools, 33,* 133-172.

Genesee, F., Paradis, J., & Crago, M. B. (2004). *Dual language development and disorders: A handbook on bilingualism and second language learning.* Baltimore, MD: Paul E. Brookes.

Girolametto, L., & Weitzman, E. (2002). Responsiveness of child care providers in interactions with toddlers and preschoolers. *Language, Speech and Hearing Services in Schools, 33,* 268-281.

Giralometto, L., Weitzman, E., Wiigs, M., & Pearce, P. (1999). The relationship between maternal language measures and language development in toddlers with expressive vocabulary delays. *American Journal of Speech-Language Pathology, 8,* 364-374.

Gleitman, L. R., Newport, E. I., & Gleitman, H. (1984). The current status of the motherese hypothesis. *Journal of Child Language, 11,* 43-79.

Glista, D., Scollie, S., Bagatto, M. Seewald, R., Parsa, V., & Johnson, A. (2009). Evaluation of nonlinear frequency compression: Clinical outcomes. *International Journal of Audiology, 48*(9), 632-644.

Goldin-Meadow, S. (2007). Pointing sets the stage for learning language—and creating language. *Child Development, 78*(3), 741-745.

Golinkoff, R. M. (Ed.). (1983). *The transition from prelinguistic to linguistic communication.* Hillsdale, NJ: Lawrence Erlbaum.

Golz, A., Netzer A., Westerman, S. T., Westerman, L. M., Gilbert, D. A., Joachims, H. Z., et al. (2005). Reading performance in children with otitis media. *Otolaryngology Head and Neck Surgery, 132,* 495-499.

Gordon, K. A., & Harrison, R. V. (2005). Hearing research forum: Changes in human central auditory development caused by deafness in early childhood. *Hearsay, 17,* 28-34.

Gordon, K. A., Papsin, B. C., & Harrison, R. V. (2003). Activity-dependent developmental plasticity of the auditory brain stem in children who use cochlear implants. *Ear and Hearing, 24*(6), 485-500.

Gordon, K. A., Papsin, B. C., & Harrison, R. V. (2004). Thalamocortical activity and plasticity in children using cochlear implants. *International Congress Series, 1273,* 76-79.

Gorga, M. P., Neely, S. T., Hoover, B. M., Dierking, D. M., Beauchaine, K. L., & Manning, C. (2004). Determining the upper limits of stimulation for auditory steady-state response measurements. *Ear and Hearing, 25*(3), 302-307.

Greenfield, P., & Smith, J. (1976). *The structure of communication in early language development.* New York, NY: Academic Press.

Grice, H. (1975). Logic and conversation. In M. Cole & J. Morgan (Eds.), *Syntax and semantics* (Vol. 3, pp. 41–58). New York, NY: Academic Press.

Grieco-Calub, T. M., Saffran, J. R., & Litovsky, R. Y. (2009). Spoken word recognition in toddlers who use cochlear implants. *Journal of Speech, Language, and Hearing Research, 52,* 1390–1400.

Griffiths, C. (1955). *The utilization of individual hearing aids on young deaf children.* Unpublished doctoral dissertation, University of Southern California, Los Angeles.

Griffiths, C. (1964). The auditory approach for preschool deaf children. *Volta Review, 66*(7), 387–397.

Hall, J. W. & Swanepoel, D. (2010). *Objective assessment of hearing.* San Diego, CA: Plural.

Halpin, K. S., Smith, K. Y., Widen, J .E., & Chertoff, M. E. (2010). Effects of universal newborn hearing screening on an early intervention program for children with hearing loss, birth to 3 yr of age. *Journal of the American Academy of Audiology, 21*(3), 169–175.

Harding, C. G. (1983). Setting the stage for language acquisition: Communication development in the first year. In R. M. Golinkoff (Ed.), *The transition from prelinguistic to linguistic communication* (pp. 93–113). Hillsdale, NJ: Lawrence Erlbaum.

Harrison, R. (2006, May). *Factors that shape the development and plasticity of the central auditory system: The balance of "nature and nurture."* Paper presented at the Fourth Widex Congress of Paediatric Audiology, Ottawa, Canada.

Hart, B. (2004). What toddlers talk about. *First Language, 24,* 91–106.

Hart, B., & Risley, T. R. (1999). *The social world of children learning to talk.* Baltimore, MD: Brookes.

Hayes, H., Geers, A. E., Treiman, R., & Moog, J. S. (2009). Receptive vocabulary development in deaf children with cochlear implants: Achievement in an intensive auditory-oral educational setting. *Ear and Hearing, 30*(1), 128–135.

Hirsch, I. (1970).Auditory training. In H. Davis & S. Silverman (Eds.). *Hearing and deafness* (pp. 346–359). New York, NY: Holt, Rinehart, & Wilson.

Hoff-Ginsberg, E. (1990). Maternal speech and the child's development of syntax: A further look. *Journal of Child Language, 17,* 85–100.

Holden, P. K., & Linthicum, F. H. (2005). Mondini dysplasia of the bony and membranous labyrinth. *Otology and Neurotology, 26,* 133.

Hood, L. (2009). Variation among individuals with auditory neuropathy/dys-synchrony and implications for management. *Educational Audiology Review, 27*(1), 10–11, 23.

Horton, K. (1974). Infant intervention and language learning. In R. L. Schiefelbusch & L. L. Lloyd (Eds.), *Language perspectives: Acquisition, retardation, and intervention* (pp. 469-491). Baltimore, MD: University Park Press.

Hymes, D. (1972). On communicative competence. In J. B. Pride & J. Holmes (Eds.), *Sociolinguistics* (pp. 269-293). New York, NY: Penguin Books.

Johnson, S. (1998). *Who moved my cheese?* New York, NY: Putnam's Sons.

Joint Committee on Infant Hearing. (2007). Year 2007 position statement: Principles and guidelines for early hearing detection and intervention programs. *Pediatrics, 120*(4), 898-921.

Kaiser, A., & Hancock, T. (2003). Teaching parents new skills to support their young children's development. *Infants and Young Children, 16*, 9-21.

Karass, J., Braungart-Reiker, J. M., Mullins, G., & Lefever, J. B. (2002). Process in language acquisition: The roles of gender, attention, and maternal encouragement of attention over time. *Journal of Child Language, 29*, 529-543.

Kaye, K. (1980). Why we don't talk "baby talk" to babies. *Journal of Child Language, 7*, 489-507.

Kaye, K. (1982). *The mental and social life of babies: How parents create persons.* Chicago, IL: Chicago University Press.

Kaye, K., & Charney, R. (1980). How mothers maintain "dialogue" with two-year-olds. In D. Olson (Ed.), *The social foundations of language and thought* (pp. 211-230). New York, NY: Norton.

Kaye, K., & Charney, R. (1981). Conversation asymmetry between mothers and children. *Journal of Child Language, 8*, 35-50.

Kaye, K., & Wells, A. (1980). Mothers' jiggling and the burst-pause pattern in neonatal sucking. *Infant Behavior and Development, 3*, 29-46.

Kenna, M. A., Feldman, H. A., Neault, M. W., Frangulov, A., Wu, B. L., Fligor, B., & Rehm, H. L. (2010). Audiologic phenotype and progression in *GJB2* (Connexin 26) hearing loss. *Archives of Otolaryngology–Head and Neck Surgery, 136*(1), 81-87.

Kent, R. D., & Read, C. (2001). *Acoustic analysis of speech* (2nd ed.). San Diego, CA: Singular Publishing Group.

Kilgard, M. P., Vazquez, J. L., Engineer, N. D., & Pandya, P. K. (2007). Experience dependent plasticity alters cortical synchronization. *Hearing Research, 229*, 171-179.

Killion, M. C., & Mueller, H. G. (2010). Twenty years later: A NEW count-the-dots method. *Hearing Journal, 63*(1), 10-17.

Kirk, K. I., Miyamoto, R. T., Lento, C. L., Ying, E., O'Neill, T., & Fears, B. (2002). Effects of age at implantation in young children. *Annals of Otology, Rhinology and Laryngology, 189*(Suppl.), 69-73.

Knightly, L. M., Jun, S. A., Oh, J. S., & Au, T. K. (2003). Production benefits of childhood overhearing. *Journal of the Acoustical Society of America, 114*(1), 465-474.

Knittel, M. A. L., Myott, B., & McClain, H. (2002). Update from Oakland schools sound field team: IR vs. FM. *Educational Audiology Review, 19*(2), 10-11.

Kolpe, V. (2003). Earmold evolution. *Hearing Health, 19*(2), 39-41.

Kouwen, H. B., & DeJonckere, P. H. (2007). Prevalence of OME is reduced in young children using chewing gum. *Ear and Hearing, 28*(4), 451-455.

Kramer, S., Dreisbach, L., Lockwood, J., Baldwin, K., Kopke, R., Scranton, S., et al. (2006). Efficacy of the antioxidant N-acetylcysteine (NAC) in protecting ears exposed to loud music. *Journal of the American Academy of Audiology, 17*, 265-278.

Kretschmer, L., & Kretschmer, R. (2001). Children with hearing impairment. In T. Layton, E. Crais, & L.Watson (Eds.), *Handbook of early language impairment in children: Nature* (pp. 56-84). Albany, NY: Delmar.

Kretzmer, E. A., Meltzer, N. E., Haenggeli, C. A., & Ryugo, D. K. (2004). An animal model for cochlear implants. *Archives of Otolaryngology-Head and Neck Surgery, 130*(5) 499-508.

Krishnan, L.A. (2009). Universal newborn hearing screening follow-up: A university clinic perspective. *American Journal of Audiology, 18*, 89-98.

Kubler-Ross, E. (1969). *On death and dying.* New York, NY: Macmillan.

Kuhl, P. K. (1987). Perception of speech and sound in early infancy. In P. Salapatek & L. Cohen (Eds.), *Handbook of infant perceptions: From perception to cognition* (Vol. 2, pp. 275-381). New York, NY: Academic Press.

Kuhn-Inacker, H., Weichbold, V., Tsiakpini, L., Coninx, S., & D'Haese, P. (2003). *Little ears: Auditory questionnaire.* Innsbruck, Austria: MED-EL.

Kuk, F., & Marcoux, A. (2002). Factors ensuring consistent audibility in pediatric hearing aid fitting. *Journal of the American Academy of Audiology, 13*, 503-520.

Lahey, M. (1988). *Language disorders and language development.* New York, NY: Macmillan.

Lai, C. C., & Shiao, A. S. (2004). Chronological changes of hearing in pediatric patients with large vestibular aqueduct syndrome. *Laryngoscope, 114*, 832-838.

Latham, N. M., & Blumsack, J.T. (2008). Classroom acoustics: A survey of educational audiologists. *Journal of Educational Audiology, 14*, 58-68.

Lasky, E. Z., & Klopp, K. (1982). Parent-child interactions in normal and language-disordered children. *Journal of Speech and Hearing Disorders, 47*, 7-18.

Laugesen, S., Nielsen, C., Maas, P., & Jensen, N. S. (2009). Observations on hearing aid users' strategies for controlling the level of their own voice. *Journal of the American Academy of Audiology, 20*(8), 503-513.

Launer, S. (2003, November) *Wireless solutions—The state of the art and future of FM technology for the hearing impaired consumer.* Paper presented at ACCESS Conference, Chicago, IL.

Law, J., Garrett, Z., & Nye, C. (2004). The efficacy of treatment for children with developmental speech and language delay/disorder: A meta-analysis. *Journal of Speech, Language, and Hearing Research, 47,* 924-943.

Leavitt, R. J., & Flexer, C. (1991). Speech degradation as measured by the rapid speech transmission index (RASTI). *Ear and Hearing, 12,* 115-118.

Levitt, H. (2004). Assistive listening technology: What does the future hold? *Volta Voices, 11*(1), 18-21.

Liden, G., & Kankkunen, A. (1969). Visual reinforcement audiometry. *Acta Otolaryngologica, 67,* 281-292.

Lieu, J. E. C. (2004). Speech-language and educational consequences of unilateral hearing loss in children. *Archives of Otolaryngology-Head and Neck Surgery, 130,* 524-530.

Ling, D. (1981). Keep your hearing-impaired child within earshot. *Newsounds, 6,* 5-6.

Ling, D. (1986). Devices and procedures for auditory learning. In E. B. Cole & H. Gregory (Eds.), *Auditory learning* (pp. 19-28).Washington, DC: Alexander Graham Bell Association for the Deaf and Hard of Hearing.

Ling, D. (2002). *Speech and the hearing impaired child* (2nd ed.). Washington, DC: Alexander Graham Bell Association for the Deaf and Hard of Hearing.

Litovsky, R. (2010). Bilateral cochlear implants: Are two ears better than one? *ASHA Leader, 12*(2), 14-17.

Litovsky, R. Y., Johnstone, P. M., Godar, S., Agrawal, S., Parkinson, A., Peters, R., et al. (2006). Bilateral cochlear implants in children: Localization acuity measured with minimum audible angle. *Ear and Hearing, 27*(1), 43-59.

Litovsky, R. Y., Parkinson, A., & Arcaroli, J. (2009). Spatial hearing and speech intelligibility in bilateral cochlear implant users. *Ear AND Hearing, 30*(4), 419-431.

Lonsbury-Martin, B. L., & Feeney, M. P. (2009). A journey for otoacoustic emissions—from the research bench to the clinic. *Audiology Today, 21,* 34-40.

Lowell, E., Rushford, G., Hoversten, G., & Stoner, M. (1956). Evaluation of pure-tone audiometry with pre-school age children. *Journal of Speech and Hearing Disorders, 21,* 292-302.

Lowy, L. (1983). Social work supervision: From models toward theory. *Journal of Education for Social Work, 19,* 55-62.

Luterman, D. (1984). *Counseling the communicatively disordered and their families.* Boston, MA: Little, Brown.

Luterman, D. M. (2001). *Counseling persons with communication disorders and their families* (4th ed.). Austin, TX: Pro-Ed.

Luterman, D. (Ed.). (2006). *Children with hearing loss: A family guide.* Sedona, AZ: Auricle Ink.

Luterman, D. M., & Maxon, A. (2002). *When your child is deaf: A guide for parents* (2nd ed.). Austin, TX: Pro-Ed.

MacDonald, J. (1989). *Becoming partners with children: From play to conversation.* San Antonio, TX: Special Press.

Madell, J.R. (2008). Evaluation of speech perception in infants and children. In J. R. Madell & C. Flexer, (Eds.), *Pediatric audiology: Diagnosis, technology, and management* (pp. 89–105). New York, NY: Thieme.

Madell, J. R., & Flexer, C. (2008). *Pediatric audiology: Diagnosis, technology and educational management.* New York, NY: Thieme.

Madell, J. R., & Flexer, C. (in press). *Pediatric audiology: Cases in childhood hearing loss.* New York, NY: Thieme.

Markides, A. (1986). The use of residual hearing in the education of hearing impaired children: A historical perspective. In E. B. Cole & H. Gregory (Eds.), *Auditory learning* (pp. 57–66). Washington, DC: Alexander Graham Bell Association for the Deaf and Hard of Hearing.

Martin, R.L. (2008). "More 2K." *Hearing Journal, 61*(3), 64–65.

Mayer, T. E., Brueckmann, H., Siegert, R., Witt, A., & Weerda, H. (1997). High-resolution CT of the temporal bone in dysplasia of the auricle and external auditory canal. *American Journal of Neuroradiology, 18*(1), 53–65.

Mazlan, R., Kei, J., & Hickson, L. (2009). Test-retest reliability of the acoustic stapedial reflex test in healthy neonates. *Ear and Hearing, 30*(3), 295–301.

McDonald, L. & Pien, D. (1982). Mother conversational behaviors as a function of conversational intent. *Journal of Child Language, 9*, 337–358.

McKay, S. (2008). Managing children with mild and unilateral hearing loss. In J. R. Madell & C. Flexer, (Eds.), *Pediatric audiology: Diagnosis, technology, and management* (pp. 291–298). New York, NY: Thieme.

McNeil, J., & Fowler, S. (1999). Let's talk: Encouraging mother-child conversations during story reading. *Journal of Early Intervention, 22*, 51–69.

Meltzer, L. (2007). *Executive function in education: From theory to practice.* New York, NY: Guilford Press.

Mendel, L. L., Roberts, R. A., & Walton, J. H. (2003). Speech perception benefits from sound field FM amplification. *American Journal of Audiology, 12*, 114–124.

Mercer, N. (2007). *Words & minds: How we use language to think Together.* New York, NY: Routledge.

Meyer, K. (2003). Mild? Moderate? Any hearing loss is a big deal. *Educational Audiology Review, 20*(4), 22–24.

Milne, A. A. (1926). *Winnie-the-Pooh.* New York, NY: Dutton.

Mitchell, R. E., & Karchmer, M. A. (2004). Chasing the mythical ten percent: Parental hearing status of deaf and hard of hearing students in the United States. *Sign Language Studies, 4*(2), 138–163.

Mlot, S, Buss, E., & Hall III, J.W. (2010). Spectral integration and bandwidth effects on speech recognition in school-aged children and adults. *Ear and Hearing, 31*(1), 56–62.

Moeller, M. P. (2007). Current state of knowledge: Psychosocial development in children with hearing impairment. *Ear and Hearing, 28(6),* 729–739.

Moeller, M. P., Donaghy, K. F., Beauchaine, K. L., Lewis, D. E., & Stelmachowicz, P. G. (1996). Longitudinal study of FM system use in nonacademic settings: Effects on language development. *Ear and Hearing, 17*(1), 28–41.

Moeller, M. P., Hoover, B., Peterson, B., & Stelmachowicz, P. (2009). Consistency of hearing aid use in infants with early-identified hearing loss. *American Journal of Audiology, 18*(1), 14–23.

Moog, J. S. (2002). Changing expectations for children with cochlear implants. *Annals of Otology, Rhinology and Laryngology, 111,* 138–142.

Moog, J. S., & Geers, A. E. (2003). Epilogue: Major findings, conclusions and implications for deaf education. *Ear and Hearing, 24*(1S), 121S–125S.

Moses, K. (1985). Infant deafness and parental grief: Psychosocial early intervention. In F. Powell, T. Finitzo-Hieber, S. Friel-Patti, & D. Henderson (Eds.), *Education of the hearing-impaired child* (pp. 86–102). San Diego, CA: College-Hill Press.

Moses, K., & Van Hecke-Wulatin, M. (1981). The socio-emotional impact of infant deafness: A counselling model. In G. T. Mencher & S. E. Gerber (Eds.), *Early management of hearing loss* (pp. 243–278). New York, NY: Grune & Stratton.

Musiek, F. E. (2009). The human auditory cortex: Interesting anatomical and clinical perspectives. *Audiology Today, 21*(4), 26–37.

Musiek, F. E., & Chermak, G. D. (2006). *Handbook for central auditory processing disorders: Satisfying the 10 cravings of a new generation of consumers.* San Diego, CA: Plural.

Myklebust, H. (1954). *Auditory disorders in children.* New York, NY: Grune & Stratton.

Myklebust, H. (1960). *The psychology of deafness.* New York, NY: Grune & Stratton.

Nelson, E. L., Smaldino, J., Erler, S., & Garstecki, D. (2008). Background noise levels and reverberation times in old and new elementary school classrooms. *Journal of Educational Audiology, 14,* 12-18.

Nelson, K. E. (1973). Structure and strategy in learning to talk. *Monographs of the Society for Research in Child Development, 38* (Serial No. 149).

Newport, E. L. (1977). Motherese: The speech of mothers to young children. In N. Castellan, D. Pisoni, & G. Potts (Eds.), *Cognitive theory* (Vol. II, pp. 69-84). Hillsdale, NJ: Lawrence Erlbaum.

Newport, E. L., Gleitman, H., & Gleitman, L. R. (1977). Mother, I'd rather do it myself: Some effects and non-effects of maternal speech style. In C. E. Snow & C. A. Ferguson (Eds.), *Talking to children: Language input and acquisition* (pp. 109-149). Cambridge, UK: Cambridge University Press.

Newson, J. (1977). The growth of shared understanding between infant and caregiver. In M. Bullowa (Ed.), *Before speech: The beginning of interpersonal communication* (pp. 207-222). Cambridge, UK: Cambridge University Press.

Nicholas, J. G., & Geers, A. E. (2006). Effects of early auditory experience on the spoken language of deaf children at 3 years of age. *Ear and Hearing, 27*(3), 286-298.

Nicholas, J. G., & Geers, A. (2007). Will they catch up? The role of age at cochlear implantation in the spoken language development of children with severe to profound hearing loss. *Journal of Speech, Language, and Hearing Research, 50,* 1048-1062.

Niparko, J. K. (2004). Cochlear implants: Clinical application. In F. G. Zeng, A. Popper, & R. Fay (Eds.), *Cochlear implants: Auditory prosthesis and electric hearing* (pp. 53-100). New York, NY: Springer-Verlag.

Nittrouer, S., & Burton, L. T. (2001). The role of early language experience in the development of speech perception and language processing abilities in children with hearing loss. *Volta Review, 103*(1), 5-37.

Nixon, M. (2005). Classroom acoustics. *Educational Audiology Review, 22*(2), 3-5.

Nohara, M., McKay, S., & Trehub, S. (1995). Analyzing conversations between mothers and their hearing impaired and deaf adolescents. *Volta Review, 97,* 23-134.

Northcott, W. (1972). *Curriculum guide: Hearing impaired children—birth to three years.* Washington DC: The Alexander Graham Bell Association for the Deaf and Hard of Hearing.

Northcott, W. H. (Ed.). (1978). *I heard that! A development sequence of listening activities for the young child.* Washington, DC: Alexander Graham Bell Association for the Deaf and Hard of Hearing.

Northern, J. L., & Downs, M. P. (2002). *Hearing in children* (5th ed.). Baltimore, MD: Lippincott Williams & Wilkins.

Nott, P., Cowan, R., Brown, P. M., & Wigglesworth, G. (2009). Early language development in children with profound hearing loss fitted with a device at a young age: Part II. Content of the first lexicon. *Ear and Hearing, 30*(5), 541-551.

Nozza, R. (2006, May). *Developmental psychoacoustics: Auditory function in infants and children.* Paper presented at the Fourth Widex Congress of Paediatric Audiology, Ottawa, Canada.

Nyffeler, M., & Dechant, S. (2010). The impact of new technology on mobile phone use. *Hearing Review, 17*(3), 42-49.

Oliveira, R., Kolpe, V., Parish, B., Babcock, M., Oliveira, D., & Venem, M. (2006, June). *Advances in earmold compatibility. . . . Or "reinventing the earmold."* Paper presented at the Alexander Graham Bell Association for the Deaf and Hard of Hearing International Convention and Research Symposium, Pittsburgh, PA.

Oller, D. K. (1995). The development of vocalizations in infancy. In H. Winitz (Ed.), *Human communication and its disorders: A review* (Vol. IV, pp. 1-30). Timonium, MD: York Press.

Oller, D. K. (2000). *Emergence of the speech capacity.* Mahwah, NJ: Lawrence Erlbaum and Associates.

Olsen-Fulero, L., & Conforti, J. (1983). Child responsiveness to mother questions of varying type and presentation. *Journal of Child Language, 10,* 495-520.

Oomen, K. P., Rovers, M. M., van den Akker, E. H., vanStaaij, B. K., Hoes, A. W., & Schilder, A. G. (2005, April). Effect of adenotonsillectomy on middle ear status in children. *Laryngoscope, 115*(4), 731-734.

Owens, R. (2004). *Language disorders: A functional approach to assessment and intervention* (4th ed.). Boston, MA: Allyn & Bacon.

Owens, R. (2005). *Language development: An introduction* (6th ed.). Boston, MA: Allyn & Bacon

Palmer, C. V., & Grimes, A. M. (2005). Effectiveness of signal processing strategies for the pediatric population: A systematic review of the evidence. *Journal of the American Academy of Audiology, 16,* 505-514.

Patton, J. B., Hackett, L., & Rodriguez, L. (2004). *The listening age formula.* San Antonio, TX: Sunshine Cottage School for the Deaf.

Paul, R. (2007). *Language disorders from infancy through adolescence: Assessment and intervention* (3rd ed.). St. Louis, MO: Mosby.

Pepper, J., & Weitzman, E. (2004). *It takes two to talk: A practical guide for parents of children with language delays.* Toronto, Canada: The Hanen Center.

Perkell, J. S. (2008). *Auditory feedback and speech production in cochlear implant users and speakers with typical hearing.* Paper presented at the 2008 Research Symposium of the Alexander Graham Bell Association International Convention, Milwaukee, Wisconsin, June 29, 2008.

Peters, A. M., & Boggs, S. T. (1986). Interactional routines as cultural references upon language acquisition. In B. B. Schiefflelin & B. Ochs (Eds.), *Language socialization across cultures*. Cambridge, UK: Cambridge University Press.

Peterson, C. F., Donner, F., & Flavell, J. (1972) Developmental changes in children's responses to three indications of communication failure. *Child Development, 43,* 1463-1468.

Peterson, P. (2004). Naturalistic language teaching procedures for children at risk for language delays. *The Behavior Analyst Today, 5,* 404-424.

Peterson, P., Carta, J., & Greenwood, C. (2005). Teaching enhanced milieu language teaching skills to parents of multiple risk families. *Journal of Early Intervention, 27,* 94-109.

Phillips, J. (1973). Syntax and vocabulary of mother's speech to young children: Age and sex comparisons. *Child Development, 44,* 182-185.

Pickering, M. (1987). Interpersonal communication and the supervisory process: A search for Ariadne's thread. In M. Crago & M. Pickering (Eds.), *Supervision in human communication disorders: Perspectives on a process* (pp. 203-225). Boston, MA: Little, Brown.

Pickett, J. M. (1998). *The acoustic analysis of speech communication: Fundamentals, speech perception theory, and technology.* Needham, MA: Allyn & Bacon.

Pirzanski, C. (2006). Earmolds and hearing aid shells: A tutorial—pediatric impressions. *Hearing Review, 13*(6), 50-55.

Pittman, A. L. (2008). Short-term word-learning rate in children with normal hearing and children with hearing loss in limited and extended high-frequency bandwidths. *Journal of Speech-Language and Hearing Research, 51*(3), 785-797.

Poehlmann, J., & Fiese, B. (2001). Parent-infant interaction as a mediator of the relations between neonatal risk stats and 12-month cognitive development. *Infant Behavior and Development, 24,* 171-188.

Pollack, D. (1970). *Educational audiology for the limited-hearing infant* (1st ed.). Springfield, IL: Charles C. Thomas.

Pollack, D. (1985). *Educational audiology for the limited-hearing infant and preschooler* (2nd ed.). Springfield, IL: Charles C. Thomas.

Pollack, D., Goldberg, D., & Caleffe-Schenck, N. (1997). *Educational audiology for the limited-hearing infant and preschooler: An auditory-verbal program.* Springfield, IL: Charles C. Thomas.

Powers, T. (2010). The pediatric device. *Advance for Audiologists, 12*(1), 24-27.

Price, L., Hitchcock, J., Breneman, A., Peterson, A., & Shallop, J. (2005). Diagnosing auditory neuropathy: Lessons learned along the way. *Educational Audiology Review, 22*(1), 8-10.

Prieve, B. A., Hancur-Bucci, C. A., & Preston, J. L. (2009). Changes in transient-evoked otoacoustic emissions in the first month of life. *Ear and Hearing, 30*(3), 330-339.

Proctor-Williams, K., Fey, M., & Loeb, D. (2001). Parental recasts and production of copulas and articles by children with specific language impairment and typical development. *American Journal of Speech-Language Pathology, 10*, 155-168.

Pugh, K. (2005, November). *Neuroimaging studies of reading and reading disability: Establishing brain/behavior relations.* Presentation at the Literacy and Language Conference of the Speech, Language and Learning Center, New York, NY.

Pugh, K. R., Sandak, R., Frost, S. J., Moore, D. L., & Menci, W. E. (2006). Neurobiological investigations of skilled and impaired reading. In D. Dickinson & S. Neuman (Eds.), *Handbook of early literacy research* (Vol. 2, pp. 64-76). New York, NY: Guilford.

Purdy, S. C., Farrington, D. R., Moran, C. A., Chard, L. L., & Hodgson, S. A. (2002). A parental questionnaire to evaluate children's auditory behavior in everyday life (ABEL). *American Journal of Audiology, 11*, 72-82.

Ramirez Inscoe, J. M., & Nikolopoulos, T. P. (2004). Cochlear implantation in children deafened by cytomegalovirus: Speech perception and speech intelligibility outcomes. *Otology & Neurotology, 25*, 479-482.

Rance, G., McKay, C., & Grayden, D. (2004). Perceptual characterization of children with auditory neuropathy. *Ear and Hearing, 25*(1), 34-46.

Raphael, Y. (2006). *Strategies for prevention and cure of inner ear disease.* Paper presented at the Alexander Graham Bell Association for the Deaf and Hard of Hearing International Convention and Research Symposium, Pittsburgh, PA.

Red Book. (2006). *2006 Report of the committee on infectious diseases.* Elk Grove Village, IL: American Academy of Pediatrics.

Regional and National Summary Report of Data from 2005-2006 Annual Survey of Deaf and Hard of Hearing Children and Youth. (2006) Washington, DC: Gallaudet University.

Rehabilitation Act Amendments of 1992, P. L. 102-569. (1992, October). *United States Statutes at Large, 106*, 4344-4488.

Rehabilitation Act of 1973, P. L. 93-112. (1973, September). *United States Statutes at Large, 87*, 355-394.

Rehm, H. L., & Madore, R. (2008). Genetics of hearing loss. In J. R. Madell & C. Flexer, (Eds.), *Pediatric audiology: Diagnosis, technology, and management* (pp. 13-24). New York, NY: Thieme.

Rehm, H. L., Williamson, R. E., Kenna, M. A., Corey, D. P., & Korf, B. R. (2003). *Understanding the genetics of deafness: A guide for patients and families*. Cambridge, MA: Harvard Medical School Center for Hereditary Deafness.

Retherford, K. S., Schwartz, B. C., & Chapman, R. S. (1981). Semantic roles and residual grammatical categories in mother and child speech: Who tunes in to whom? *Journal of Child Language, 8*, 583–608.

Rice, M. (2004). Growth models of developmental language disorders. In M. Rice & F. Warren (Eds.), *Developmental language disorders: From phenotypes to etiologies* (pp. 207–240). Mahwah, NH: Lawrence Erlbaum.

Riesen, A. H. (1974). Studies of early sensory deprivation in animals. In C. Griffiths (Ed.), *Proceedings of the International Conference on Auditory Techniques* (pp. 33–38). Springfield, IL: Charles C Thomas.

Rini, D., & Hindenlang, J. (2006). Family-centered practice for children with communication disorders. In R. Paul & P. Casaella (Eds.), *Introduction to clinical methods in communication disorders* (pp. 317–336). Baltimore, MD: Paul H. Brookes.

Robbins, A. M., Green, J., & Waltzman, S. B. (2004). Bilingual oral language proficiency in children with cochlear implants. *Archives of Otolaryngology-Head and Neck Surgery, 130*, 644–647.

Robbins, A. M., Koch, D. B., Osberger, M. J., Zimmerman-Philips, S., & Kishon-Rabin, L. (2004). Effect of age at cochlear implantation on auditory skill development in infants and toddlers. *Archives of Otolaryngology-Head and Neck Surgery, 130*(5), 570–574.

Robbins, A. M., Renshaw, J. J., & Berry, S.W. (1991). Evaluating meaningful integration in profoundly hearing impaired children (MAIS). *American Journal of Otolaryngology, 12*(Suppl.), 144–150.

Robertson, L. (2009). *Literacy and deafness: Listening and spoken language*. San Diego, CA: Plural.

Rocissano, L., & Yatchmink, Y. (1983). Language skill and interactive patterns in prematurely born toddlers. *Child Development, 54*, 1229–1241.

Roeser, R. J., & Downs, M. P. (2004). *Auditory disorders in school children: The law, identification, remediation* (4th ed.). New York, NY: Thieme.

Rogers, C. (1951). *Client-centered therapy*. Boston, MA: Houghton Mifflin.

Rosenberg, G. G., Blake-Rahter, P., Heavner, J., Allen, L., Redmond, B. M., Phillips, J., et al. (1999). Improving classroom acoustics (ICA): A three-year FM sound field classroom amplification study. *Journal of Educational Audiology, 7*, 8–28.

Ross, M. (2005). Fitting hearing aids and evidence-based audiology. *Hearing Loss, 26*(4), 30–33.

Ross, M., Brackett, D., & Maxon, A. (1991). *Assessment and management of mainstreamed hearing-impaired children*. Austin, TX: Pro-Ed.

Rossetti, L. (2001). *Communication intervention: Birth to three* (2nd ed.). San Diego, CA: Singular Publishing Group.

Rossi, K. (2003). *Learn around the clock: A professional's early interven-tion toolbox.* Washington, DC: Alexander Graham Bell Association for the Deaf and Hard of Hearing.

Sabbagh, M. A., & Moses L. J. (2006). Executive functioning and preschool-ers' understanding of false beliefs, false photographs, and false signs. *Child Development, 77*(4), 1034–1049.

Sachs, J. (1983). The adaptive significance of linguistic input to prelinguis-tic infants. In C. E. Snow & C. A. Ferguson (Eds.), *Talking to children: Language input and acquisition.* Cambridge, UK: Cambridge Univer-sity Press.

Saxton, M. (2005). 'Recasts' in a new light: Insights for practice from typ-ical language studies. *Child Language Teaching and Therapy, 21,* 23–38.

Schafer, E. C., & Thibodeau, L. M. (2003). Speech-recognition performance in children using cochlear implants and FM systems. *Journal of Educa-tional Audiology, 11,* 15–26.

Schaub, A. (2009). *Digital hearing aids.* New York, NY: Thieme.

Schauwers, K., Gillis, S., & Govaerts, P. (2005). Language acquisition in children with a cochlear implant. In P. Fletcher & J. Miller (Eds.). *Devel-opmental theory and language disorders* (pp. 95–120). Philadelphia, PA: John Benjamin.

Schein, J. D., & Miller, M. H. (2010). Genetics and deafness: Implications for education and life care of students with hearing loss. *Hearing Review, 17*(4), 38–42.

Scherer, N., & Olswang, L. (1984). Role of mothers' expansions in stimu-lating children's language production. *Journal of Speech and Hearing Research, 27,* 387–396.

Scholl, J. R. (2006). Unilateral hearing loss and babies: Finding the right mix. *Hearing Journal, 59*(7), 47.

Schneider, W., Schumann-Hengsteler R., & Sodian, B. (2005). *Young chil-dren's cognitive development: Interrelationships among executive functioning, working memory, verbal ability, and theory of mind.* Mahwah, NJ: Lawrence Erlbaum.

Scholl, J. R. (2010). Happy ideas for the pint-sized set. *Advance for Audi-ologists, 12*(1), 10.

Schum, D. J. (2010). Wireless connectivity for hearing aids. *Advance for Audiologists, 12*(2), 24–26.

Scollie, S. (2006, May). *Current issues in paediatric amplification: Roles for technology and for prescriptive methods.* Paper presented at the Fourth Widex Congress of Paediatric Audiology, Ottawa, Canada.

Seitz, S., & Stewart, C. (1975). Imitation and expansion: Some developmen-tal aspects of mother-child conversation. *Developmental Psychology, 11,* 763–768.

Sexton, J. (2003). FM as a component of primary amplification. *Educational Audiology Review, 20*(4), 4-5.

Sharma, A., Dorman, M. F., & Kral, A. (2005). The influence of a sensitive period on central auditory development in children with unilateral and bilateral cochlear implants. *Hearing Research, 203*, 134-143.

Sharma, A., Dorman, M. F., & Spahr, A. J. (2002). A sensitive period for the development of the central auditory system in children with cochlear implants: Implications for age of implantation. *Ear and Hearing, 23*(6), 532-539.

Sharma, A., Martin, K., Roland, P., Bauer, P., Sweeney, M. H., Gilley, P., et al. (2005). P1 latency as a biomarker for central auditory development in children with hearing impairment. *Journal of the American Academy of Audiology, 16*, 564-573.

Sharma, A., & Nash, A. (2009). Brain maturation in children with cochlear implants. *ASHA Leader, 14*(5), 14-17.

Sharma, A., Tobey, E., Dorman, M., Bharadwaj, S., Martin, K., Gilley, P., et al. (2004). Central auditory maturation and babbling development in infants with cochlear implants. *Archives of Otolaryngology-Head and Neck Surgery, 130*(5), 511-516.

Shaywitz, S. E., & Shaywitz, B. A. (2004). Disability and the brain. *Educational Leadership, 61*(6), 7-11.

Sheng, L., McGregor, K., & Xu, Y. (2005). Prosodic and lexical syntactic aspects of the therapeutic register. *Clinical Linguistics and Phonetics, 17*, 355-363.

Sherrer, K. R. (1974). Acoustic concomitants of emotional dimensions: Judging affect from synthesized tone sequences. In J. Weitz (Ed.), *Nonverbal communication* (pp. 145-180). Oxford, UK: Oxford University Press.

Sheridan, D. J., & Cunningham, L. L. (2009). Music to my ears: Enhanced speech perception through musical experience. *Audiology Today, 21*(6), 56-57.

Shprintzen, R. J. (2001). *Syndrome identification for audiology: An illustrated pocket guide.* San Diego, CA: Singular Thomson Learning.

Siem, G., Fruh, A., Leren, T. P., Heimdal, K., Teig, E., & Harris, S. (2008). Jervell and Lange-Nielsen syndrome in Norwegian children: Aspects around cochlear implantation, hearing and balance. *Ear and Hearing, 29*(2), 261-269.

Simmons, D. D. (2003). The ear in utero: An engineering masterpiece. *Hearing Health, 19*(2), 10-14.

Sindrey, D. (2002). *Listening games for littles* (2nd ed.). London, Canada: WordPlay Publications.

Sininger, Y. S., Grimes, A., & Christensen, E. (2010). Auditory development in early amplified children: Factors influencing auditory-based communication outcomes in children with hearing loss. *Ear and Hearing*, *31*(2), 166-185.

Sininger, Y. S., Martinez, A., Eisenberg, L., Christensen, E., Grimes, A., & Hu, J. (2009). Newborn hearing screening speeds diagnosis and access to intervention by 20-25 months. *Journal of the American Academy of Audiology*, *20*(1), 49-57.

Sjoblad, S., Harrison, J., & Roush, J. (2004). Parents' experiences and perceptions regarding early hearing aid use. *Volta Voices*, *11*(4), 8-9.

Skinner, B. F. (1957). *Verbal behavior.* New York, NY: Appleton-Century-Crofts.

Skinner, B. F. (1964). New methods and new dimensions in teaching. *New Scientist*, *22*(392), 483-484.

Sloutsky, V. M., & Napolitano, A. C. (2003). Is a picture worth a thousand words? Preference for auditory modality in young children. *Child Development*, *74*, 822-833.

Smaldino, J. (2004). Barriers to listening and learning in the classroom. *Volta Voices*, *11*(4), 24-26.

Smaldino, J. J., & Crandell, C. C. (Eds.). (2004). Classroom acoustics. *Seminars in Hearing*, *25*(4), 113-206.

Snow, C. E. (1972). Mother's speech to children learning language. *Child Development*, *43*, 549-565.

Snow, C. E. (1977). The development of conversation between mothers and babies. *Journal of Child Language*, *4*, 1-22.

Snow, C. E. (1984). Parent-child interaction and the development of communicative ability. In R. L. Schiefelbusch & J. P. Pickar (Eds.), *The acquisition of communicative competence* (pp. 69-107). Baltimore, MD: University Park Press.

Snow, C. E., de Blauw, S., & van Roosmalen, G. (1979). Talking and playing with babies: The role of ideologies of childrearing. In M. Bullowa (Ed.), *Before speech: The beginning of interpersonal communication* (pp. 269-288). Cambridge, UK: Cambridge University Press.

Snow, C. E., & Gilbreath, B. J. (1983). Explaining transitions. In R. M. Golinkoff (Ed.), *The transition from prelinguistic to linguistic communication* (pp. 281-296). Hillsdale, NJ: Lawrence Erlbaum.

Snow, C. E., Midkiff-Borunda, S., Small, A., & Proctor, A. (1984). Therapy as social interaction: Analyzing the context of language remediation. *Topics in Language Disorders*, *4*, 72-85.

Snow, C. E., Perlman, R., & Nathan, D. (1987). Why routines are different: Toward a multiple-factors model of the relation between input and language acquisition. In K. E. Nelson & A. Van Kleeck (Eds.), *Children's language* (Vol. 6, pp. 65-97). Hillsdale, NJ: Lawrence Erlbaum.

Snow, C. E., Tabors, P., & Dickinson, D. (2001). Language development in the preschool years. In D. Dickinson & P. Tabors, *Beginning literacy with language*. Baltimore, MD: Brookes.

Spiker, D., Boyce, G., & Boyce, L. (2002). Parent-child interactions when young children have disabilities. *International Review of Research in Mental Retardation, 25*, 35-70.

Stach, B. A. (2008). Reporting audiometric results. *Hearing Journal, 61*(9), 10-16.

Stach B. A., & Ramachandran, V. S. (2008). Hearing disorders in children. In J. R. Madell & C. Flexer, (Eds.), *Pediatric audiology: Diagnosis, technology, and management* (pp. 3-12*)*. New York, NY: Thieme.

Stedler-Brown, A., & Johnson, D. C. (2003). Functional auditory performance indicators: An integrated approach to auditory development. Retrieved on October 16, 2006 from http://www.csdb.org/chip/resources/docs/fapi6_23.pdk .

Stern, D. N. (1974). Mother and infant at play: The dyadic interaction involving facial, vocal, and gaze behaviors. In M. L. Lewis & L. A. Rosenblum (Eds.), *The effects of the infant on its caregiver* (pp. 187-213). New York, NY: John Wiley and Sons.

Stern, D. N., Spieker, S., Barnett, R. K., & MacKain, K. (1983). The prosody of maternal speech: Infant age and context-related changes. *Journal of Child Language, 10*, 1-16.

Strickland, D. S., & Shanahan, T. (2004). Laying the groundwork for literacy. *Educational Leadership, 61*(6), 74-77.

Strom, K. (2010). Why we should get looped. *Hearing Review, 17*(2), 8.

Sugarman, S. (1984). The development of communication: Its contribution and limits in promoting the development of language. In R. L. Schiefelbusch & J. P. Pickar (Eds.), *The acquisition of communicative competence* (pp. 23-67). Baltimore, MD: University Park Press.

Sun, W. (2009). The biological mechanisms of hyperacusis. *ASHA Leader, 14* (11), 5-6.

Suzuki, T., & Ogiba, Y. (1961). Conditioned orientation audiometry. *Archives of Otolaryngology, 74*, 192-198.

Sweetow, R. W., Rosbe, K. W., Philliposian, C., & Miller, M. T. (2005). Considerations for cochlear implantation of children with sudden fluctuating hearing loss. *Journal of the American Academy of Audiology, 16*, 770-780.

Sylvester, J. (2006). Noisy toys: Annoying or harmful? *Hearing Review, 13*(1), 58-60.

Tallal, P. (2004). Improving language and literacy is a matter of time. *Nature Reviews Neuroscience, 5*, 721-728.

Tallal, P. (2005, November). *Improving language and literacy*. Paper presented at the Literacy and Language Conference of the Speech, Language and Learning Center, New York, NY.

Tannock, R., & Girolometto, L. (1992). Re-assessing parent-focused language interventions programs. In S. F. Warren & J. Reichle (Eds.), *Causes and effects in communication and language intervention* (pp. 49-80). Baltimore, MD: Paul H. Brookes.

Tees, R. C. (1967). Effects of early auditory restrictions in the rat on adult pattern discrimination. *Journal of Comparative and Physiological Psychology, 63*, 389-393.

Tervoort, B. (1964). Development of language and "the critical period" in the young deaf child: Identification and management. *Acta Otolaryngologica, 206*(Suppl.), 247-251.

Thal, D., & Clancy, B. (2001). Brain development and language learning: Implications for nonbiologically based language learning disorders. *Journal of Speech-Language Pathology and Audiology, 25*, 52-76.

Tharpe, A. M. (2004). Who has time for functional auditory assessments? We all do! *Volta Voices, 11*(4), 10-12.

Tharpe, A. M. (2006, May). *The impact of minimal and mild hearing loss on children.* Paper presented at the Fourth Widex Congress of Paediatric Audiology, Ottawa, Canada.

Tharpe, A. M. (2008). Unilateral and mild bilateral hearing loss in children: Past and current perspectives. *Trends in Amplification, 12*(1), 7-15.

Tharpe, A. M. (2009). Closing the gap in EHDI follow-up. *ASHA Leader, 14*(4), 12-14.

Thoman, E. B. (1981). Affective communication as the prelude and context for language learning. In R. L. Schiefelbusch & D. D. Bricker (Eds.), *Early language: Acquisition and intervention* (pp. 181-200). Baltimore, MD: University Park Press.

Thomas, E., El-Kashlan, H., & Zwolan, T.A. (2008). Children with cochlear implants who live in monolingual and bilingual homes. *Otology and Neurology, 29*(2), 230-234.

Tjellstrom, A. (2005). Baha in children—An overview. *Bone-anchored applications.* Goteborg, Sweden: Entific Medical Systems.

Tobey, E. (2010). The changing landscape of pediatric cochlear implantation: Outcomes influence eligibility criteria. *ASHA Leader, 12*(2), 10-13.

Tomasello, M. (2008). *The origins of human communication* (pp. 57-72). Cambridge, MA: MIT Press.

Trevarthen, C. (1977). Descriptive analyses of infant communicative behavior. In H. R. Schaffer (Ed.), *Studies in mother-infant interaction* (pp. 227-270). London, Canada: Academic Press.

Tye-Murray, N. (2003). Conversational fluency of children who use cochlear implants. *Ear and Hearing, 24*(Suppl. 2) 82S-89S.

Tyler, R. S., Parkinson, A. J., Wilson, B. S., Witt, S., Preece, J. P., & Nobel, W. (2002). Patients utilizing a hearing aid and a cochlear implant: Speech perception and localization. *Ear and Hearing, 23*, 98-105.

Uchanski, R. M., & Geers, A. (2003). Acoustic characteristics of the speech of young cochlear implant users: A comparison with normal hearing age mates. *Ear and Hearing, 24*(Suppl. 1), 90S–105S.

Van Camp, G. (2006, May). *Deafness in children: The role of genes unraveled.* Paper presented at the Fourth Widex Congress of Paediatric Audiology, Ottawa, Canada.

Vouloumanos, A., & Werker, J. F. (2007). Listening to language at birth: Evidence for a bias for speech in neonates. *Developmental Science, 10*(2), 159–164.

Vygotski, L. (1978). *Mind in society.* Cambridge, MA: University Press.

Wallber, J. (2009). Audiologists' role in early diagnosis of Usher syndrome. *ASHA Leader, 14*(16), 5–6.

Waltzman, S. (2005). Expanding patient criteria for cochlear implantation. *Audiology Today, 17*(5), 20–21.

Wanska, S. K. & Bedrosian, J. L. (1985). Conversational structure and topic performance in mother-child interaction. *Journal of Speech and Hearing Research, 28*, 579–584.

Warren, S., & Yoder, D. (1998). Facilitating the transition from preintentional to intentional communication. In A. Wetherby, S. Warren, & J. Riechle (Eds.), *Transitions in prelinguistic communication* (pp. 365–384). Baltimore, MD: Paul H. Brookes.

Waseem, M., & Aslam, M. (2006, June). *Otitis media.* Retrieved August 13, 2006, from http://www.eMedicine.com

Weber, P., Bluestone, C. D., & Perez, B. (2003). Outcome of hearing and vertigo after surgery for congenital perilymphatic fistula in children. *American Journal of Otolaryngology, 24*(3), 138–142.

Weismer, S. (2000). Intervention for children with developmental language delay. In D. Bishop & L. Leonard (Eds.), *Speech and language impairments in children: Causes, characteristics, intervention and outcome* (pp. 157–176). New York, NY: Psychology Press.

Weizman, Z. & Snow, C. (2001). Lexical input as related to children's vocabulary acquisition: Effects of sophisticated exposure and support for meaning. *Developmental Psychology, 37*, 265–279.

Werker, J. (2006, May). *Infant speech perception and early language acquisition.* Paper presented at the Fourth Widex Congress of Paediatric Audiology, Ottawa, Canada.

Werker, J. F., & Byers-Heinlein, K. (2008). Bilingualism in infancy: First steps in perception and comprehension. *Trends in Cognitive Sciences, 12*(4), 144–151.

Whetnall, E. (1958). Clinics for children handicapped by deafness. In A. Ewing (Ed.), *The modern educational treatment of deafness* (pp. 16/1–16/11). Manchester, UK: Manchester University Press.

White, K. (2008). Newborn hearing screening. In J. R. Madell & C. Flexer, (Eds.), *Pediatric audiology: Diagnosis, technology, and management* (pp. 31-41). New York, NY: Thieme.

Williams, C. (2003). The children's outcome worksheets (COW): An outcome measure focusing on children's needs (ages 4-12). *News from Oticon.* Retrieved January 30, 2005 from http://www.oticon.com

Wills, T., & Goodrich, J. M. (2006, August). *Cytomegalovirus.* Retrieved on August 29, 2006, from WebMD, http://www.eMedicine.com

Windmill, S., & Windmill, I. M. (2006). The status of diagnostic testing following referral from universal newborn hearing screening. *Journal of the American Academy of Audiology, 17,* 367-378.

Winegert, P., & Brant, M. (2005, August). Reading your baby's mind. *Newsweek, 15,* 33-39.

Wolfe, J., & Schafer, E. (2010). *Programming cochlear implants.* San Diego, CA: Plural.

Wolfe, J., & Scholl, J.R. (2009). Ensuring well-fitted earmolds for infants and toddlers. *Hearing Journal, 62*(10), 56.

Wright, C. G. (1997). Development of the human external ear. *Journal of the American Academy of Audiology, 8,* 379-382.

Wu, C. C., Chen, Y. S., Chen, P. J., & Hsu, C. J. (2005). Common clinical features of children with enlarged vestibular aqueduct and Mondini dysplasia. *Laryngoscope, 115,* 132-137.

Yoder, P., McCathren, R., Warren, S., & Watson, A. (2001). Important distinctions in measuring maternal responses to communication in prelinguistic children with disabilities. *Communication Disorders Quarterly, 22,* 135-147.

Yoder, P., & Warren, S. (1998). Maternal responsivity predicts the prelinguistic communication intervention that facilitates generalized intentional communication. *Journal of Speech, Language, and Hearing Research, 41,* 1207-1219.

Yoder, P., & Warren, S. (2001). Prelinguistic milieu teaching. In H. Goldstein, L. Kaczmarek, & K. English (Eds.), *Promoting social communication: Children with developmental disabilities from birth to adolescence* (pp. 98-135). Baltimore, MD: Paul H. Brookes.

Yoder, P., & Warren, S. (2002). Effects of prelinguistic milieu teaching and parent responsivity education on dyads involving children with intellectual disabilities. *Journal of Speech, Language, and Hearing, 45,* 1158-1175.

Yoshinaga-Itano, C. (1998). Early identification and intervention: It does make a difference. *Audiology Today, 10*(Suppl. 11), 20-22.

Yoshinaga-Itano, C. (2004, September). *Issues and outcomes of early intervention.* Presentation at the Consensus Conference on Early Intervention, Washington, DC.

Yoshinaga-Itano, C., Sedey, A. L., Coulter, D. K., & Mehl, A. L. (1998). Language of early- and later-identified children with hearing loss. *Pediatrics, 102,* 1161-1771.

Young, A., & Tattersall, H. (2007). Universal newborn hearing screening and early identification of deafness: Parents' responses to knowing early and their expectations of child communication development. *Journal of Deaf Studies and Deaf Education. 12*(2), 209-220.

Zhang, T., Spahr, A. J., & Dorman, M.F. (2010). Frequency overlap between electric and acoustic stimulation and speech-perception benefit in patients with combined electric and acoustic stimulation. *Ear and Hearing 31*(2), 195-201.

Zeng, F. G., Popper, A., & Fay, R. (Eds.). (2004). *Cochlear implants: Auditory prosthesis and electric hearing.* New York, NY: Springer-Verlag.

Zimmerman-Phillips, S., Osberger, M. F., & Robbins, A. M. (1997). *Infanttoddler: Meaningful auditory integration scale (IT-MAIS).* Sylmar, CA: Advanced Bionics.

Zupan, B., & Sussman, J. E. (2009). Auditory preferences of young children with and without hearing loss for meaningful auditory–visual compound stimuli. *Journal of Communication Disorders,* 42, 381-396.

Zwolan, T. A., Ashbaugh, C. M., Alarfaj, A., Kileny, P. R., Arts, H. A., El-Kashlan, H. K., et al. (2004). Pediatric cochlear implant patient performance as a function of age at implantation. *Otology and Neurotology, 25*(2), 112-120.

Glossary of Terms

Accommodations: Services or equipment to which the student with a disability legally is entitled for the purpose of providing an adequate and equitable education.

Acoustic: Sound, its physical nature.

Acoustic filter effect of hearing loss: Hearing loss acts like an invisible acoustic filter that distorts, smears, or eliminates incoming sounds; the negative impact of this filter effect on spoken communication, reading, academics, and independent function causes the problems associated with hearing loss.

Acoustic phonetics: The study of speech sounds as they are perceived by the ear of the listener; objective study and measurement of the sounds waves produced when speech sounds are spoken.

Acoustic saliency: An acoustically salient phoneme (speech sound) or word is one that is obvious and prominent in an utterance. In a sentence context, acoustically nonsalient morphemes are shorter in duration and softer than louder phonemes in adjacent portions of the utterance.

Acoustical treatment: Using a material or process for changing the absorptive or reflective characteristics of a surface in a room.

Acoustically modified earmolds: Specifically shaped earmolds that change the output of the hearing aid (e.g., horn-shaped earmold that improves high-frequency amplification).

Acquired hearing loss: Hearing losses that occur after speech and language have been developed.

Affect: Pertaining to feelings, emotions.

Aided thresholds: Represented by the symbol A on an audiogram, they are the softest tones that a person can hear while wearing hearing aids.

Air conduction: Sound travels through the air from a source, reaches the ear, enters the auditory system through the ear canal, and progresses through the eardrum, middle ear, inner ear, and then to the brain. Air conduction thresholds are obtained by using the earphones (or ear inserts) of an audiometer, with the symbol *O* representing right ear sensitivity and the symbol *X* representing left ear sensitivity on an audiogram.

Alveolar: A speech sound produced with involvement of the ridge in the mouth just behind the upper teeth, such as /t/ or /d/.

Ambient noise: Sounds in the environment that are not part of the desired acoustic signal.

Amplification: To make sounds louder; may also refer to a piece of equipment used to make sounds louder, such as a hearing aid.

Amplifier: A device that increases the intensity of an electrical signal.

Amplitude: The intensity of a sound.

Assistive listening device (ALD): Any of a number of pieces of equipment used to augment hearing or to assist the hearing aid in difficult listening situations; through the use of a remote microphone, assistive listening devices provide a superior signal-to-noise ratio that enhances the clarity (intelligibility) of the speech signal.

Atresia: Absence or complete closure of the ear canal, causing a conductive-type hearing loss.

Attenuation: A reduction or decrease in magnitude; a sound made softer.

Audibility: Being able to hear but not necessarily distinguish among speech sounds.

Audiogram: A graph of a person's peripheral hearing sensitivity with frequency (pitch) on one axis and intensity (loudness) on the other.

Audiologist: An individual who holds a doctoral degree, state license, and optional professional certification for the diagnosis and treatment of hearing and balance problems. See the American Academy of Audiology Web site for more information: http://www.audiology.org

Audiometer: An instrument that delivers calibrated pure-tone or speech stimuli for the measurement of sound detection, speech detection, speech recognition, and word identification.

Auditory background: An unconscious (primitive) function of hearing that allows identification of sounds that are consistent with specific locations (e.g., schools, grocery stores, hospitals) and biological functions.

Auditory behaviors: Behaviors displayed by infants and children in response to acoustic stimulation; may be categorized as being attentive or reflexive in nature.

Auditory brainstem response test (ABR): An objective test that measures the tiny electrical potentials produced in response to sound stimuli; the synchronous discharge of the first- through sixth-order neurons in the auditory nerve and brainstem.

Auditory processing disorder (APD): Not really a hearing loss relative to a reduction of sound reception, central auditory problems cause difficulty with perception or deriving meaning from incoming sounds. The source of the problem is in the central auditory nervous system (brainstem or cortex), not in the peripheral hearing mechanism (outer, middle, or inner ear).

Auditory system: A term used to describe the entire structure and function of the ear.

Autoimmune: This term refers to a disordered immunologic response in which the body produces antibodies against its own tissues; may occur in the inner ear.

Background noise: Any unwanted sound that may or may not interfere with listening depending on the speech-to-noise ratio in the environment.

Behavioral observation audiometry (BOA): The "lowest" developmental level test procedure whereby a controlled, calibrated sound stimulus is presented, and an infant's or child's *unconditioned* response behaviors are observed.

Behavioral tests: Hearing tests that elicit a behavior, measure that behavior, and infer function of the auditory system.

Bilabial: A speech sound produced with involvement of the lips, such as /b/ or /m/.

Bilateral: A disorder or hearing loss that involves both ears.

Binaural: Hearing with both ears; wearing a separate hearing aid on each ear.

Bone conduction: A pathway by which sounds directly reach the inner ear primarily through skull vibration, thereby bypassing the outer and middle ears.

Bone oscillator: The piece of audiometric equipment that looks like a small black box attached to a headband and is used to obtain bone conduction thresholds.

Calibrate: To check or adjust a piece of equipment until it accurately conforms to a predetermined, standard measure.

Caregiver: Any adult who takes care of a child.

Central mechanism: The part of the ear structure that includes the brainstem and cortex.

Certified auditory-verbal therapist (Cert. AVT): Audiologists, speech-language pathologists, or teachers of children with hearing loss who have obtained additional supervised training beyond their typical degrees and who have passed a special certification examination for auditory-verbal therapists; a registry of Cert. AVTs may be obtained from http://www.agbellacademy.org .

Cerumen: Also called earwax, cerumen is a normal, protective secretion of the ear canal. Approximately 30% of infants and young children in early intervention programs have so much earwax that it causes a hearing loss that interferes with the learning of language (spoken communication).

Classroom acoustics: The noise and reverberation (echo) characteristics of a classroom as determined by sound sources inside and outside the classroom, including classroom size, shape, surface, material, furniture, persons, and other physical characteristics.

Clear speech: Speech that is spoken at a moderately loud conversational level; characterized by precise but not exaggerated articulation, pausing at appropriate places, and speaking at a somewhat slower rate; clear speech is easier for people with hearing loss to understand.

Cochlea: The inner ear where the reception of sound actually occurs. The organ of Corti (end-organ for hearing) and hair cells (sensory receptors for sound) are located in the cochlea.

Cochlear implant: A biomedical device that delivers electrical stimulation to the eighth cranial nerve (auditory nerve) via an electrode array that is surgically implanted in the cochlea.

Complementation: A grammatical term for a particular way of inserting new verbal relationships into sentences.

Complex sound: A sound made up of two or more frequencies.

Compression (in hearing aid circuitry): Nonlinear amplifier gain used to determine the output of the signal from the hearing aid as a function of the input signal.

Conductive hearing loss: Hearing loss caused by damage or disease (pathology) located in the outer or middle ear that interferes with the efficient transmission of sound into the inner ear where sound reception occurs.

Conductive mechanism: The part of the auditory system that includes the outer and middle ear.

Congenital hearing loss: A hearing loss that occurs prior to the development of speech and language, usually before or at birth.

Conjoining: A grammatical term for putting together or combining.

Consonant: A speech sound formed by restricting, channeling, or directing air flow with the tongue, teeth, and/or lips (e.g., *th, s, p, f, m*, and so on).

Continuates: Caregiver talk that narrates the obvious.

Coupled: The connecting or attaching of one object to another, for example, a hearing aid to an assistive listening device.

CV syllable: A consonant-vowel syllable.

CVC syllable: A consonant-vowel-consonant syllable.

Decibel (dB): The standard unit for measuring and describing the intensity of a sound; the logarithmic unit of sound intensity or sound pressure; one-tenth of a Bel.

Diagnostic audiologic assessment (hearing test): The collection of tests given to an individual who wants his or her hearing evaluated, typically including: case history, speech tests (threshold and word identification), pure-tone air and bone conduction testing, immittance, and counseling.

Differential diagnosis: Separating peripheral hearing loss from other problems that present with symptoms similar to hearing loss (e.g., lack of appropriate spoken language development and/or lack of appropriate and observable auditory behaviors).

Direct audio input (DAI): Direct transmission of a sound signal into a hearing aid without being changed from one form of energy to another.

Disability: Impairment or loss of function of whole or parts of body systems.

Discrimination: Ability to differentiate among sounds of different frequencies, durations, or intensities.

Distance hearing: The ability to monitor environmental events and to overhear conversations, an ability that is severely reduced by hearing loss of any type or degree.

Distortion: Adding to or taking away from the original form or composition of the acoustic signal.

Dynamic range compression circuits: Circuits in hearing aids designed to provide more amplification for soft sounds than for loud sounds to meet the needs of many hearing aid wearers who primarily need more amplification of soft sounds.

Dysplasia (of the inner ear): Incomplete development or malformations of the inner ear (cochlea).

Ear canal: The canal between the pinna and eardrum, also called the external auditory meatus.

Earmold: The part of a hearing aid or ALD that fits into the ear and functions to conduct sound from the hearing aid into the ear.

Earshot: The distance over which (speech) sounds are intelligible; this distance is reduced when someone has a hearing loss of any type or degree.

Echo: A reflected sound that is perceived after the direct sound that initiated it.

EduLink: This personal FM system was designed specifically for listeners with normal hearing sensitivity. It is a miniaturized FM receiver that can be used with a variety of FM transmitters. Its primary purpose is to improve listening and attention skills, and perhaps the academic abilities of children with attention and processing difficulties.

Efficacy: Efficacy can be defined as the extrinsic and intrinsic value of a treatment. Every technology or treatment that we institute for a baby or child should have some associated efficacy measure in order to determine if the treatment is effective.

Electroacoustic: Pertains to the electronic processing of sound.

Electrophysiologic tests: Tests that measure the electrical activity of the brainstem and brain in response to acoustic stimulation.

Embedded: A grammatical term for inserting additional information into a sentence.

Endogenous hearing loss: A hearing loss caused by genetic factors that have various probabilities of being passed on to children or to grandchildren.

Environmental sounds: Nonspeech sounds such as a fire engine, a siren, a telephone ringing, the garage door opening, or a doorbell ringing.

Etiology: Cause of the hearing loss.

Exogenous hearing loss: A hearing loss caused by environmental factors such as a virus, medications, or lack of oxygen; it cannot be passed on to offspring.

Feedback (acoustic): A high-pitched squeal produced by a hearing aid and caused most often by a poorly fitting earmold. Feedback also can be caused by cracked earmold tubing, earwax in the earmold, or a crack in the earhook or hearing-aid case.

Frequency: The number of times that any regularly repeated event, such as sound vibration, occurs in a specified period of time, usually measured in cycles per second. Also called pitch and measured in hertz (Hz) along the top of an audiogram from low- to high-frequency sounds; low-frequency sounds are most commonly associated with vowel sounds and high-frequency sounds with consonants.

Frequency modulation (FM): The frequency of transmitted waves is alternated in accordance with the sounds being sent; radio waves.

Frequency response: The way that each hearing aid or ALD shapes the incoming (speech) sounds to best reach the person's hearing loss; the amount of amplification provided by the hearing aid at any frequency.

Fricatives: Speech sounds such as /f/ and /th/ that have turbulent breath flow.

Functional assessment: Functional measures of efficacy are typically accomplished by having the teacher, student, or parent complete a questionnaire before and after use of a hearing aid, cochlear implant, personal FM, or sound field system.

Functional hearing loss: A hearing problem with no physiological basis.

Fundamental frequency: The rate at which an individual speaker's vocal cords vibrate in speaking.

Gain: The amount by which the output level of the hearing aid or ALD exceeds the input level; how much louder sounds are made by an amplification device.

Hearing age (also called listening age): The relationship between the age of the child when he or she first receives amplification and that child's chronological age; for example, a 3-year-old child is 1 day old relative to listening, language, and information learning when his or her hearing aids or cochlear implants are first fit.

Hearing aids (also called hearing instruments): Miniature public address systems that amplify and shape the incoming sounds to make them audible to an ear that would not otherwise detect them; the first step in an early intervention treatment paradigm.

Hearing aid adjustment: Varying the program of a hearing aid or the acoustics of an earmold to improve its capability to assist a specific person with a particular hearing loss.

Hearing aid fitting: Trying a hearing aid and earmold on a person using specific formula, programs, and procedures, until it is suitable for the person acoustically, physically, and cosmetically.

Hearing aid programmability: Refers to a hearing aid's adjustment capability. If a hearing aid is *programmable*, its amplification characteristics can be fine-tuned via a special computer program to the hearing aid wearer's needs. If the hearing aid user's hearing changes, the hearing aid can be easily and quickly reprogrammed.

Hearing aid stethoscope: An instrument that allows one to listen to the output of a hearing aid or an ALD to detect a malfunction.

Hearing loss: Lessened or loss of hearing sensitivity caused by disease or damage to one or more parts of one of both ears.

Hertz (Hz): The standard unit for measuring and describing the frequency of a sound; a unit of frequency measurement equal to 1 cycle per second.

Horn, acoustic (of an earmold): Progressive increase of the internal diameter of the earmold sound channel resulting in a "horn effect" that enhances certain sounds. A common use is to restore some of the high frequency sound energy associated with ear canal resonance that may be lost when a conventional earmold is inserted into the ear.

Idiopathic: No known cause (of the hearing loss).

Impedance (immittance) testing: An objective measure of middle-ear function, not hearing sensitivity; measures how well the eardrum moves.

Inner ear: Comprised of the cochlea, which contains hair cells (the thousands of tiny receptors of sound), the vestibular or balance system, and the acoustic nerve that transmits nerve impulses from the inner ear to the brain.

Intelligibility: The ability to detect differences among speech sounds (e.g., to hear words such as *vacation* and *invitation* as separate and distinct words).

Intensity: Intensity also is referred to as loudness and is measured in dB.

Internal noise: Noise generated within a sound system such as a hearing aid or assistive listening device.

Intonation: Variations in pitch patterns (melody) and stress in an utterance that add meaning to the message; the melody carried in the voice when speaking.

Inverse square law: The intensity or loudness of a sound decreases by 6 dB as the distance between the sound source and the listener is doubled.

Jack: An electrical device that can receive a plug to make a connection in a circuit (e.g., an amplifier that has a specific place where earphones can be attached to the unit).

Labiodental: A speech sound produced with involvement of the lips and teeth, such as /f/ or /v/.

Labiolingual: A speech sound produced with involvement of the lips and tongue, such as children's "raspberries."

Language: A structured symbolic system used to communicate ideas in the form of words, with rules for combining and sequencing these words into thoughts, experiences, or feelings. An oral language system is comprised of a sound system, a vocabulary or concept system, a word ordering and grammar system, and rules for effectively using this symbolic system.

Learning disability: The lack of a skill in one or more areas of learning that is inconsistent with the child's overall intellectual capacity.

Lexicon: Vocabulary; understanding the meaning(s) of words.

Listening: Understanding speech and environmental sounds by attending to auditory clues; detection, discrimination, recognition, identification, and comprehension of speech and environmental sounds; being able to determine where a sound is coming from.

Listening age: *See* Hearing age.

Live signal: An unrecorded sound or voice.

Localization: The ability to determine where a sound is coming from; to associate a sound with its source by finding the source.

Loudness: The perception of sound intensity; marked by high volume.

Loudspeaker: An electroacoustic transducer that changes electrical energy into acoustical energy at the output stage of a sound system so that the acoustic event can be heard by many people at the same time.

Mainstreaming: The process that promotes integration into a general educational setting using a typical curriculum for a child with a disability, to the maximum extent possible in accordance with federal laws. Integration with typical children ranges from full-time placement to integration in some classes like music, art, or gym.

Masking: A procedure often used in hearing testing where a static-like noise is presented to the nontest ear through headphones to keep it from responding to the test stimuli.

Microphone/transmitter: An electroacoustic transducer that changes a sound stimulus to electrical energy.

Middle ear: The part of the auditory mechanism that functions to conduct sound efficiently into the inner ear; made up of the eardrum, a small air-filled space, and the three smallest bones in the body.

Minimum response level (MRL): The lowest or softest dB hearing level (dB HL) where a baby displays identifiable behavioral change to sound, usually considerably above or louder than his or her actual threshold—may also be called minimal response level (MRL).

Mixed hearing loss: A hearing loss caused by the presence of more than one pathology in different parts of the ear at the same time; it can be thought of as having two hearing losses in the same ear, usually conductive and sensorineural.

Modality: Sensory channel, such as audition, vision, touch.

Motherese: The way that many mothers (and other caregivers) talk with small children.

Multifactorial inheritance: This means that there are additive effects of several minor gene-pair abnormalities in association with nongenetic environment interactive factors or "triggers" that cause hearing loss in a child.

Multiple-memory hearing aids: These hearing aids offer different settings or memories for various listening environments. One memory may be used for quiet listening and another for listening in a noisy restaurant; a remote control is usually used to access the various memories. Ideally, each memory is adjusted to provide the hearing aid wearer with optimum hearing in that particular environment. Note that children *must* additionally have the remote microphone of an FM unit when in a class-room learning situation.

Nasals: Speech sounds produced with air emitted from the nose, such as /m/ or /n/.

Neuropathy, auditory: A disorder of the auditory neural pathways including the eighth cranial (auditory) nerve, brainstem, and cortex.

Noise: Any unwanted or unintended sound or electrical signal that interferes with communication or transmission of energy; it may be disturbing and/or hazardous to hearing health.

Noise reduction: A process of acoustical treatments and structural modifications whereby the intensity in dB of unwanted sound is reduced in a room.

Objective tests: Objective tests provide some direct measurement of the auditory system (e.g., eardrum and middle ear mobility, middle ear muscle reflex action, outer hair cell function,or transmission of sound up the auditory pathways of the lower brainstem).

Occupied classroom: A classroom when the teacher and students are present.

Orosensory: Tactile sensation in the mouth.

Otitis media: Also known as middle ear infection, otitis media is the most common cause of conductive hearing loss in children. It is an inflammation of the middle ear, typically with fluid present in the normally air-filled middle ear space.

Otoacoustic emissions (OAEs): Soft, inaudible sounds produced by vibratory motion of the (outer) hair cells in the cochlea. To measure evoked otoacoustic emissions, a small probe is inserted in the ear canal, sounds are presented, and response tracings are recorded.

Otologist: A physician who specializes in the diagnosis and treatment of diseases of the ear; also known as an otolaryngologist or an ear-nose-throat (ENT) specialist.

Ototoxicity: A "poisoning" of the delicate inner ear by high doses of certain drugs and medications.

Outer ear: The part of the hearing mechanism made up of the pinna and external auditory meatus (ear canal) that functions to protect and channel sounds into the middle ear.

Pediatric audiologic test battery: The use, with infants and children, of several, developmentally appropriate behavioral and objective hearing tests to avoid drawing conclusions from a single test, allow detection of multiple pathologies, and provide a framework for observation of auditory behaviors.

Perception: Understanding the meaning of incoming sounds; occurs in the central auditory system (brainstem and cortex).

Perilymphatic fistula: A leak in the oval or round windows, both being points of communication between the middle and inner ear; causes a sudden or degenerative hearing loss.

Peripheral auditory mechanism: The part of the ear that includes the outer, middle, and inner ear; it functions to receive incoming sounds.

Peripheral ear: External, middle, and inner ear (not the auditory cortex).

Personal-worn FM systems: They are like individual, private radio stations where the talker (typically the teacher or parent) wears the wireless microphone transmitter, and the child wears the radio-like receiver coupled to the ears via headphones, ear buds, or personal hearing aids.

Phonation: voicing, vocalizing

Phoneme: the smallest meaningful unit of sound in a language.

Phonemic: Pertaining to speech sounds, usually in isolation or in nonsense syllables.

Phonetic: Having to do with phonemes; the distinctive sounds that make up the words of a language.

Phonologic: Relating to the production and use of speech sounds in meaningful language.

Phonological awareness (phonemic awareness): The explicit awareness of the speech sound structure of language units that forms the basis for reading. It is demonstrated by a variety of skills that include generating rhyming words, segmenting words into syllables and into discrete sounds, and categorizing groups of words based on a similarity of sound segments.

Pinna: The auricle or outer flap of the ear; one located on each side of the head.

Pitch: The overall highness or loudness of a person's voice or of a speech sound; it can be measured, but in this context, it is usually a perceptual estimation.

Play audiometry: The highest level of pediatric task in hearing testing, play audiometry involves the active cooperation of the child while an auditory stimulus is paired with an operant task, such as dropping a block in a bucket. It's also called the "listen and drop" test.

Plosives: Speech sounds such as /p/, /t/, or /k/ which are produced with a sudden burst of air.

Pragmatics: The study of how language is used.

Prognosis: A prediction of the course of outcome of a disease or treatment.

Programmable hearing aid: *See* Hearing aid programmability.

Pronominal: Pertaining to pronouns.

Propagation: Act of extending, projecting, or traveling through space.

Prosodic: Stress, intonation, or melodic features of spoken language.

Prosody: The melody and rhythm of speaking; features of prosody include pitch, intonation, intensity, and duration.

Pure tone: A tone that has energy at only one frequency. Pure tones are useful for evaluating hearing sensitivity because they permit measurement of the contour or configuration of the hearing loss.

Rapid speech transmission index (RASTI): A number between zero and one that quantifies speech intelligibility. RASTI is derived from measurement of the modulation transfer function of the two octave bands of pink noise modulations that mimic the long-term speech spectrum.

Real-ear measurements: Measurement of amplified sound in the ear canal through the use of a probe microphone.

Reception: The detection of sound that occurs in the inner ear.

Receptive language: Skills involving the ability to receive and comprehend the language one hears in the environment.

Redundancy: The part of a message that can be eliminated without loss of information.

Reflected sound: Propagated sound after it has struck one or more objects or surfaces in a room.

Remote microphone: A microphone that can be placed close to the desired sound source, thereby improving the speech-to-noise ratio (S/N ratio); a key feature of personal-worn FM systems, sound field FM or IR systems, and some hardwired assistive listening devices.

Residual hearing: The hearing that remains after damage or disease in the auditory mechanism; there is almost always some residual hearing, even with the most profound hearing losses.

Residual hearing can be accessed through the use of amplification technology.

Resonant voice: A voice that is strong and rich in overtones.

Reverberant sound: Sound that reaches a given location in a room only after being reflected from one or more barriers or partitions within a room.

Reverberation: The amount of echo in a room; the more reverberant the room, the poorer the speech-to-noise ratio and the less intelligible the speech.

Secondary language: Skills that involve higher level language functions such as reading and writing versus listening and speaking.

Segmental(s): Pertaining to the sounds of speech; consonants and vowels.

Semantic: Related to the meaning of words or groups of words in a language system.

Sensation: The conscious awareness of the arrival of the auditory signal.

Sensorineural hearing loss: Often called a *nerve loss*, a sensorineural hearing loss results from disease or damage located in the inner ear; usually a permanent hearing loss.

Sensorineural mechanism: The part of the ear structure that includes the inner ear and acoustic nerve.

Sensory deprivation: Lack of auditory sensory input to the brain, caused by a hearing loss, which can cause delayed and/or deviant behaviors.

Signal: Sounds that carry information to listeners.

Signal-to-noise ratio (also called speech-to-noise ratio): S/N ratio is the relationship between a primary signal such as the teacher's or parent's speech and background noise. The quieter the room and the more favorable the S/N ratio, the clearer the auditory signal will be for the brain.

Signal warning: The function of hearing that enables one to monitor the environment, including other people's interactions.

Sine wave: A periodic wave related to simple harmonic motion.

Site of lesion: The location in the auditory system where disease or damage occurs, causing hearing loss.

Sound field: A space where sound is propagated.

Sound field systems (also called classroom amplification systems): The teacher wears a wireless microphone transmitter, just like the one worn for a personal FM unit, and her voice is sent via radio waves (FM), or light waves (infrared—IR) to an amplifier that is connected to loudspeakers. It looks like a wireless public address system, but it is designed specifically to ensure that the entire speech signal, including the weak high frequency consonants, reaches every child in the room no matter where the children and the teacher are located.

Sound field testing: Calibrated auditory signals are presented through loudspeakers into the sound-isolated room rather than through headphones to test hearing; represented by the symbol *S* on an audiogram.

Sound-isolated room: An acoustically treated room where hearing tests should be performed to obtain accurate results.

Sound level: The intensity of sound in decibels.

Spectrogram: A graphic illustration of speech sounds displaying intensity, frequency, and duration.

Speech intelligibility: The percentage of the speech of a talker that is understood by a listener(s).

Speech-language pathologist: A specialist who has a graduate degree in speech and language disorders and how to alleviate them, and holds a state license and certification from the American Speech-Language-Hearing Association (ASHA).

Speech recognition or reception threshold (SRT): An audiologic test that determines the softest level that a person can just barely understand speech 50% of the time.

Speech sound improvement: Therapy directed at improving the production of specific sounds such as *r, s, l, sh, ch*.

Static: Electrical discharges in a hearing aid, cochlear implant, radio, etc., that causes crackling sounds, interferes with signal reception, and can damage the electronic device.

Stenosis: An abnormally small ear canal.

Stimulus: Something, such as a sound, that can evoke or elicit a response.

Support services: Ancillary services that are provided to assist a child in achieving academic success; services can include speech-language therapy, occupational therapy, aural habilitation, tutoring.

Suprasegmentals: Prosodic aspects of speech; variations in the pitch, loudness, rate, and duration of speech patterns.

Syndrome: A collection of anomalies that co-occur; hearing loss often accompanies other disabilities or abnormalities, such as skeletal malformations or endocrine disorders.

Telecoil: A series of interconnected wire loops in a hearing aid that respond electrically to a magnetic signal.

Telecoil switch: An external control (switch or program) on a hearing aid that turns off the microphone and activates a telecoil in the hearing aid, which picks up magnetic leakage from a telephone or the loop of an ALD; hearing aids for children need to come equipped with a telecoil.

Threshold: The intensity at which an individual can just barely hear a sound 50% of the time; all sounds louder than threshold can be heard, but softer sounds cannot be detected.

Tinnitus: Any of a number of internal head noises that can accompany hearing loss; also called *ringing in the ears.*

Topicalize: Establish topics in conversations.

Transducer: A device such as a microphone or loudspeaker that changes sound into electricity (microphone) or changes electricity into sound (loudspeaker).

Transformer: A two-coil, induction device for increasing or decreasing the voltage or alternating current.

Transition time: The time required to move from a consonant to a vowel or from a vowel to a consonant in speaking, usually measured in milliseconds.

Transmitter: An apparatus that sends out electromagnetic rays; the FM system component that modulates the frequency of the radio signal in an audio frequency signal and sends the radio waves through the air to the antenna of the amplifier/receiver.

Treatment paradigm for recommending (sound field) technology: If viewed as a treatment, technology is recommended for a particular child and managed through the special education system.

Troubleshooting (hearing aids or ALDs): Performing various visual and listening inspections to determine whether an amplification unit is malfunctioning and, if so, evaluating the nature and severity of the malfunction.

Tympanostomy tubes: Tiny ventilating tubes that are surgically inserted through the eardrum to replace a malfunctioning eustachian tube in allowing ventilation of the middle ear space.

Unilateral hearing loss: Hearing loss in one ear; the other ear has normal hearing sensitivity. A unilateral hearing loss can have a negative impact on a child's behavior, social skills, and development of spoken communication (language), due in large part to the reduction of incidental learning caused by the hearing loss.

Universal design paradigm for recommending sound field technology: This concept means that the assistive technology is not specially designed for an individual student but rather for a wide range of students. Universally designed approaches are implemented by general education teachers rather than by special education teachers.

Velar: Speech sounds made with the tongue elevated near or touching the velum.

Vent: A small hole or opening that serves as an outlet for sound in an earmold.

Vertigo: Dizziness that includes a sensation of spinning or whirling.

Vestibular system: Composed of the saccule, utricle, and semicircular canals, the vestibular system is located in the inner ear and functions to regulate balance. Specifically, it coordinates changes in head position, acceleration and deceleration, and gravitational effects.

Vibrotactile: Pertains to the detection of vibrations through the sense of touch; sounds that are felt rather than heard.

Vibrotactile hearing aid: An assistive listening device that converts acoustic energy into vibratory patterns that are delivered to the skin.

Visual reinforcement audiometry (VRA): A pediatric behavioral hearing test in which a child's auditory behaviors (usually localization) are conditioned to and rewarded by a visual display.

Vocalizations: Babbling sounds produced by infants.

Volume control: A wheel or knob for adjusting the intensity of sound produced by a sound system.

Vowel: A speech sound identified by its unrestricted voice flow.

Wavelength: The distance between one peak of a sine wave and the next peak of the same wave.

Word discrimination testing (also called word identification testing): Part of a diagnostic audiologic assessment where one determines how well words can be distinguished when they are presented at a typical conversational level of loudness and at an additional level loud enough to overcome the individual's hearing loss.

Wireless system: An FM transmitter and FM receiver; radio waves, not wires, connect the talker and listener.

Index